Smart textiles for medicine and healthcare

Related titles:

Intelligent textiles and clothing
(ISBN-13: 978-1-84569-005-2; ISBN-10: 1-84569-005-2)
Intelligent textiles and clothing can be defined as those that react to exterior or physiological stimuli. This important book brings together recent research in the area. The book is divided into parts, each one containing an overview chapter followed by specific research and applications. Its main focus is on phase change materials, shape memory textiles, chromic and conductive materials. It is an essential read for anyone wanting to know more about intelligent textiles.

Handbook of nonwovens
(ISBN-13: 978-1-85573-603-0; ISBN-10: 1-85573-603-9)
Given their rapid development and diverse markets, understanding and developing nonwovens is becoming increasingly important. This comprehensive review discusses the development of the industry and the different classes of nonwoven material. The book then reviews methods of manufacture such as dry-laid, wet-laid and polymer-laid web formation. Other techniques analysed include mechanical, thermal and chemical bonding as well as chemical and mechanical finishing systems. The book concludes by assessing the characterisation, testing and modelling of nonwoven materials.

Thermal and moisture transport in fibrous materials
(ISBN-13: 978-1-84569-057-1; ISBN-10: 1-84569-057-5)
The transfer of heat and moisture through textiles is vital to the manufacture and design of clothing as well as technical and protective textiles. The first part of this important book summarises the structure, geometry and stereology of fibrous materials. The fundamentals of wetting and its dynamics are also discussed. Part II analyses thermal and liquid interactions in textiles and offers insights into the thermodynamic behaviour of moisture as well as heat and moisture coupling. The book concludes with chapters on the human thermoregulatory system, interfacing between fibrous materials and the human body and modelling techniques.

Details of these books and a complete list of Woodhead's titles can be obtained by:

- visiting our web site at www.woodheadpublishing.com
- contacting Customer Services (e-mail: sales@woodhead-publishing.com; fax: +44 (0) 1223 893694; tel.: +44 (0) 1223 891358 ext. 130; address: Woodhead Publishing Ltd, Abington Hall, Abington, Cambridge CB21 6AH, England).

Smart textiles for medicine and healthcare

Materials, systems and applications

Edited by

L. Van Langenhove

The Textile Institute

CRC Press
Boca Raton Boston New York Washington, DC

WOODHEAD PUBLISHING LIMITED
Cambridge, England

Published by Woodhead Publishing Limited in association with The Textile Institute
Woodhead Publishing Limited, Abington Hall, Abington
Cambridge CB21 6AH, England
www.woodheadpublishing.com

Published in North America by CRC Press LLC, 6000 Broken Sound Parkway, NW, Suite 300, Boca Raton FL 33487, USA

First published 2007, Woodhead Publishing Limited and CRC Press LLC

British Library Cataloguing in Publication Data
A catalogue record for this book is available from the British Library.

Library of Congress Cataloging in Publication Data
A catalog record for this book is available from the Library of Congress.

Woodhead Publishing ISBN-13: 978-1-84569-027-4 (book)
Woodhead Publishing ISBN-10: 1-84569-027-3 (book)
Woodhead Publishing ISBN-13: 978-1-84569-293-3 (e-book)
Woodhead Publishing ISBN-10: 1-84569-293-4 (e-book)
CRC Press ISBN-13: 978-1-4200-4448-5
CRC Press ISBN-10: 1-4200-4448-6
CRC Press order number: WP4448

The publishers' policy is to use permanent paper from mills that operate a sustainable forestry policy, and which has been manufactured from pulp which is processed using acid-free and elementary chlorine-free practices. Furthermore, the publishers ensure that the text paper and cover board used have met acceptable environmental accreditation standards.

Project managed by Macfarlane Production Services, Dunstable, Bedfordshire, England (macfarl@aol.com)
Typeset by Replika Press Pvt Ltd, India
Printed by T J International Limited, Padstow, Cornwall, England

Contents

Contributor contact details

(* = main contact)

Editor

Professor Dr Ir Lieva Van Langenhove
Universiteit Gent
Vakgroep Textielkunde
Technologiepark 907
9052 Zwijnaarde
Belgium

E-mail:
lieva.vanlangenhove@ugent.be

Chapter 1

Sandy Black
London College of Fashion
University of the Arts London
20 John Princes Street
London W1G 0BJ
UK

E-mail: s.black@fashion.arts.ac.uk

Chapter 2

Dr Yimin Qin
Department of Chemical Engineering
Jiaxing College
56 Yuexiu Road South
Jiaxing 314001
Zhejiang Province
China

E-mail: yiminqin1965@126.com

Chapter 3

V.A. Nierstrasz
Textile Technology Group
Department of Science and Technology
University of Twente
P.O. Box 217
7500 AE Enschede
The Netherlands

E-mail: v.a.nierstrasz@utwente.nl

Chapter 4

Barbara Pause
Textile Testing & Innovation, LLC.
7161 Christopher Court
Longmont CO 80503
USA

E-mail: pause@textile-testing.com

Chapter 5

Michael Catrysse,* Fabrice Pirotte and Robert Puers
Centexbel
Rue Montoyer, 24
Montoyerstraat, 24
1000 Brussels
Belgium

E-mail:
michael.catrysse@centexbel.be

Chapter 6

Professor Dr Ir Lieva Van Langenhove,* Carla Hertleer, Jorgos Priniotakis and Philippe Westbroek
Universiteit Gent
Vakgroep Textielkunde
Technologiepark 907
9052 Zwijnaarde
Belgium

E-mail:
lieva.vanlangenhove@ugent.be
Carla.Hertleer@UGent.be

Chapter 7

Tatjana Rijavec* and Sabina Bračko
University of Ljubljana
Faculty of Natural Sciences and Engineering
Department of Textiles
Snezniska 5
1000 Ljubljana
Slovenia

E-mail: Tatjana.rijavec@ntf.uni-lj.si

Chapter 8

Niina Lintu,* Dr M. Mattila and Dr O. Hänninen
Department of Physiology
University of Kuopio
P.O. Box 1627
70211 Kuopio
Finland

E-mail: lintu@messi.uku.fi

Chapter 9

Jane McCann
E-mail:
Jane.McCann@newport.ac.uk

Chapter 10

Penny Bougia, Evaggelas Karvounis and D.I. Fotiadis
University of Ioannina
Department of Computer Science
Unit of Medical Technology and Intelligent Information Systems
45110 Ioannina
Greece

E-mail: pbougia@cc.uoi.gr
ekarvuni@cc.uoi.gr

Chapter 11

Professor Dr Ir Lieva Van Langenhove,* Carla Hertleer and Robert Puers
Universiteit Gent
Vakgroep Textielkunde
Technologiepark 907
9052 Zwijnaarde
Belgium

E-mail:
lieva.vanlangenhove@ugent.be
Carla.Hertleer@UGent.be

Chapter 12

Professor Guido Belforte,*
Professor Giuseppe Quaglia,
Professor Franco Testore, Ing.
Gabriella Eula and Ing.
Silvia Appendino

E-mail: guido.belforte@polito.it
giuseppe.quaglia@polito.it

Chapter 13

Dr Tünde Kirstein,*
Professor Gerhard Tröster,
Ivo Locher and Christof Küng
Wearable Computing Lab
ETH Zürich
Gloriastrasse 35
CH-8092 Zürich
Switzerland

E-mail: Kirstein@ife.ee.ethz.ch

Chapter 14

Oliver Amft*
Electronics Laboratories (IfE), ETZ
H61.1
Wearable Computing Laboratory
Gloriastrasse 35
CH-8092 Zürich
Switzerland

E-mail: oam@ife.ee.ethz.ch

Jörg Habetha
Philips Research Laboratories
Germany

Introduction

The original function of textiles was to shield man from cold and rain. Later on in history aesthetic aspects also came to play a role in clothing. Much more recently a new generation of textiles has arisen; smart or intelligent textiles. Intelligent textiles are a relatively new discipline in the textile sector. They are active materials that have sensing and actuation properties. Their potential is enormous. One could think of smart clothing that makes us feel comfortable at all times, during any activity and in any environmental conditions, a suit that protects and monitors, that warns in case of danger and even helps to treat diseases and injuries. Such clothing could be used from the moment we are born till the end of our life, particularly in healthcare applications.

The potential impact of smart textiles for healthcare is significant; risk assessment and diagnosis will be faster and more accurate, treatment and care will be more effective. Intelligent suits fit in with societal trends; the ageing population increasingly requires health monitoring and support which smart clothing could provide. These new textiles are knowledge based with high added value. They can be custom made for specific end uses. Consequently their economic impact is expected to be extremely high as well.

Many aspects need to be addressed when designing intelligent clothing. Several disciplines must be combined such as material science, medicine and electronics. An intelligent suit, for example, must be fully self-sufficient, comfortable, durable and reliable, easy to use and with low care requirements. The challenges are at least as big as the potential benefits. The way to successful commercial development is long but many steps have already been taken.

This book addresses intelligent textiles for health care applications. It includes contributions from material designers, system manufacturers and end users. This gives the reader a broad introduction to all aspects of the potential, development and use of intelligent textiles for medicine and healthcare.

Professor Dr. Ir. Lieva Van Langenhove, dr. h.c.

Part I

Types of smart medical textile

1 Trends in smart medical textiles

S BLACK, University of the Arts London, UK

1.1 Introduction

Much has been written about the accelerating pace of human development and change: from isolated pre-industrial agricultural societies, through the industrial revolution and development of transport and communication systems, and now to the exponentially developing information or knowledge age with its global connectivity through networked technologies – 'a degree of connectivity previous generations of engineers could only dream of' (Bhattacharyya 2006:52).

Textiles originated in the first of these eras; early manual production of woven cloth was rapidly developed with the machine age to become literally 'the fabric of our lives'. Textiles occupy a unique and universal position across societies and cultures being the material form which creates the interface between the naked body and the potentially hostile environment. Textiles cushion our personal and public spaces; in the home and at work, in transportation or in hospital, with a ubiquity that is now being harnessed for positive uses. The evolution and maturity of sophisticated information and communication technologies, together with microelectronics and systems developments, provide an incomparable opportunity for functional electronic integration with textiles in a manner which breaks down the norms of computing hardware and embeds computer functions into the soft textile interface.

The last ten years have seen the emergence of new multi-disciplinary approaches to textile research. As micro-, nano-, bio- and information technologies and biomaterials have continued to evolve to new stages of maturity there is an extraordinary array of new possibilities for enhanced functionalities within textiles, from new fibre structures, composite materials and coatings at the nano and micro levels to the visible integration of wearable electronic assemblies into clothing. Now, as a range of previously disparate technologies converge, for instance, biochemistry and polymer chemistry meet computer processor miniaturisation to produce so-called 'lab-on-a-chip' diagnostics, and new forms of textile sensors, actuators and other components become available, previous dreams for truly functional and intuitively wearable computing can start to become a reality via the medium of textiles.

Since its rudimentary beginnings, pioneered by Steve Mann in the 1980s in the experimental labs of Massachusetts Institute of Technology (MIT), wearable computing has escaped from the confines of the rigid box and beyond the distribution of elements in clothing or on the body to now merge with textile technology. New conductive yarns have been developed which can be woven, knitted and even embroidered into electronically enabled textiles to provide innovative soft textile interfaces that are highly acceptable to the end user. Acceptance of products and devices is especially significant within the medical context where direct intervention is required, opening up opportunities for textiles to meet genuine needs and facilitate clinical interaction and monitoring through enhanced comfort, mobility and convenience.

1.2 Advantages of textiles in medical and healthcare

The key properties of textiles that are mobilised in smart applications are flexibility to conform to the body, comfort to touch, softness and wearability, plus the intrinsic familiarity and acceptability of textiles to the patient. However, because textile technology is very old – weaving and knitting can draw upon centuries of manufacturing knowledge – it is important not to discount existing technologies for innovation: novel application of 'old' technology can prove to be as fruitful as a newly emerging technology; the use of existing technologies with new materials can propel an established process into an unforeseen avenue. For example, TWI (The Welding Institute) have established a centre for materials joining technology, based on an adaptation of a Prolast sewing machine to utilise laser beams (Jones and Wise, 2005) Further examples of these permutations of old and new are evident throughout this book – see, for example, section 1.4 regarding the uses of embroidery in medical implants.

As the global population continues to increase, the prevailing demographic profile moves towards greater life expectancy and an ageing populace whose expectations for enhanced healthcare continue to grow. Together these factors exert ever greater pressures on medical care systems. One important avenue by which these issues are currently being addressed is research into the use of 'smart' textile systems which integrate responsive and enhanced functionalities to textiles in the medical environment, be they garments, bandages, dressings, surgical implants, bedding, screens or hospital furnishings. These smart systems aim to provide a seamless relationship between textiles and technology for therapeutic care, to aid diagnostics and monitoring of vital signs, and provide aids to recovery and recuperation which can function in diverse locations, enabling remote monitoring of patients through wireless communication technologies. The direct advantage of remote monitoring (see examples in section 1.4.1) is envisaged as streamlining and freeing hospital resources by returning patients to their home environment earlier, whilst they are still being carefully monitored through telecommunications systems from which medical professionals can harvest and interpret data.

Research is taking place on an unprecedented international scale in North America, Europe and Asia, and its spin-off product developments are now emerging at an increasing rate. As the first products start to become available the expectations of the new smart textiles will continue to rise, challenging research to move ever onward. Smart textiles is a hybrid research area crossing many disciplines that, having learnt from early attempts at wearable computing, is moving into another generation of technologies which are designed to solve specific problems in particular contexts. It is poised to have tremendous impact within the medical sector and beyond to everyday life.

The following chapters cover in detail the materials, technologies, systems and applications that are now emerging from this exciting trans-disciplinary collaborative research area to provide cutting edge solutions to problems and scenarios within the entire spectrum of medical applications.

1.2.1 What are smart textiles?

As a newly emergent field there is no one accepted definition, with various terms such as 'intelligent', 'smart' or 'active' materials and textiles often used interchangeably. However, as more research literature and product prototypes appear, definitions are converging and coming into accepted use. According to Xiaoming Tao, whose publication *Smart Fibres, Fabrics and Clothing* is becoming a key reference text for technologies in the field 'Smart materials and structures can be defined as the materials and structures that sense and react to environmental conditions or stimuli, such as those from mechanical, thermal, chemical, electrical, magnetic or other sources.' She further subdivides smart materials into

> ... passive smart, active smart and very smart materials. Passive smart materials can only sense the environmental conditions or stimuli; active smart materials will sense and react to the conditions or stimuli; very smart materials can sense, react and adapt themselves accordingly (Tao 2001: 2).

These definitions can clearly be applied directly to the textiles arena, perhaps equating intelligent with 'very smart'. Other researchers argue that passive cannot by definition be smart, whereas Gonzalez at the University of Alberta USA distinguishes between 'very smart' and 'intelligent' adding the definition: 'intelligent materials are those capable of responding or being activated to perform a function in a pre-programmed manner' (www.ualberta.ca/~jag3/smart_textiles). Baurley, in *Wearable electronics and photonics* (Tao 2005: 236), adopts a less precise definition: 'smart is a term used to define a material that reacts in a particular way when exposed to stimuli such as environmental changes, for example, temperature or electronic currents'. However, some equate 'smart textiles' only with the integration of electronic functionality, whilst others include chemical and mechanical responses in the definition of 'smart'.

At the symposium on Smart Textiles held at the *Plastic Electronics* conference in Frankfurt October 2005, 'smart' and 'intelligent' were differentiated:

> 'smart textiles' utilise integrated or applied electronics such as sensors, actuators, etc., whereas 'intelligent textiles' produce predictable effects and phenomena by interacting with the environment and the wearer. (Peijs 2005).

This agrees with the definition from Strese *et al.* 2004 who define smart textiles as 'textiles with integrated electronics and microsystems which could be in clothes and in technical textiles'. They further define three levels of integration but without specific names:

- solutions adapted to clothes, e.g., mobile phone in a pocket
- electronics and micro systems integrated into clothes or textiles with connectable modules, e.g., with textile conductors
- functions integrated into the textile via direct insertion into textile fibres, e.g., woven displays (Strese, *et al.* 2004).

The Venture Development Corporation (VDC), a USA-based technology market research company, define 'smart fabrics and intelligent textiles' in their report of January 2005 as 'fabrics and textiles that cognitively respond or interact to environmental or electrical stimuli'. With a focus on applications that utilise electrical stimuli, they further outline these responses as

- conducting, transferring or distributing various properties through the material or across the material's membrane; such properties include electrical current, light energy, molecular or particulate matter, and thermal energy
- changing physical characteristics or phase, such as colour, permeability, porosity, rigidity, shape, size (VDC 2005).

The Foresight Smart Materials taskforce, a UK government initiative, recently reviewed the potential for wealth creation and strategies for UK industry and academia, concluding that competitive advantage will depend on products with increasing levels of functionality. Their report defined 'smart materials' as 'materials that form part of a smart structural system that has capability to sense its environment and the effects thereof, and if truly smart, to respond to that external stimulus via an active control mechanism'.

There appear then to be clear 'degrees of smartness' defined for materials which can be transposed to a textile system. The Foresight report goes on to say:

> The terms 'smart', 'functional', 'multifunctional', and 'intelligent' are often used interchangeably. This is reasonable, if confusing, for the first three terms but the last certainly suggests a degree of consciousness that does not exist in any non-biological system. There is arguably no such thing as a 'smart material' *per se* – only materials that exhibit interesting intrinsic characteristics which can be exploited within systems or structures that, in turn, can exhibit 'smart' behaviour (Hooper *et al.* 2003).

This is similar to El-Sherif's definition:

> smart textiles are an interesting class of electronic and photonic textiles ...defined as textiles capable of monitoring their own 'health' conditions and structural behaviour, as well as sensing external environmental conditions and sending the information to other locations (Tao 2005: 105).

There is clearly a need for a standard definition to be adopted throughout this growing niche sector of the textile industry. A consensus has recently been proposed in the UK through the setting up of a smart materials network SMART.mat by the government, regional development offices and the research councils, part of a larger materials knowledge transfer network. (www.materialsktn.net, www.SMARTmat.org). Whatever the nuances interpreted, the fundamental property expected of smart textiles is a measurable, reliable and useful responsiveness to environmental conditions and stimuli, such as heat, light and moisture. This may include changes in properties such as physical shape and length – as in textiles made from shape memory polymers (see chapter 4) or changes in colour or surface as in textiles incorporating phase change materials such as hydrogel, or the integration of optical or conductive fibres into textiles structures to create new textile sensors. These subjects are covered in detail in later chapters of the book, together with smart polymers and smart dyes incorporating nano-scale technologies.

Other functions that may be expected of 'intelligent textiles' and 'smart clothes' in addition to environmental responsiveness are location, entertainment, information, and biophysical monitoring. These are achieved through sensor and actuator technologies, (see chapter 6), switches, transponders and touch pads, sensors for pressure and temperature, and global positioning system (GPS) modules communicating with a server system. Some or all of these elements will be formed of textiles elements themselves. 'Smart' is a recently adopted term in the context of materials and textiles, which can also cover earlier technologies in its wider definition. Conversely not all material properties may be regarded as smart, for example, the expected phase change of a metal at its melting point is not generally regarded as a smart property (Hooper *et al.* 2003, p. 11).

1.3 Drivers for smart textiles in medical care

The drivers for the rapid current development of smart textiles have traditionally come from military research and space exploration where rigorous performance under extreme conditions is paramount. The protection of the individual in hostile environments, and the necessity for communication and monitoring have provided impetus both for materials and textile research, which then transfer to civilian use. The drivers for specific development in medical application as referred to in section 1.2 are both the pressure of a growing world population and greater longevity, creating an urgent need for improvements in administering nursing care, delivery of drugs, surgical and other medical procedures, including monitoring and diagnosis, therapeutic treatments and professional interactions in patient recovery. This leads to products driven by stringent performance and standards criteria which test the parameters and will provide the new paradigms for the future. Textiles (woven, non-woven or knitted) are already widely utilised in medical care in a range of contexts from wipes and bandages to clean room protection, with most textiles used being disposable, therefore by necessity, cheap. Rajendran and Anand (2002) identify key areas as textiles for wound care and bandages for support, dressing retention and compression, especially for varicose veins and leg ulcers, the most frequently occurring chronic wound. New research into textiles with specific functionalities could meet both patient and hospital needs in major areas such as prevention of pressure sores and chronic wound care.

The enablers for smart textiles are therefore both technological and commercial – the potential market for smart products has been estimated to become a multi-billion dollar business over the next ten years, of which a substantial proportion will be in the medical area, making research and development a viable investment, the results of which will also have cross-over benefits to non-medical situations.

1.3.1 Wearable computing

In the 1990s a great deal of research activity was expended in the field known as wearable computing which attempted to integrate the interactive functions of a computer firstly onto the body (via data gloves and head sets) and then into clothing. The initial forays into wearable computing applications for outdoor and sports clothing, such as Levi's and Philips' ICD+ jacket (2000), Burton's snowboarding jacket (2001) (see Fig. 1.1) and France Telecom's Create wear (2004) were relatively short-lived due to their niche appeal, rather cumbersome nature and expense, although new designs have recently been released. Imperatives provided by medical needs have given stimulus to the resolution of these problems in new ways. Smart textiles represent the latest generation of research into functional and performance textiles. The transfer of computing and processing functionalities directly embedded into textiles via a range of technologies has taken this research into areas of particular interest and benefit to medical usage. Researchers in Belgium working on a smart suit for monitoring children regard smart textiles as 'one step beyond' wearable computing, which will provide distinct advantages. (Puers *et al.* 2005).

1.3.2 Benefits of smart textiles in medical contexts

The potential benefits of smart textiles in medical use can be summarised as follows:

- integration of functionality into textile interface
- flexible materials which conform to the body

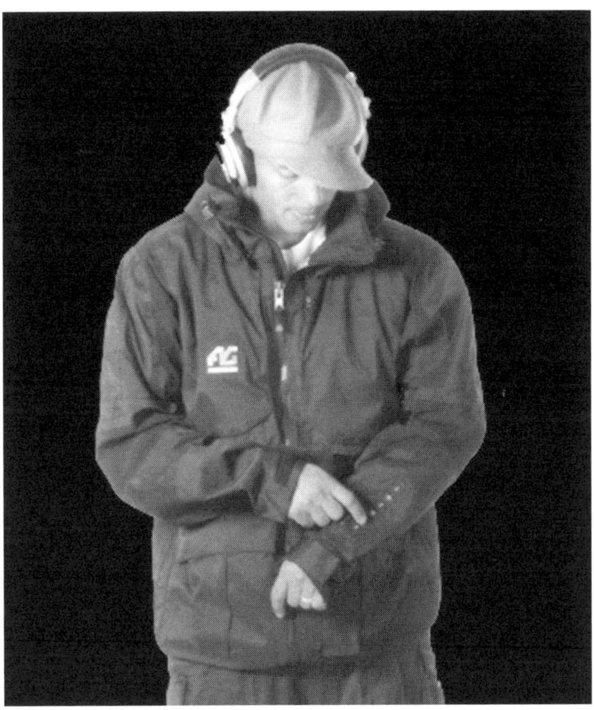

1.1 Burton Jacket (2001 version).

- wearable materials suitable for clothing or bedding
- familiar interface providing more comfortable and acceptable products
- versatile in design, materials and structures
- enable patient mobility whilst undergoing monitoring
- continuous monitoring of vital signs for post-operative recuperation, premature or chronically ill babies, elderly patients
- reduction of invasive procedures
- inclusive design solutions for all users
- remote or at-home monitoring of activity through clothing, bedding, upholstery or carpets
- low power needs linked to communication network
- cost-effective solutions appropriate for disposable usage
- facilitate preventative healthcare
- enable integration of feedback and therapies into monitoring.

With the advent of ubiquitous (or pervasive) computing (Weiser 1991, 1999), sensors, antennae, miniature processor chips, radio frequency identification (RFID) tags and readers embedded in the domestic or hospital environment will be able to interact with sensors on the body or clothing, recognising pre-programmed parameters or biometric data. The concept of the 'smart home' for the elderly then becomes a reality – enabling a greater degree of independence and dignity whilst still being cared for. Sensors in carpets, for example, with integrated electronics – currently being developed by Infineon for airports and other public spaces (Lauterbach 2004) – could detect whether movement was taking place, or if there had been a fall and automatically alert the ambulance services. With all such monitoring procedures and devices ethical issues are raised regarding surveillance and control of data – who has access to the information?

1.3.3 Technology enablers and drivers

Current and emerging technologies for the development of smart materials are specifically adapted for use in the manufacture of textile products. Interdisciplinary collaboration is an essential feature to enable product development – the electronics industry is learning about textile production and fabric architecture; clothing manufacturing techniques are applied to products to specifically solve problems in wearable electronics; and standard commercial textile production methods from the mature textile manufacturing sector are adapted to create smart textiles at mass-produced affordable costs.

Established technologies which are currently being developed for specific medical and textile applications include:

- phase change materials
- thermochromic materials

- shape memory alloys and polymers
- conductive fibres and yarns – metals, wires and conductive polymers
- quantum tunnelling composites for switching devices
- piezoelectric resistance
- organic or plastic electronics
- biomaterials
- light-emitting polymers;
- light-emitting diodes
- fibre optics
- photovoltaics and solar cells
- photoluminescence
- photochromic materials
- holography
- plasma technologies
- nano technologies for fibre and fabric coating
- micro encapsulation for therapy delivery
- global positioning and wireless communications
- radio frequency identification (RFID) tags
- micro-electronic mechanical systems (MEMS).

Individual technologies are combined in systems comprising the sensing mechanisms, which respond to different external stimuli, the conversion of those responses to electrical signals, and the transmission of information within the system to actuate an effect which is received either by the user or a third party. Great progress has been made in the past ten years to bring prototypes and products very close to or actually into commercial markets. Research to develop useful products is necessarily a collaborative affair between many disciplines; the required building blocks must appropriately combine materials, technologies and design, together with expertise from the healthcare and psychology dimensions, before any user trials and marketing can take place. A failure on any one of these areas results in an unsuccessful product or a product which will not be accepted by the user. Therefore, testing prototypes with potential users is the most effective way in which to predict success or failure. VDC predicts the global market for electronically enabled smart fabrics and intelligent textiles will grow from a level of $304 million at the start of 2005 to $642 million dollars by 2008 (VDC 2005). All estimates propose an almost exponential growth in this market.

There are inevitably a number of barriers to be overcome before electronic smart textiles become universally usable and acceptable, one of which is the lack of global standards due to divergent strategies and cultures of research and development, and another the issue of power supply. Power sources remain a key issue for smart textiles, which will only be resolved when relevant enabling technologies converge in their development stages, to create smaller, lighter, longer lasting batteries, or to be able to generate and harvest energy from an individual's motion or the environment. This will provide the true breakthrough anticipated and transport products into mainstream commerce.

1.4 Examples of research and product development

Effective development of smart textile solutions to medical problems and procedures can be achieved only through a combination of several areas of expertise and research: several research groups now exist which combine medical knowledge and requirements with those of material scientists, textile technologists, information and communication technology experts, software developers and clothing designers and manufacturers. New alliances and new hybrid technologies are emerging from these collaborations. The union of the electronics industry with textiles has bred the new field of electronic textiles or e-textiles (also known as textronics, see chapter 5) to provide the next generation of wearable computing. This research process starts from user requirements and needs, and takes a human centred product development approach focused on design solutions, thus avoiding the cyborg-like effect of earlier wearable computing such as the MiThril vest developed by MIT in 2000 in which computer parts in pouches were distributed externally over a vest.

A number of technology platforms have now been established, based on different underlying technologies, by pioneering companies such as Softswitch and Eleksen, which integrate electronic functionality into textiles and clothing, primarily for sportswear, portable entertainment and lifestyle products. However, power supply for all electronic solutions still remains a fundamental problem when attempting to impart electronic functionality into clothing whilst simultaneously remaining completely portable. The development of a personal or body area network has been a key goal, particularly in military research to enable a soldier to collect, process and transmit data regarding his medical and security status. In the USA the Georgia Institute of Technology created the 'wearable motherboard' technology which was developed into the SmartShirt® by Sensatex in 2001 (Fig. 1.2). Here a supple textile of natural fibre with very thin wires and optical fibres was devised for monitoring biometric data continuously. This provided a versatile framework for sensing, monitoring and data processing devices, whereby patented sensors could be attached to any part of the person's body and plugged into the motherboard, becoming a flexible data bus transmitting information in and out. (www.sensatex.com, www.startupjournal.com 10 Aug 2001).

Solutions for smart textiles in medical care need to be more context-specific and the examples which follow indicate the wide range of approaches

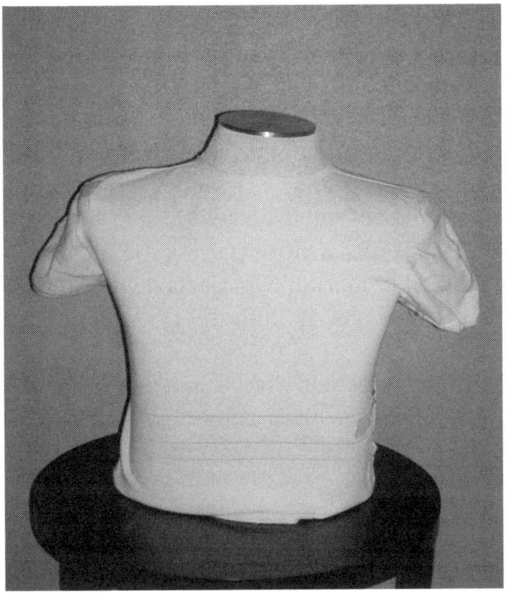

1.2 Sensatex SmartShirt.

currently being undertaken in research, together with the detailed case studies of prototypes and products in the final section of the book. Development of functionality is on many levels, but two classes of products can be defined: those that already have textile components, and those in which textiles will replace hard components.

Embroidery is an unexpected area of traditional textiles which is proving invaluable in developing medical implants, for example, in cardiovascular surgical procedures (where sewing in the form of sutures has long been a vital part of activities) using either specially developed bio-compatible and biodegradable materials or polyester. Building on earlier research (Ellis 1997), Ellis Developments have recently brought to market a range of embroidered textile implants (Tao, 2001; 222) utilising a novel adaptation of a standard sewing machine. The advantages of embroidery over woven or knitted structures in these circumstances include the ability to orientate fibres in any direction, and to build up layers on a substrate to exact shape specifications through computer-aided design. As in industrial lace manufacturing, the substrate can be dissolved away, leaving the threads as reinforcement where required.

Conductive polymer fibres and metallic wires spun with natural or standard synthetic fibres form conductive yarns which, with little adaptation, can be used in the normal textile processes of embroidery, knitting and weaving. The technical textiles field has seen rapid recent growth (Horrocks and Anand 2000; xiii) with applications to all aspects of society including in particular automotive and aerospace industries plus utilisation in architectural tensile structures and geo-textiles for civil construction. Much of this established textiles expertise is now being applied to medical uses. For example, knitting machinery specifically adapted for knitting metallic wires for automotive components are now used for knitting stainless steel electrodes such as those used in the Wealthy project, a collaborative EU-funded project which created a prototype health-monitoring bodysuit with textile interface utilising the piezoresistive effect and transferring data to a wireless communication system (Fig. 1.3). Both the Wealthy and SmartShirt projects demonstrate the levels of strategic funding recently available in both the USA and EU to support research into health monitoring.

The use of conductive fibres together with seamless knitting technology builds on the textile knowledge of the Textronics™ company founders who previously worked for Invista (formerly DuPont) fibres. This collaboration

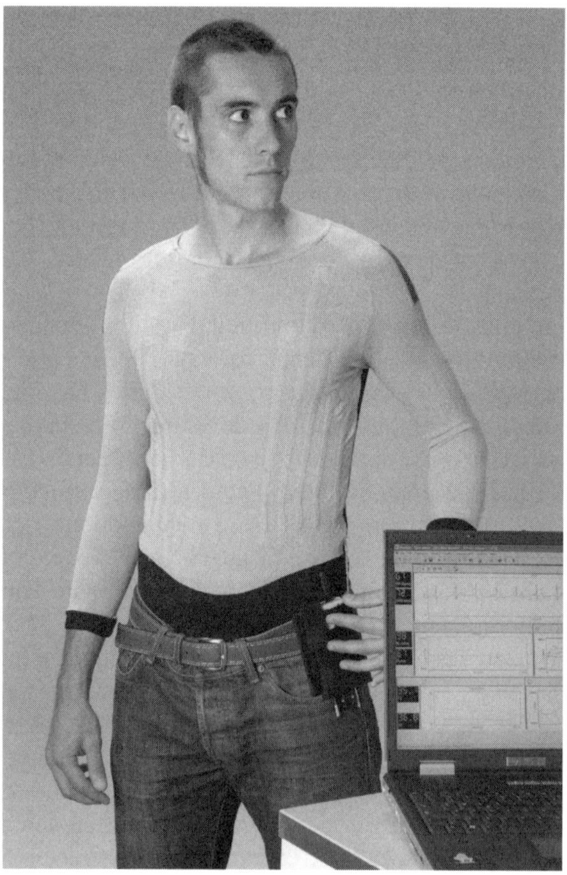

1.3 Wealthy healthcare system.

has produced an engineered seamless sports bra Numetrex™, recently launched on the commercial market, which contains totally integrated knitted sensors in specific areas incorporating silver-coated nylon with cotton covered Lycra™ fabric. The sensors detect heart rate directly through the pressure of the knitted fabric in contact with the body, utilising precise measurements of the degree of stretch in the fabric. The monitoring data is processed by the Polar™ heart rate monitoring unit which is inserted into the lower band of the bra, and read back from a watch-shaped monitor worn on the wrist. Although this product is designed for sports use, the potential for preventative healthcare is enormous, as comfort, washability (around 100 times) and ease of use are key features. (Fig. 1.4)

A similar technology is utilised for a different purpose in the WarmX® undershirt which is a knitted sleeveless vest incorporating two heated areas around the kidneys at the front and back, made from Shieldex™ yarn of silver coated polyamide, powered by a mobile phone sized 12 V battery pack held in a knitted pocket, which can be removed for washing. This product has been developed by a classic knitwear company of 100 years experience adapting and developing technologies for wellbeing, and is now available on the commercial market. (Fig. 1.5).

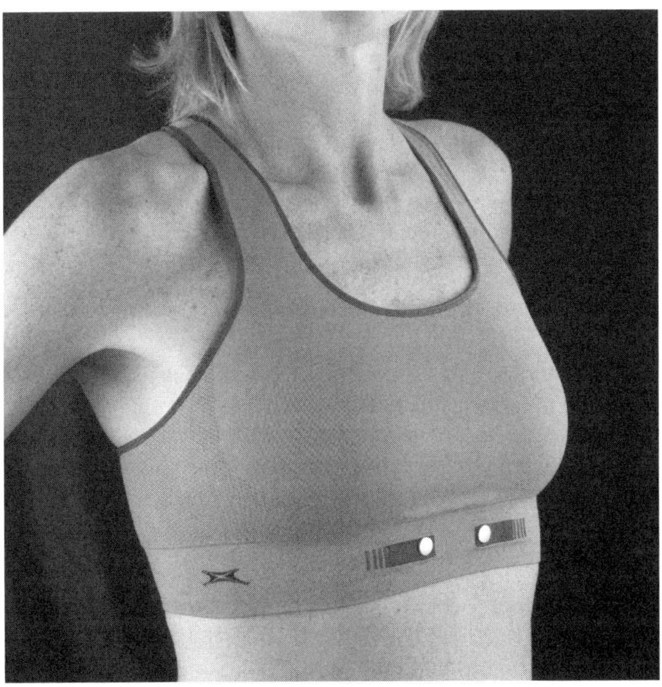

1.4 Numetrex sports bra (source: Textronics).

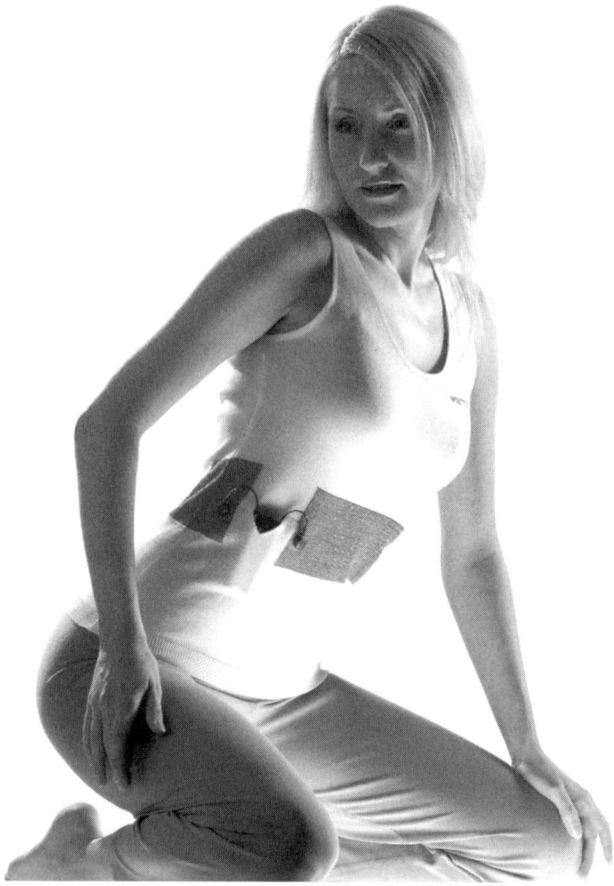

1.5 WarmX vest (source: WarmX).

1.4.1 Wearable technologies

A definition of 'wearable' in the context of electronics is offered in *Wearable Electronics and Photonics:*

> A device that has the functions of generation, transmission, modulation and detection of electrons and photons, is always attached to a person, and is comfortable and easy to keep and use. In other words it is apparel with unobtrusively built-in electronic and photonic functions (Tao 2005:1).

It is useful to note that 'wear*ing* technology is not the same as wear*able* technology', as stated by Stuart Collie of Softswitch (Collie 2004) and therefore the user experience is a vital component of success. Several companies have developed different patented technologies to integrate electronic functionality into textiles. Softswitch was one of the pioneering wearable technology companies, originating in the UK, and is now a subsidiary of Peratech, whose technology combines electrically conductive polymers, yarns and fabrics, based on the quantum tunnelling effect (www.peratech.co.uk/textech) which produces variable electrical resistance in response to pressure. Many prototypes and a limited number of final products have been developed such as the Burton jacket (see Fig. 1.1), updated in 2003 with iPod® technology, and a prototype of a formal business suit exhibited at Avantex 2005. Future concepts proposed include a pressure sensitive disposable bed sheet that would allow a nurse to quickly identify when a patient is in danger of getting a bedsore; an under layer which can detect moisture, and heated textile technology for sufferers of circulatory diseases (Collie 2004).

Eleksen has marketed portable electronic products based on their pressure sensitive layered textile interface ElekTex™, particularly the soft, flexible and portable keyboard comprising entirely fabric components orientated at 90° to each other which become conductive under pressure. Switches and buttons can therefore be incorporated into clothing as the technology is claimed to be washable. Although most applications to date are in lifestyle products and exclusive sportswear such as the Spyder Ski Jacket with integrated iPod™, the planned launch of standard Eleksen components may bring the technology into a more mass-market arena, more appropriate to medical uses (Jordan, 2005). The company's new collaboration with Microsoft for 'ultra-mobile' computing, with first products launched in 2006, will no doubt accelerate this process.

Intelligent Textiles, a UK company combining electrical engineering with textile design, have developed integrated electronic circuitry through traditional textile weaving technology. The textiles are mass produced industrially and cut and sewn as normal fabric. The company aims to 'make electrical products soft and soft products unobtrusively electronic'. Product concepts include a single layer woven keyboard and two fabrics, Heat and Detect, which are resistant to abrasion, can be washed at least 30 times and feel and perform as normal textiles. Heat incorporates low voltage heating elements and has been developed for heated glove linings to replace cumbersome circuitry, and features non-homogeneous heated functionality, directing warmth where required, with many potential applications such as heated bandages. Detect has a surface comprising thousands of small switches which are pressure sensitive, enabling a range of potential medical applications such as blankets sensing potential pressure sores in wheelchair users (Fig. 1.6), intelligent bedding, upholstery and carpets to monitor prolonged inactivity, posture, and falls or to incorporate easy to use alarm buttons, and to provide feedback in recuperation. Work is under way to develop a communication textile tag for sufferers of conditions such as cerebral palsy, in which pre-recorded simple messages can be played back.

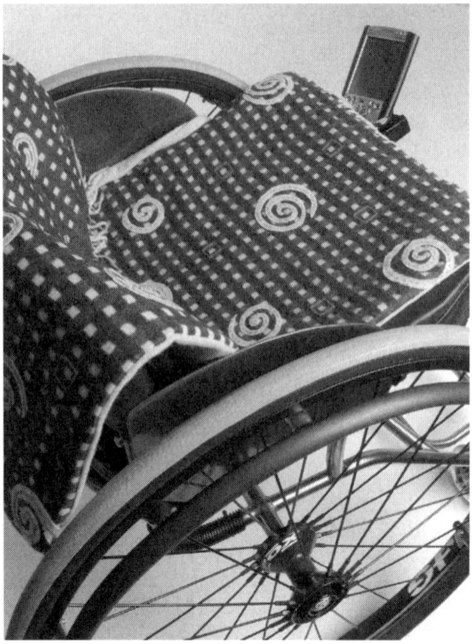

1.6 Wheelchair blanket prototype (source Intelligent Textiles).

Elsewhere in Europe, a collaboration between the Wearable Computing Lab of ETH Zürich, a Swiss research group, and Sefar AG is developing an e-fabric sensor consisting of a woven polyester fabric substrate with an embedded homogeneous insulated copper wire grid. The grid is thus insulated from short circuits and protected from environmental stresses, and can be used for the assembly of electrical components onto the cloth for specific functions, or potentially for temperature profiling and detection of 'hot spots' through measurement of changes in resistance. The technology is suitable for large area applications in clothing and interiors.

Research is also thriving in Asia. In Japan, there has been a growing trend in developing functional synthetic fibres and textiles with large investments in research, driven not by military research, but focused on consumer-related areas, with products such as temperature-modifying shoe insoles readily available. However, collaborations between the electronic and textiles industries (often the same parent company) are now developing wearable electronics applications for 'direct relay of visual and life sign data to hospitals from paramedics at accident sites, assistance to the visually impaired by direct visual link to a carer, or for medical training with direct links to databases and personnel' (Stylios 2004).

In Taiwan e-texcare®, a wearable technology physiological measurement system, is in development by Feng Chia University, integrating technologies of 'information technology, electrical engineering, electronics, communications, biomedical engineering, textiles, material science and aesthetics'. Prototype product concepts are tee shirts, vests and tracksuit tops which will carry their own power source supply in the form of a thin film battery or 'hot nanobattery', and are said to have potential for diagnosis and treatment of cardiovascular diseases. (NSC International Cooperation Science and Technology Newsbrief Feb 2005 http://stn.nsc.gov.tw)

The need to closely monitor infants born prematurely, or with medical problems, has led to a number of initiatives using smart textiles, such as the Mamagoose sleep suit developed by Verhaert, Belgium, which is designed to assist in continued research on sudden infant death syndrome. A British company, Intelligent Clothing, is developing a tele-monitoring device for babies which is inserted into a miniature textile teddy bear with a 'smart patch' and placed in a pocket on the chest of a specially designed garment. It is claimed that up to 25 patients could be monitored simultaneously in real time and garments are undergoing testing to meet hospital standards. The sensors measure heart rate through displacement of the vest and will communicate with a PDA or mobile phone, as does another device called 'Smart band' placed on the foot to measure oxygen saturation, temperature and heart rate.

Another example of a preventative device currently being tested is produced by researchers at ITV in Denmark, which integrates sensors into standard vests, to measure heart rate, respiration, temperature and humidity, with an alarm for life threatening situations, but is so far not as elegant as either of the other solutions. From these examples it is clear that deep integration of functional technologies into textiles will allow such technologies to become ubiquitous, and wearable healthcare systems to be successfully implemented.

1.4.2 Textiles in surgical implants, tissue engineering and wound care

Broadening the definition of smart textiles away from electronic textiles to functional textiles utilising other responses, there is extensive research being conducted into novel uses of textiles in surgical procedures, reaching 'a new quality of interactivity between biological tissues and textiles' (Wollina *et al.* 2003; 1) Examples can be found in textile scaffolds for tissue growth and regeneration, and woven, knitted, embroidered and braided structures for stents, replacement ligaments, arteries and blood vessels, or mesh grafts for hernia repairs, using biocompatible natural materials such as silk, catgut, chitin and collagen, or synthetic polymers (Rajendran and Anand 2002). Full reference material on these subjects can be found in two companion publications: the *Handbook of Technical Textiles* (2000) and *Medical Textiles and Biomaterials for Healthcare* (2005).

Mechanical functionality is the subject of interesting research for future applications. Shape memory materials are potentially used as actuators or 'muscle wires' in several applications. A new type of smart bandage is proposed by the Auxetic Materials group at the University of Bolton which utilises the highly unusual properties of auxetic fibres that have a negative Poisson ratio, and have been developed to expand when stretched (e.g., with swelling of the leg) to potentially release impregnated medication (Anderson and Anderson 2004). Micro-encapsulation of active materials into textiles has long been established, fibres coated using silver particles have been in medical use since the 1990s for antimicrobial, and anti-fungal functionality in bandages, dressings and medical devices. Both silver coated and carbon fibre fabrics are also used to absorb odours. The latest smart textiles for drug delivery and wound care are discussed in Chapter 3.

1.5 Future trends

The traditional processes of screen printing, (already used in printed circuits) and digital inkjet printing, have taken on new importance in the rapidly developing field of printed electronics, also termed plastic electronics, in which electro-active polymer layers are printed onto flexible substrates in the manner of inks, enabling light-emitting diodes to create electronic displays for smart packaging and flexible displays. Organic semi-conductive materials are key in many developments, enabling ease of processing although their short life is currently a major constraint, which will be overcome in time through continued research. These materials will become highly significant over the next 20 years as products reach the market and will greatly impact the medical sector along with retail and consumer goods, enabling coded wearable tags or other time-sensitive indicators, which may produce colour change or other visual responses to stimuli, to be reliably and cheaply produced.

As miniaturisation of consumer electronic devices reaches its limits and devices such as mobile phones and PDAs become difficult to use (with very small keyboard interfaces and screens), attention has turned to the molecular level of engineering and nanotechnologies, still highly controversial and producing much debate. Government initiatives in the USA and Europe have created a research environment which is now focusing on nanotechnology of all kinds, seen as having vast commercial potential, and already familiar to the medical profession through human biology and immunology for example. The science fiction writers have long envisaged the future filled with 'nanobots' – tiny nano-scale robots – that will clean and repair materials and cellular tissue, form particles which can travel through our skin (already available in cosmetic products and sun screens) and create changes in form, colour and structure within materials, clothing and the built environment. In the scientific community around the developed world, fundamental research is under way in nanocomposite structures and carbon nanotubes (CNTs) such as formation of 'the ultimate textile yarn' from CNTs with an exciting combination of properties: conductivity, strength, lightness, and fineness compared with carbon fibres, which could lead the way to controlled release of drugs, and other medications (Atkinson 2004).

Holographic and lenticular technologies on the micro level are very familiar through security coding devices on credit cards and graphic packaging materials. New research is taking place into applications of holographic printing technology at the nano scale to create colour and image responsive smart holograms sensitive to humidity and temperature, For enhanced functionality, a hologram is created in a polymer layer which can be controlled by variations in the wavelength of diffracted light patterns. This creates a simple visual indicator as colour changes in response to moisture or temperature changes. Further controlled changes are achieved from holograms in environments that are sensitive to changes in pH values, or to different enzymes, or to glucose levels in tear fluid. The latter is leading to the development of smart contact lenses as a diagnostic tool for diabetic patients. As a generic technology which is a combined sensor and transducer, with visual indication which is remotely interrogateable, and is potentially mass producible, disposable and cheap, there is no doubt that smart holograms will be integrated into many products in the next 10–20 years, and will have a great impact on medical uses for real-time monitoring (Lowe, 2006).

Another technology which is in development includes the integration into textiles of optical fibres to link light-emitting diodes (LEDs) to the light source, or the use of photovoltaics for incorporating flexible solar cells into textiles, a current subject of research by Centexbel in Belgium, the Hohenstein Institute in Germany and others. Challenges here to be resolved before products can be suitable are miniaturisation, interconnection methods, packaging and washability – a key issue with all electronic textile applications for clothing applications. However, there is less importance attached to washability in many medical uses where the majority of textiles are used only once.

Fibretronics, a UK company, are of the opinion that it is the availability of cheap components ready to be applied in electronic textiles which has so far prevented commercial take up and exploitation of wearable electronics (Leftly 2005). Now, with the merging of technologies so important to this field, and the collaborative approaches to research problems together with the commercial push to fully exploit research spin out in the market place, the barriers to real and effective products being available are being rapidly torn down.

Textiles are already a key feature in all medical contexts from dressings and bandages, to surgical clothing, wipes and clean room protection – most textiles being single use and disposable to avoid cross contamination. A novel solution to immediate availability of wipes and other coverings could be provided by FabriCan™ – a spin-out company based on fashion designer Manel Torres' patented technology concept of 'spray-on fabric', (Fig. 1.7)

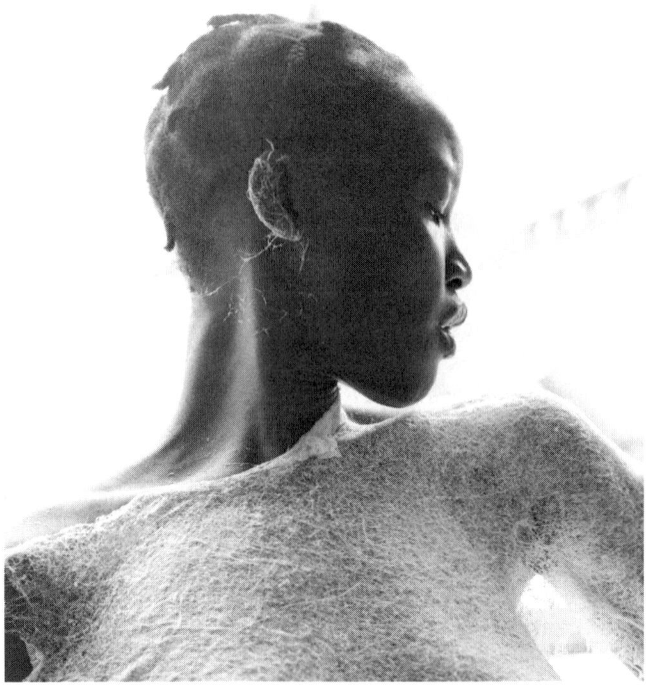

1.7 FabriCan spray-on fabric, (photo Rebecca Harman).

developed with mechanical engineers at Imperial College London, using different combinations of fibres suspended in solution. Stretchable fibres resulting in latex-like membranes or the paper-like quality of cotton fibres is ideal for disposable medical use. There is potential for targeted fibre delivery for textile scaffolds, plasters and bandages, drug delivery, applications in skin treatments, colour changing bandages and much more.

New fibre construction and fabric treatment technologies are in development to introduce the beneficial effects of microencapsulation and release of therapeutic treatments including aloe vera, anti-bacterial and anti-odour effects, such as adapted core spun yarns by Swiss company Spoerry® Functional, and Cavatex® from Germany, who produce cyclodextrin fabric finishes which can capture odours and release active ingredients in cycles, which are refreshed through washing.

There is a growing new area of research into the personal effect of self-esteem and environment on recuperation, and the part contributed by the clothing that patients may be asked to wear in hospital or for clinical reasons. Designer Rebecca Earley, commissioned by Birmingham hospital in 1999, demonstrated that breast cancer patients' self-esteem was improved when specially designed printed garments were worn (www.chelsea.arts.ac.uk/research.Chelsea3). Ulrich (1984) found patient post-operative recovery improved where they could see trees rather than a brick wall from the window, and that stress delays wound repair. This was followed by a number of other studies (Devlin and Arneill 2003). The entire 'healing environment' of the hospital and doctor's general practice is being considered in terms of design by a research group based in Kings College London to promote healthcare design for healing spaces – much of which includes textile elements (www.the-space-works.org). Smart textiles and clothing can therefore make a significant contribution to healing, as can music, which could be available to individual patients through linking their hospital clothing to personal music systems.

Dr Jenny Tillotson, a textile researcher of Sensory Design and Technology Ltd, is pioneering collaborative research for embedding microfluidics into textiles to create a personal olfactory environment or 'scent bubble', integrating sensors to provide a smart responsive environment, rather than passive, which she terms Scentsory Design® for stress relief and wellbeing. Olfactory technologies are an under-researched area which may have potential benefits to drug delivery and therapeutic and preventative care. Although microencapsulation has been available for some time and can be found commercially in lingerie and hosiery products delivering skin creams or controlling odour in socks, research is progressing rapidly at the nanotechnology scale to create hollow nanospheres and clusters designed for perfumes and flavours but which could eventually be used for controlled drug delivery or other active ingredients (Sukhorukov 2006).

Arguably the smartest known material is human skin which acts simultaneously as a protective barrier, a porous permeable membrane and is sensitive to light, heat and chemicals. The ultimate delivery of drugs and other active ingredients may become directly transmitted though the skin, which is predicted in various future scenarios based on technologies currently being researched. The integration of nanotechnology with cosmetic applications could lead to active tattoos applied to the skin that are non-invasive but can transmit medication, or change colour to indicate medical condition in a similar but more refined manner than current trans-dermal patches. Working in conjunction with telecommunications, implants under the skin could (controversially) be used to monitor movement (or lack of it) and track individuals and provide either monitoring and feedback or surveillance. In future a functional prosthetic skin will be able to withstand environments that are too extreme or hostile and transmit continuous data about a patient's condition. Certainly research is under way in Korea into the development of flexible artificial skin fabrics, with potential use by burn victims (Stylios 2004).

1.6 Conclusions

The previous technology drivers have been military or space explorations, but 'real life' commercial applications may be the ones that now create a substantial market pull. Because of the stringent requirements that are required in medical uses, the crossover potential is great – the medical market is a major driver but will have many non-medical spin-offs. With so much research activity in progress, and nearing the commercial market, it is clear that smart textiles integrated into medical devices and clothing will revolutionise the way medical and healthcare is conducted. The future will include more personalised healthcare and greater empowerment of patients to manage their health conditions in their own homes with greater mobility through biofeedback and vital signs and motion monitoring, enabling home-based diagnostics, and for preventative care through wellness monitoring. Advantages will include more inclusively designed solutions to problems and the removal of stigma associated with current, obviously visible medical devices, as functionalities are integrated further into textile interfaces and substrates. Drug delivery may eventually be accomplished through the clothes themselves, as truly smart 'second skins' which can protect, monitor, communicate and heal.

The power supply to drive the electronic and smart functionalities will eventually be derived not from batteries but from energy harvested from kinetic movement or generated from the environment through, for example, embedded solar cells. The ultimate goal of wearable technology is intelligence embedded or integrated into clothing leading to a genuine body area network or 'personalised wearable information infrastructure' (Tao 2001:227).

Finally, the holistic treatment of patients will be recognised in the total environment of the hospital; the healing hospital of the future will create a positive ambient environment through light, sound and colour responsiveness throughout the environment including walls, curtains, carpets and furniture in addition to the specific medical products discussed in this book. Psychology in health studies is beginning to gain momentum and recognises the importance of maintaining self esteem and motivation for recovery, just as emotional marketing has transformed the commercial landscape.

Many technologies relevant to smart textiles are now maturing, as others continually emerge. In the near future, products that will seamlessly integrate into many life situations, and that will be intuitive, ubiquitous and almost invisible in use will genuinely transform and even help save lives.

1.7 Sources of further information and advice

1.7.1 Further reading

Anand SC, Miraftab M, Rajendran S and Kennedy JF (eds) (2005) *Medical textiles and biomaterials for healthcare*, Cambridge, Woodhead.

Nanotechnology and the Health of the EU Citizen in 2020, *EuroNanoForum 2005 Proceedings,* Edinburgh, Institute of Nanotechnology.

Pearson I and Lyons M (2003) *Business 2010*, Spiro.
Plastic Electronics, Printing's Potential as a Manufacturing Technology (2005), I.T. Strategies Inc, Global Industry Review USA.

1.7.2 Resources

Institute of Nanotechnology www.nano.org.uk
London Centre for NanoTechnology www.lcn.ucl.ac.uk
Technitex Faraday Partnership www.technitex.org
TechTextil and Avantex symposia
Materials Knowledge Transfer Network www.materialsktn.org
Wearable Electronics and Smart Textiles Network www.smartextiles.info
EPSRC smart textiles network www.smartextiles.co.uk
www.eleksen.com
www.fabrickeyboard.com
www.intelligenttextiles.com
www.peratech.co.uk
www.wealthy-ist.com
www.numetrex.com
www.sefar.com
www.intelligentclothing.com
www.smartholograms.com
www.warmx.de

1.8 References

Anderson A and Anderson K (2004) 'Auxetic Materials: expanding materials and applications', briefing paper, University of Bolton.

Atkinson K (2004) 'Australian developments in textile and fibre technology'. CSIRO *Proceedings of New Technologies and Smart Textiles for Industry and Commerce,* London. Institute of Nanotechnology.

Bhattacharyya K (2006) 'Revolution in the Making', *RSA Journal* Feb 2006 pp 50–54.

Collie S (2004) 'Intelligent textiles: are we overlooking the basics?' *Proceedings of Technical Textiles: the innovative approach.* Manchester UK.

Devlin AS and Arneill AB (2003) 'Health care environments and patient outcomes: a review of the literature', *Environment and Behaviour* Vol 35 pp 665–694.

Ellis JG (1997) *The Manufacture of Structural Composites using the Techniques of Embroidery,* LINK project report, Ellis Developments Ltd.

Hooper A *et al.* (2003) *Smart Materials for the 21st Century*, Foresight Smart Materials Taskforce, London, Institute of Materials, Minerals and Mining. Report no FMP/03/04/IOM3.

Horrocks AR and Anand SC (2000), *Handbook of Technical Textiles*, Woodhead Publishing, Cambridge.

Jones I and Wise RJ (2005) 'Novel joining methods applicable to textiles and smart garments', *Wearable Futures* Conference presentation, Newport UK.

Jordan M (2005) 'Real products for real life'. *Wearable Futures* Conference presentation, Newport UK.

Lauterbach C (2004) 'Smart textiles: integrated microelectronics for large-area sensor and display systems', *Proceedings of New Technologies and Smart Textiles for Industry and Commerce,* London. Institute of Nanotechnology.

Leftly S (2005) 'Enabling supply of volume components to the wearable electronics industry', *Proceedings of 3rd International Avantex Symposium,* Frankfurt, Germany.

Lowe C (2006) 'Tales of the Unexpected: Smart holograms in crime, sport and medicine', Royal Society lecture, London.

Peijs T (2005) Chairman Smart Textiles Symposium (in call for papers), Plastic Electronics Conference, September, Frankfurt, www.plastictronics.org.

Puers R, Hermans B, Catrysse M, Coosemans J, Hertleer C and Langenhove L (2005) 'A smart suit for the monitoring of children'. *Proceedings of 3rd International Avantex Symposium*, Frankfurt, Germany.

Rajendran S and Anand SC (2002) 'Developments in medical textiles: a critical appraisal of recent developments', *Textile Progress* Vol 32 no 2.

Strese H, John L and Kaminorz Y (2004) *Technnical textiles and micro systems technology in market segments medicine and safety textiles: needs and requirements*, Tetlow, Germany. VDI/VDE Innovation+Technik GmbH.

Stylios GK (2004) *Interactive Smart Textiles: Innovation and Collaboration in Japan and South Korea,* London, Report of a DTI Global Watch mission.

Sukhorukov G (2006) 'Multifunctional polymer micro- and nano-sized capsules'. *Proceedings of Novel Delivery Techniques for Industrial Scents and Flavours*. London, Institute of Nanotechnology Conference.

Tao X, ed. (2001) *Smart Fibres, Fabrics and Clothing*, Cambridge, Woodhead.

Tao X, ed. (2005) *Wearable Electronics and Photonics,* Cambridge, Woodhead.

Ulrich R (1984) 'View through the window may influence recovery from surgery'. *Science*, Vol 224, No 4647, 420–421.

VDC (2005) *Smart Fabrics and Interactive Textiles. OEM and end-user requirements, preferences and solution analysis*. 2nd edn. Venture Development Corporation USA.

Weiser M (1991) 'The Computer for the 21st Century', *Scientific American*, Sept, 94–104.

Weiser M, Gold R and Brown JS (1999) 'The origins of ubiquitous computing research at PARC in the late 1980s', *IBM Systems Journal*, Vol 38, No 4, Pervasive Computing.

Wollina U, Heide M, Muller-Litz W, Obenhauf D and Ash J (2003) 'Functional Textiles in prevention of chronic wounds, wound healing and tissue engineering', in Elsner P, Hatch K, Wigger-Alberti W, (eds) *Textiles and the Skin*, Current Problems in Dermatology, Vol 31, Basel, London: Karger.

2
Smart wound-care materials

Y QIN, Jiaxing College, China

2.1 Introduction

Wounds are defined as skin defects caused by mechanical, thermal, electrical and chemical injuries, or by the presence of an underlying medical or physiological disorder. Wound dressings are materials used to cover the wounds. Many types of wounds occur in everyday life, such as mechanical injuries including abrasions, lacerations, acute bullet or knife cuts, bites and surgical wounds, and various types of burns caused by thermal, chemical, electrical and radiational injuries. Other types of wounds such as chronic ulcerative wounds including pressure sores and leg ulcers occur more commonly among elderly people.

Wound dressings have been in use for as long as conventional textile materials. The primary function of wound dressings is to avoid strikethrough and to protect the wounded site from contamination and further injuries. Wound dressings may not help accelerate the healing process but they must not in any way delay the wound repair process through a number of mechanisms, such as adherence to wound bed, leaching toxic component, causing wound maceration, etc. Wound dressings need to be easy to apply and easy to remove. These traditional requirements for wound dressings have largely been met by the various types of gauzes and various derivatives of gauze dressings, such as bandages, wax impregnated gauze, woven, nonwoven and knitted gauze, etc. Nonwoven materials laminated with perforated plastic film have been used to reduce dressing adherence and to reduce the amount of fibrous residue, thus overcoming one of the main shortcomings of traditional wound dressings [1].

In the 1960s, the science of wound dressings achieved a breakthrough, when Winter [2] reported the results of a study on the treatment of pig wounds in an occlusive condition. It was found that when the wound is kept in a moist condition as would have resulted from the application of an occlusive dressing, epithelisation of the wound surface occurred much faster than if the wound were kept in an otherwise dry condition, which was then regarded as the desirable condition. Further studies on human wounds confirmed that wound healing took place much faster when the wound is kept in a moist condition [3, 4]. These early studies provided the scientific and medical foundation for modern wound-management materials, which are designed to provide a moist healing environment for the wound. The so-called 'moist healing' dressings were developed in order to create this moist interface between the wound and the dressing [5].

It is interesting to note that much of the research that led to the development of modern wound management products was concentrated on the 'moist healing' principle, and in the 1980s and 1990s, many 'moist healing' products, such as hydrocolloids, alginates, polyurethane foams and hydrogel, were developed and launched into the European and North American health care market, where the advent of the ageing population together with the increased need for managing chronic ulcerative wounds provided a growing market for companies supplying wound care products, at the same time stimulating the research and development efforts for smart wound-care materials that are more effective and more functional than traditional materials. Figure 2.1 shows the number of new wound-care products listed in the British Drug Tariff during the 1990s. There was a clear surge in the number of new products from 1996 and onwards, when many new types of alginates, hydrogels and other smart wound-care materials became commercialised.

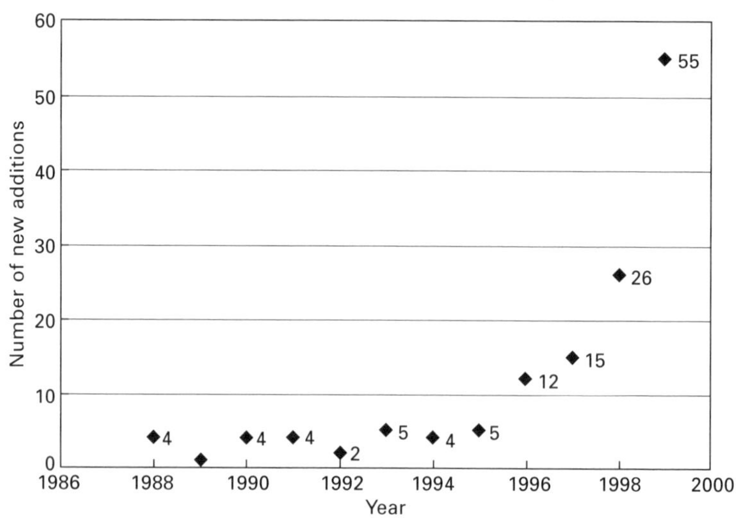

2.1 Number of new wound-care products listed on the British Drug Tariff during the 1990s.

2.2 Functional requirement for modern wound-care materials

Wounds differ from one type to another, and the functional requirement for the wound dressings can only be specified for specific types of wounds [6]. In defining the requirement of a wound dressing, it is also important to observe that for a specific type of wound, the requirement for the dressing is different at different stages of the healing process. According to their physiological condition, wounds can be classified into five types, each with a symbolic colour code, i.e., necrotic wounds (black), sloughy wounds (yellow), granulating wounds (red), epithelialising wounds (pink), and infected wounds (green). These five types of wounds differ in their physical appearances, the level of exudate, and the level of microbial contamination. Figure 2.2 shows a schematic illustration of the five types of wounds.

For the necrotic wounds, one of the main aims of applying a dressing is to facilitate the separation of the dead tissue from the underlying healthy tissue so as to enable a normal wound healing process. If exposed to a relatively dry atmosphere, as would be found in a hospital ward or in a centrally heated room, dead tissue rapidly loses moisture and becomes dehydrated. As it does so, it shrinks and progressively becomes olive-green or black in colour. It is also hard and dry to touch. In this condition, autolysis is inhibited and separation of the necrotic tissue may be delayed indefinitely. For the treatment of necrotic wounds, it is essential that the dressings must be able to prevent the dehydration process. Indeed, they should be able to facilitate a hydration process for the dead tissue so that the autolytic debridement process, in which the dead tissue is separated from healthy tissue, can take place. Necrotic wounds are ideally treated with hydrogels and/or hydrocolloid dressings [7].

For the yellow sloughy wounds, such as burns, leg ulcers, pressure sores, etc., where a necrotic covering has been removed, a glutinous yellow covering normally develops on the wound surface. This is not dead tissue, but a complex mixture of fibrin, protein, serous exudate, leucocytes and bacteria. To treat this type of wound, the sloughy mess must first be properly cleaned

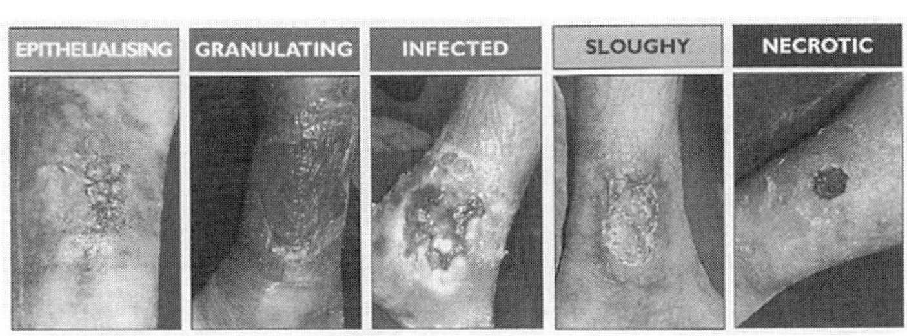

2.2 Schematic illustration of the five types of wounds.

or debrided. If the slough is moist, an alginate dressing can be used to absorb the exudate. On the other hand, if the slough is dry, hydrocolloid or hydrogel dressings may be used.

Normal wound healing progresses from necrotic and sloughy phases to granulating phase, when the wound is covered by granulation tissue composed of collagen and proteoglycan in a complex of protein and polysaccharides, with salts and other colloidal materials. These produce a gel-like matrix which is contained within the fibrous collagen network with a highly vascular nature that gives it a characteristic deep pink colour. Granulating wounds vary considerably in size, shape and the amount of exudate that they produce. As a result, no single dressing will be suitable for use in all situations. Depending on the particular shape and the amount of exudate, alginate, hydrocolloids and hydrogels may be used.

The final phase of the wound healing process is the epithelialisation of the wound surface. With a few exceptions, superficial or epithelialising wounds tend not to produce large quantities of exudate. Traditionally, these wounds have been dressed with paraffin gauze and cotton tissue but sometimes alginate and hydrocolloids can be used. It is important to recognise that at this stage the tissue is soft and fragile, and therefore any dressings used on these wounds must not adversely disturb the delicate tissue structure. In particular, dressings must not unnecessarily adhere to the wound. For epithelialising wounds, alginate, hydrocolloid, vapour-permeable film, silicon coated film and knitted viscose gauze may be used as the primary wound dressings.

Infected wounds tend to generate a large amount of exudate and also unpleasant odour. The treatment of infected wounds therefore comprises absorbing exudate, containing odour and controlling microbial contamination. Dressings that in part contain activated charcoal can be used to absorb odour, whilst the odour-generating bacteria can be controlled by using dressings with an antimicrobial function, such as those with chlorhexidine, silver compounds or iodine [8–13].

The main functions of wound dressings are summarised below.

1. **Fluid control** The ability to absorb fluid from a highly exuding wound or to donate moisture to a dry wound is one of the main functions of a wound dressing.
2. **Odour management** The wound quite often produces an unpleasant and noxious odour. When this occurs, dressings must be able to contain the odour.
3. **Microbial control** For infected wounds, it is important that bacteria is contained by appropriate methods.
4. **Physical barrier** One of the principal functions of a wound dressing is to avoid strikethrough. In addition to its aesthetic purpose of hiding the wound, wound dressings also help to separate the wound surface

from the atmosphere and prevent the wound from bacterial contamination and further physical damage to the tissue.

5. **Space filler** For deep cavity wounds, it is important that the wound is kept open by filler materials, so that the healing process can take place from bottom upwards and unnecessary closure of the wound before the whole cavity is healed can be prevented.
6. **Debridement** The removal of dead necrotic tissue is essential for facilitating the normal wound healing process. Wound dressings can accelerate the debridement process by providing the appropriate moisture, pH, temperature, and other conditions that are ideal for the autolytic debridement process.
7. **Haemostatic effect** For acute surgical wounds and traumatic wounds, it is important that bleeding is stopped as early as possible to prevent blood loss. Appropriate wound dressings can help blood clotting.
8. **Low adherence** Adherence of the whole or part of the dressing to the wound surface is a major problem in wound management, often causing trauma on removal of the dressing. A low-adherent dressing can help lower or eliminate adherence to the wound.
9. **Scar reduction** For large wounds, scar formation presents a major aesthetic problem for the patient. Any dressing that can reduce or prevent scar formation can give great benefit to the patient.
10. **Metal ion metabolism** A number of metal ions such as iron, zinc, copper, magnesium, selenium, etc., play important roles in cellular activities. Deficiency in any metal ions delays wound healing. Apart from systemic intake of these metal ions, they can be administered through the topical use of appropriate wound dressings.
11. **Wound healing acceleration** Wound healing is a complex physiological process. Wound dressing often plays a minor role in the overall rate of the wound healing process. However, when combined with a number of factors, the appropriate use of dressings can accelerate the wound healing process.

2.3 Smart materials used in modern wound-care products

Because of the similarity in their uses and functional requirements, wound dressings are often made from similar materials to those used in traditonal textile fabrics. Indeed, traditional gauze materials are made from cotton yarn, using a simple woven technique. For different applications, traditional wound dressings use many different materials and have different types of textile structures. For example, the *British Pharmacopoeia* classifies surgical dressings into four types:

- X-ray detectable absorbents
- extensible bandages
- tubular bandages
- wound dressings and medicated bandages.

It is often difficult to draw a line between the so-called traditional dressings and the modern high-tech dressings. As has been mentioned, the evolution of modern dressings began with the discovery of the 'moist healing' concept, and many high-tech wound dressings are often able to control the level of moisture at the interface between the wound and the dressing so as to create a 'moist but not wet' condition. Since the 1990s, more and more advanced wound dressings have been developed by a number of wound-care companies and launched into the western healthcare market. As an illustration of the diverse modern smart wound-care materials, the British Drug Tariff now has ten categories of wound dressings, as can be seen below.

1. low-adherence dressings
2. gauze-impregnated dressings
3. dextranomer paste pad and dressing
4. alginate dressings
5. hydrocolloid dressings
6. hydrogels
7. vapour-permeable adhesive film dressings
8. polyurethane foam dressings
9. zinc paste bandages
10. iodine-containing dressings.

These products are often used alone or in combination on wounds with many diversified physiological backgrounds and at different stages of the healing process. In order to satisfy the requirements of the healing process, many types of smart materials and technologies have also been developed; some of these are introduced below.

2.3.1 Polysaccharide fibres

Alginate fibres

Alginate is a natural polysaccharide extracted from brown seaweeds. Alginate fibres can be made by extruding the water-soluble sodium alginate solution into an aqueous calcium chloride bath, using a simple wet spinning process. The resultant calcium alginate fibres have been known for many years for their non-inflammability, due to the high concentration of metal ions in the fibres, and their solubility in dilute aqueous alkali solutions, which was utilised in the production of socks as a draw thread.

Alginate fibres have a unique ion exchange property [14]. On contact with wound exudate, the calcium ions in the fibre exchange with the sodium ions in the body fluid and as a result, part of the fibre becomes sodium alginate. Since sodium alginate is water soluble, this ion-exchange leads to the swelling of the fibre and the *in-situ* formation of gel on the wound surface. This unique property makes alginate fibre one of the ideal materials for the production of 'moist healing' wound dressings, and after much development during the 1980s and 1990s, various types of alginate fibres and dressings are now available, utilising the diversified properties of the different types of alginate extracted from different sources of seaweeds and the availability of many types of salts of alginate, such as zinc and silver alginate, which are used for zinc-deficient people and for antimicrobial properties respectively [15, 16]. Due to their unique properties and the fact that the dressings can be used in the dry form or hydrated form, alginate dressings can be used for a wide range of wounds, providing a cost-effective treatment that involves a minimum number of dressing changes.

The properties of alginate fibres can be modified in many ways. For example, in order to make the alginate fibres more absorbent, sodium ions can be introduced into the calcium alginate fibres through chemical treatment. In this process, the calcium alginate fibres can be first washed with hydrochloric acid to replace part of the calcium ions with hydrogen ions. The hydrogen ions are then replaced with sodium ions by a treatment with sodium carbonate or sodium hydroxide [17, 18]. Highly absorbent calcium sodium alginate fibres can also be made by treating the fibres with aqueous solutions containing different amount of Na_2SO_4. The Na_2SO_4 is used because the solubility of $CaSO_4$ in water is only 0.209 g per 100 ml at 30 °C, hence it can easily replace calcium ions from the alginate fibres [19].

Table 2.1 shows the composition and properties of the various calcium sodium alginate fibres. It can be seen that by replacing calcium ions with sodium ions, fibres with increasing gel swelling ratios can be made. This indicates that for the alginate fibre, its absorption capacity can be easily regulated by varying the sodium content of the fibre.

Table 2.1 Effect of Na_2SO_4 concentration on fibre calcium content and gel swelling ratio [19]

Na_2SO_4 concentration	Fibre Ca (II) content	Fibre Na (I) content	% Alginic acid as Na (I) salt	Gel swelling ratio in water
Control	8.35%	0.20%	2.0%	1.8 ± 0.15
0.1%	6.55%	1.25%	14.2%	6.5 ± 0.45
0.2%	6.45%	1.6%	17.7%	8.5 ± 0.65
0.5%	5.65%	1.85%	22.2%	11.1 ± 0.80
0.7%	5.95%	2.65%	27.9%	21.0 ± 1.50

Figures 2.3 and 2.4 show the photomicrographs of alginate fibres with different sodium content when they were placed in contact with water. It is clear that as the sodium content increases, the fibres are capable of holding more water within the fibre structure. This is important in two respects. First, as the fibres hold more water, the dressings are capable of absorbing more wound exudate, hence extending the duration of the dressing. Second, when the fibre absorbs water into the fibre structure and swells, the spaces between the fibres in the dressing are closed, thus prohibiting liquid from lateral spreading and preventing the maceration of the areas surrounding the wound surface [20]. As can be seen in Fig. 2.5, when 5 ml of normal saline is dropped onto the nonwoven structure, the sodium alginate fabric is capable

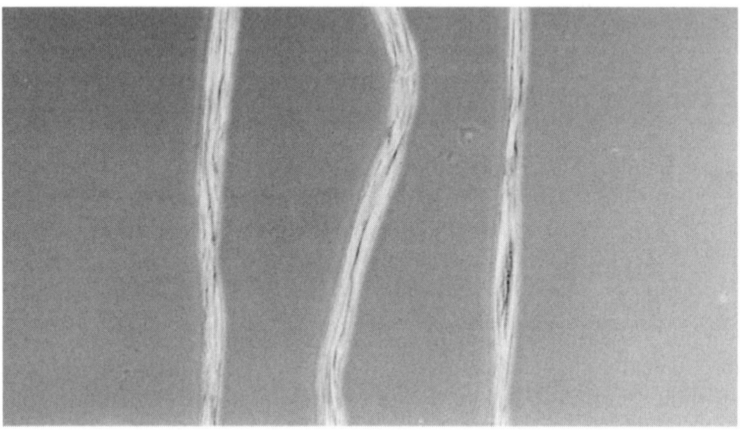

2.3 Photomicrograph of alginate fibres with 2.0% sodium alginate, wet in water (× 200) [19].

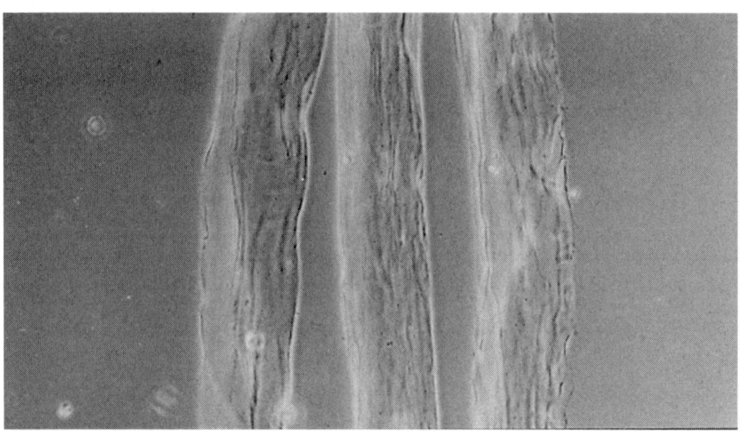

2.4 Photomicrograph of alginate fibres with 27.9% sodium alginate, wet in water (× 200) [19].

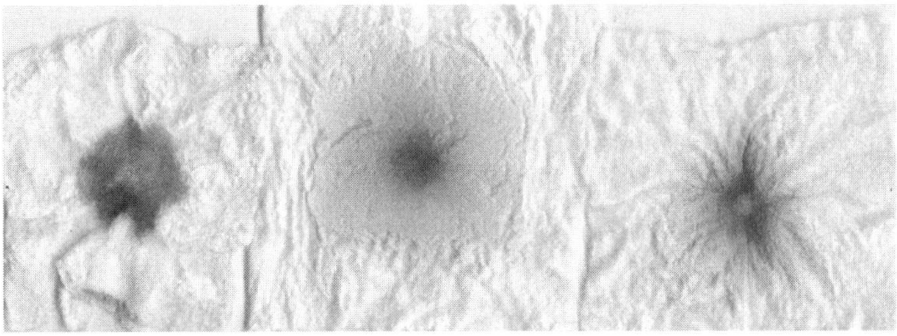

2.5 The spreading of liquid on nonwoven fabrics made of sodium alginate, alginic acid and calcium alginate fibres [21].

of holding the liquid within a very narrow area, showing a much better 'gel blocking' property than the calcium alginate and alginic acid fabric.

Chitin and chitosan fibres

Chitin, poly-1,4-2-acetamido-2-deoxy-β-D-glucose, is the second most abundant natural polymer existing widely in cell walls of fungi and crustacean shells. Chitin is commercially produced from the shell waste of crabs, shrimps and krill through a series of deproteinisation and demineralisation to remove the protein and minerals, which together with chitin, form the composite structure of the shells. The dry mass of shell waste typically contains about 15–25% of chitin.

Chitin has long been known as being able to accelerate the wound-healing process. It has been shown that by applying chitin dressings, the wound-healing process can be accelerated by up to 75% [22]. Chitin fibre was first reported in 1926 [23], when German scientists succeeded in making an artificial silk that resembles the texture of natural silk. Chitin is, however, by its chemical and physical nature, very difficult to dissolve. Although a large number of solvents such as concentrated mineral acids, trichloroacetic acid, formic acid, etc., have been used to dissolve chitin, the process is often complicated and impractical for large-scale fibre production.

In the 1980s, following extensive development on the solvent system, a new solvent for chitin was developed which offers the opportunity for easy processing of chitin into fibres. By treating chitin first with p-toluene sulphonic acid in i-propanol, chitin can be easily dissolved in dimethyl acetamide (DMAc) containing a small amount of lithium chloride [24]. The chitin solution in DMAc-LiCl can be extruded into a coagulation bath of either water or methanol solution to form fibres. Chitosan is the deacetylated derivative of chitin. Like chitin, chitosan is also known to have wound-healing acceleration properties and a number of studies have shown that chitosan fibres have unique properties as a suture and wound dressing material [25].

Chitosan can be easily dissolved in aqueous solutions of almost all the organic and inorganic acids because of the primary amine group on the C-2 position of the glucose residue. Chitosan fibres can be made by first dissolving it in an aqueous acidic solution and then extruding the solution through fine holes into a coagulation bath of a dilute alkali solution. Chitosan precipitates out in the form of a filament which can be washed, stretched and dried to form fibres for the production of wound dressings [26, 27].

Since chitosan is chemically the deacetylated form of chitin, by acetylating chitosan with acetic anhydride, it has been found that chitosan fibres can be converted to chitin fibres, which have similar properties to that of natural chitin fibre. Both the chitin and chitosan fibres have good mechanical properties, with fibre tenacities in the region of 1.5 to 2.5 g/decitex and elongation at break at about 8–20% [24, 26]. These fibres are highly hydrophilic and are biocompatible, biodegradable and non-toxic, thus providing unique raw materials for advanced wound dressings.

Superabsorbent cellulosic fibres

In order to produce highly absorbent fibres, cellulosic fibres such as cotton and viscose rayon can be treated with chloro-acetic acid to make carboxymethyl cellulose. As can be seen in Fig. 2.6, when the cellulosic fibres are partially carboxymethylated, the carboxylic group is capable of absorbing a large amount of water and the fibres are capable of a high degree of swelling when wet in water. By controlling the degree of substitution, it is also possible to maintain their fibrous form when in contact with water [28].

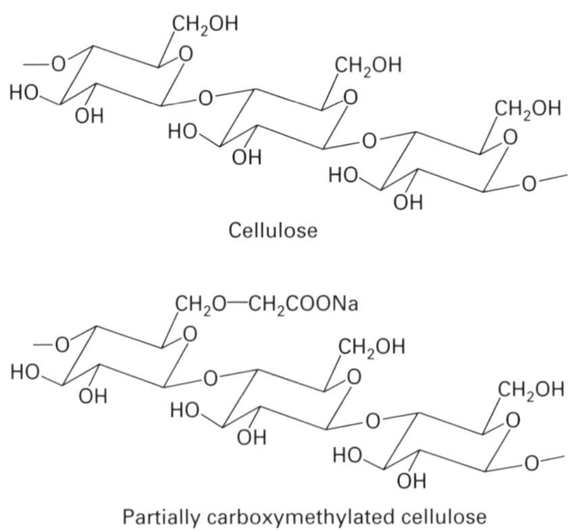

2.6 Chemical structure of cellulose and partially carboxymethylated cellulose.

This type of carboxymethylation process can be applied to the solvent spun Tencel fibres, in which case the nonwoven dressing can retain the soft and fine features of the solvent spun fibres and also at the same time possess the superabsorbency that is derived from the carboxymethylation treatment. This type of product has the ability to absorb fluid directly into the body of the fibre, thus significantly increasing the volume of fluid that can be absorbed. In clinical circumstances, the removal of a large volume of exudates may lead to a decrease in the number of micro-organisms on the wound surface. Also, in the presence of wound exudates, this type of carboxymethylated cellulosic dressing can form a cohesive gel sheet, which facilitates its use under compression bandages. The non-adherent features of these dressings leads to significantly less pain on dressing change [29, 30].

As can be seen in Fig. 2.7, upon contact with exudates, the carboxymethylated cellulosic fibres take the liquid up into the structure of the fibres themselves, instead of holding it within a web of gelled fibres. This property results in a range of clinical benefits for wound dressings made of partially carboxymethylated cellulosic fibres, including:

- superior exudate absorption and retention
- improved handling characteristics
- enhanced vertical wicking, which minimises the potential for maceration.

2.3.2 Polyurethane film and foam

Semi-permeable polymeric coatings have been used in the textile industry for making breathable clothings. As a wound-management material, a semi-

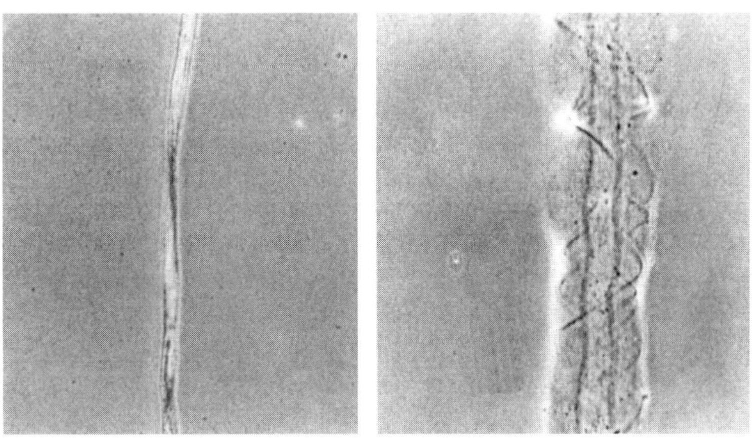

(a) (b)

2.7 The dry(a) and wet(b) structure of carboxymethylated cellulosic fibre (× 200) [28].

permeable film allows gaseous exchange between the wound and the surrounding environment, whilst preventing airborne bacteria from contaminating the wound. The semi-permeable nature of the film allows a high rate of moisture vapour transmission through the film, thereby reducing the build-up of wound exudate under the film. These films are highly comfortable and convenient to use and they can permit constant observation of the wound. They allow gaseous and moisture exchange but provide a barrier against water and micro-organisms [31, 32].

Modern semi-permeable film dressings are usually made from polyurethane of various compositions and the moisture vapour transmission rate can be modified by modifying the polymer and the film structure. Moisture vapour transmission rates of 3000 $g/m^2/24$ hrs or greater can be achieved with the latest high-tech films. Semi-permeable film dressings can be used for surgical wounds and for protecting the site of insertion and in-dwelling catheters. They are also used in the treatment of superficial partial thickness burns and early decubitus ulcers. These dressings are light and resilient, ideal for the prevention of skin damage against friction. They are also widely used as a secondary dressing in conjunction with hydrogels, hydrocolloids and alginates.

Polyurethane foams are soft and porous materials that can be used for wound-contacting primary dressings or as secondary dressings, utilising their relatively high strength and flexibility. The polyurethane can be made from hydrophobic or hydrophilic monomers, resulting in foams with varying characteristics of porosity and fluid handling capability. When placed on wet wounds, fluid is absorbed into the foam by capillary action and transferred across the dressing. When placed on a relatively dry wound, the polyurethane backing layer reduces moisture vapour loss and helps to prevent dehydration of the wound surface [33].

2.3.3 Hydrogels

Hydrogels are cross-linked polymeric networks swollen in biological fluid. They are widely used in drug delivery and tissue/organ repairs. Two types of hydrogels are usually available, i.e., sheet hydrogels and amorphous hydrogels. With the sheet hydrogel, the hydrophilic polymers, typically polyacrylamide or polyethylene oxide, are partially cross-linked to form a membrane with sufficient water-holding hydrophilic sites. Typically a hydrogel contains about 96% water. When applied to wound sites such as dermabrasion, minor burns and skin donor sites, they relieve pain and reduce trauma both on application and the removal of the dressings. Hydrogels can be dried to form the dehydrated hydrogel, which has a higher absorption capacity than the hydrated film. These dressings are ideal carriers for antibiotics and placental growth factors.

Amorphous hydrogels can be made from a number of water-soluble polymers such as cross-linked carboxymethyl cellulose, modified starches, alginate, pectin, etc. Unlike the sheet hydrogel, which takes up a three-dimensional structure, these gels are thick viscous fluids. When absorbing wound exudate, they swell until they lose all the cohesive properties. Amorphous hydrogels are excellent donors for water. They are ideally used for dry and sloughy wounds whereby the water-donating properties assist the autolysis process for the debriding and cleansing of slough and black necrotic tissue from the underlying healthy tissue. Amorphous hydrogels are also widely used in the treatment of cavity wounds, where their easy flowing properties can be used for the packing of a deep cavity to avoid wound closure from side to side [34, 35].

2.3.4 Hydrocolloids

Hydrocolloids wound dressings are among the first type of high-tech modern dressings. These dressings are typically made of hydrophilic polymeric granules dispersed in an elastic adhesive matrix. Typically, the hydrophilic granules are hydrophilic polymers such as sodium carboxymethyl cellulose, pectin, gelatin and sodium alginate, whilst the adhesive matix is typically polyisobutylene. The hydrocolloid and the adhesive form a homogeneous mixture such that the granules are uniformly dispersed in the adhesive matrix. The final dressing is usually composed of the hydrocolloid matrix cast on a sheet of polymeric membrane or film (occlusive or semi-permeable for different applications). On contact with wound exudate, the hydrophilic granules absorb the fluid to form a hydrogel, while the adhesive material provides a tack that keeps the dressing adhered to the wound. Since the moisture transportation is relatively slow through the hydrocolloid matrix, the wound surface is covered by a moist contacting layer which assists the healing of the wound. The dressing is easy to remove and provides good protection against bacterial contamination of the wound [36, 37].

2.3.5 Activated carbon

The production of wound odour can represent a major problem for patients and their carers. Wounds most commonly associated with odour production include leg ulcers and fungating (cancerous) lesions of all types. The smell from these wounds is caused by a cocktail of volatile agents that includes short chain organic acids, such as n-butyric, n-valeric, n-caproic, n-haptanoic and n-caprylic acids, produced by anaerobic bacteria, together with a mixture of amines and diamines such as cadaverine and putrescine that are produced by the metabolic processes of other proteolytic bacteria.

The most effective way of dealing with malodorous wounds is to prevent or eradicate the infection responsible for the odour. This may be achieved in a number of ways. The administration of systemic antibiotics or antimicrobial agents may be effective in some cases, but often the nature of the wound is such that it is not possible to achieve an effective concentration of the antibiotic at the site of infection by this method, particularly in the presence of slough or necrotic tissue. If the formation of the odour cannot be prevented, it may be necessary to use a dressing that can absorb the smell. Dressings containing activated carbon fibres can be used for the treatment of these malodorous wounds [38–40].

Activated charcoal cloth is produced by carbonising a suitable cellulose fabric by heating it under carefully controlled conditions. During this process, the surface of the carbon breaks down to form small pores. These greatly increase the effective surface area of the fibres and hence their ability to remove unpleasant smells, since the molecules that are responsible for the production of the odour are attracted to the surface of the carbon and are held there by electrical forces.

2.3.6 Low adherent dressings

One of the major problems with the traditional gauzes is the difficulty in removing the gauzes upon healing of the wound. Fibrous matters from the dressing tend to mix up with exudate and blood. When the wound heals and dries, the fibres often get stuck with the dry escar. Bleeding of the new tissue is common in these cases and the trauma in removing traditional gauze from large wounds often poses a serious problem. Low adherent dressings were developed in order to prevent the above problem by placing a primary wound contacting layer that separates the exuding wound with the absorbent dressing layer. A typical low adherent dressing is the so-called 'tulle gras', invented during the First World War. These dressings are usually made of cotton gauzes impregnated with a coating of paraffin, which provides a low adherence to the wound surface. Quite often, the paraffin gauzes can be medicated to enhance their performances.

For heavily exuding wounds, the poor absorption properties of the tulle gras tend to reduce the fluid uptake and skin maceration occurs as a result of the build-up of the fluid under the dressing. Other forms of low adherent dressings were developed in order to improve this problem. Most of the modern low adherent dressings are perforated polymeric films, with the pores acting as the channel for the exudate to pass through to the absorbent layer. Knitted gauzes made of continuous viscose rayon filament (see Fig. 2.8) are also used as a low adherent dressings for the treatment of such heavy exuding wounds as leg ulcers. It is, however, usually a problem area for these dressings when the new tissue grows into the pores of the perforated film or knitted structure, causing tissue damage on removal of the dressing. In these respects, modern dressings such as hydrogels, hydrocolloids and alginate offer far superior properties both as high absorbent dressings and

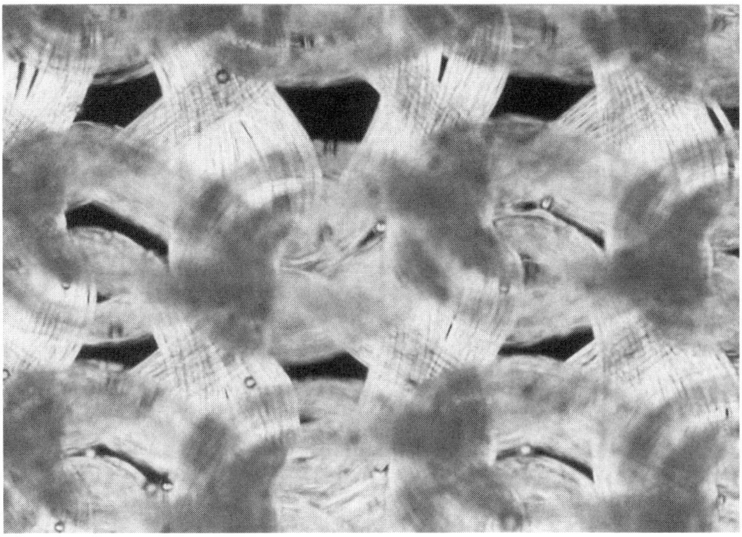

2.8 Photomicrograph of a low adherent dressing made of knitted viscose rayon fabric.

for their low adherent properties. Silicone coated fabric can also be used to reduce adherence [41–43].

2.4 Composite wound-care products

After many years of research and development, especially since the widespread use of 'moist healing' products in the 1990s, modern wound dressings are now much more functional and smart than the traditional products such as cotton gauzes and absorbent swabs. Compared to traditional products, the new generation of smart wound care products tend to be easy to use and cost effective. In achieving these functionalities, the modern wound care products also adopt many novel composite structures. For example, in the management of leg ulcers, the four-layer system has proven to be effective in applying compression as well as exudate management to chronic leg ulcers, which is achieved by first applying a wool bandage from the base of the toes to just below the knee joint, followed by the application of a crepe bandage and then an elastic compression bandage, and finally wrapping in a cohesive layer [44].

Many other types of composite wound care products have also emerged. In general, these products are composed of three key components, i.e., the wound contact layer, the functional layer and the retention layer. Figure 2.9 shows the schematic illustration of modern composite wound care products. In three-layered modern composite wound dressings, the contact layer serves to provide a low or non-adherent interface between the wound surface and

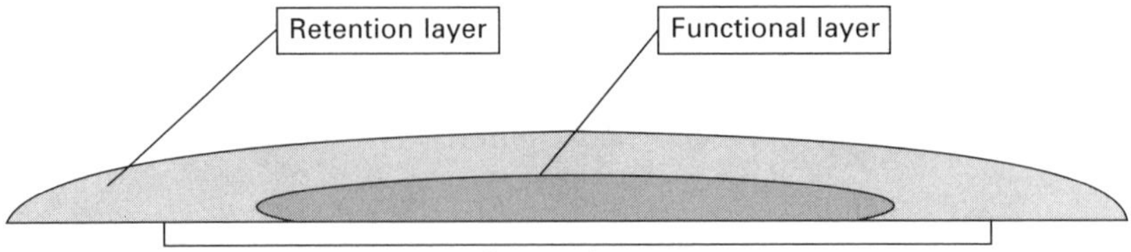

2.9 Schematic illustration of modern composite wound care products.

the dressing. This should allow wound exudate to pass into the functional layer whilst being able to prevent the adherence of the dressing to a drying surface at the end of the healing process. At the same time, the contact layer also stops the release of loose fibres or particles from the dressing into the wound site. Polyamide nonwoven and polyurethane foam materials can be used for the wound contact layer. Other materials that have been used include perforated plastic films, knitted viscose filament yarn, silicone gel, etc.

The functional layers vary greatly for different products because of the variations in their intended uses. For the majority of wounds, the main issues in wound management are to contain wound exudate, control microbial growth and to combat odour. In these cases, a layer of superabsorbent material, antimicrobial substance and activated carbon fabric respectively can be laminated into the wound dressing to provide the functional layer.

The retention layer is used for two main purposes, i.e., to secure the dressing onto the wound edge and to provide physical protection of the wound surface. Polyurethane films and hydroentangled nonwoven fabrics are often used as retention layers. These materials are soft and flexible, thus making it easy to apply the dressings onto curved areas of the body, such as around the shoulders and elbow. In addition, these materials are breathable, thus allowing oxygen to penetrate into the wound, and allow moisture to evaporate from under the dressing, thereby extending the duration of the product. Figure 2.10 shows an example of an absorbent layer secured by a retention layer made of hydroentangled nonwoven fabric.

2.5 Current developments and future trends

Today, wound care practitioners have at their disposal a wide range of smart wound dressings. These can be grouped under different product technologies, such as hydrocolloid dressings, alginate dressings, hydrogels and foam dressings. Each of these product groups contains various brands that often have markedly different performance characteristics. As part of an overall wound management plan, these smart wound dressings can help facilitate fast wound healing by providing the optimal environment for healing to proceed. They are also able to deal with the odour, leakage, maceration,

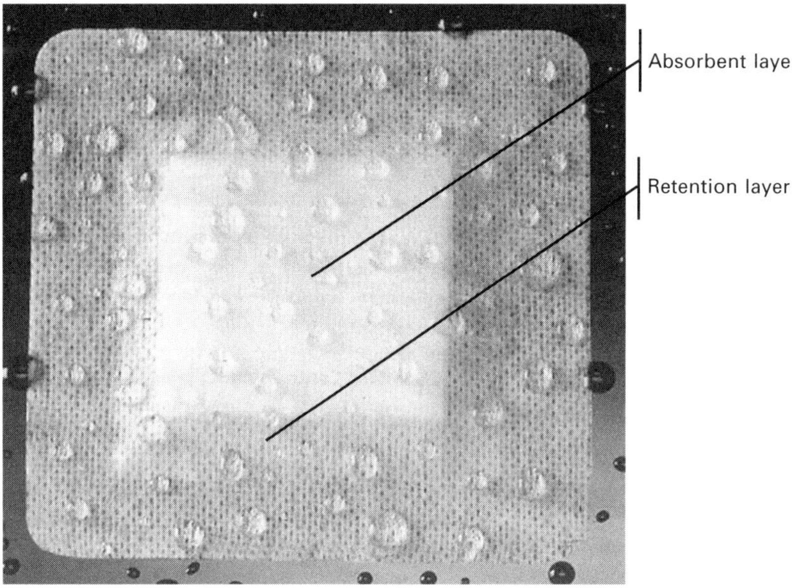

2.10 Examples of functional and retention layers.

pain, infection and other problems for the wounded patients. It should be pointed out that although wound dressings may not be able significantly to promote the healing process, the use of inappropriate dressings can often cause delayed wound healing, resulting in complications caused by poor wound management such as:

- delayed healing and/or wound deterioration
- increased risk of local or systemic infection
- increased demand for nursing time and increased dressing costs
- damage to the wound surface
- damage to the surrounding skin
- failure to control odour
- detrimental effect on the quality of patients' lives.

In order to provide the best solutions for wound care practioners, new types of advanced wound dressings and wound management materials are being developed to provide the means to ensure the best possible patient outcome. The aims of the new developments can be summarised into the following three areas:

- **E**fficacy of the material
- **E**ffectiveness of the product
- **E**fficiency of the treatment.

These three 'E's symbolise the goal-orientated approach for the current and future development for wound management materials and products. Some of these new developments are outlined briefly below.

2.5.1 Antimicrobial wound dressings

The spread of antibiotic-resistant strains of micro-organisms such as methicillin-resistant Staphylococcus aureus (MRSA) represents an ever-increasing threat to the health of vulnerable people throughout the world who are obliged to spend extended periods in healthcare facilities. The organism is also responsible for increasing the financial burden placed on such centres and the wider community at large, with the result that precious financial resources are diverted from other areas of need to deal with the consequences of infection. In order to overcome microbial infection, many dressings now incorporate 'bioactive' ingredients such as iodine and silver ions that can be released sustainably when the dressings are in contact with wound exudates. For example, Inadine (from Johnson & Johnson) contains povidone iodine, whilst Actisorb Plus (also from Johnson & Johnson) is an activated charcoal cloth impregnated with silver. During application, the activated charcoal cloth can absorb the bacteria in wound exudate, whilst the silver ions released from the dressing further inactivate the bacteria [45].

Another new generation product, Acticoat, utilises novel silver-coating technologies in a dressing designed to prevent wound adhesion, control bacterial growth and facilitate burn wound care. The Acticoat dressing consists of a rayon/polyester nonwoven core, laminated between layers of silver-coated high-density polyethylene mesh. This product can provide an effective antimicrobial barrier for up to 3–5 days against 150 pathogens, including both methicillin-resistant Staphylococcus aureus (MRSA) and Vancomycin-resistant Enterococci (VRE) [46].

As can be seen in Fig. 2.11, novel antimicrobial wound dressings can also be made by blending calcium alginate fibres with the silver-containing X-static fibres. In this system, the calcium alginate fibres provide the high absorbency and gelling ability, whilst the silver-containing fibres provide the sustained release of silver ions and hence the antimicrobial properties of the product. Because of the broad-spectrum antimicrobial efficacy and the relatively low toxicity of silver ions, there have been many attempts to combine silver ions into wound dressings, resulting in a number of commercial products now available in Europe and North America. In addition to the products mentioned above, some of these silver-containing products are introduced below [47, 48].

Arglaes. Arglaes comprises a mixture of an alginate powder and an inorganic polymer containing ionic silver. In the presence of moisture, the alginate

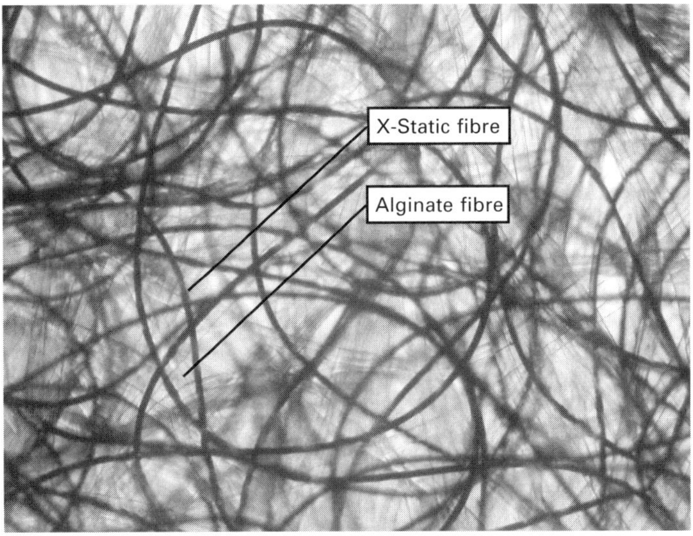

2.11 A composite dressing made of alginate and X-Static fibres.

absorbs liquid to form a gel and the silver complex breaks down in a controlled fashion, releasing ionic silver into the wound.

Aquacel Ag. Aquacel Ag consists of a fleece of sodium carboxymethylcellulose fibres containing 1.2% ionic silver. In the presence of exudate, the dressing absorbs liquid to form a gel, at the same time releasing silver ions.

Calgitrol. Calgitrol consists of an absorbent foam sheet, one surface of which is coated with an alginate matrix containing ionic silver together with a 'cleanser, moisturizer and a superabsorbent starch co-polymer'.

Contreet Foam. Contreet is a polyurethane foam dressing that contains silver, which is released as the foam absorbs exudate.

Contreet Hydrocolloid. The Contreet Hydrocolloid dressing, which is based on established standard hydrocolloid technology, also contains a silver complex that is released by wound fluid absorbed by the dressing. This mechanism ensures a sustained release of silver ions as long as the dressing continues to absorb fluid.

Silverlon. Silverlon is a knitted fabric dressing that has been silver plated by means of a proprietary autocatalytic electroless chemical plating technique. This technique coats the entire surface of each individual fibre from which the dressing is made, resulting in a very large surface area for the release of ionic silver.

SilvaSorb. SilvaSorb is composed of a synthetic, polyacrylate hydrophilic matrix in which is dispersed or suspended microscopic silver-containing particles. On exposure to moisture, the silver is released into the wound in a controlled fashion.

Urgotul SSD. Urgotul SSD consists of a polyester mesh impregnated with carboxymethylcellulose, white soft paraffin and silver sulfadiazine (SSD).

2.5.2 Interactive dressings

Interactive dressings are the product that can interact with cells or matrix proteins in the wound bed to promote healing. As has been mentioned above, alginates are highly absorbable biodegradable dressings derived from seaweed. As well as controlling exudate by ion exchange, alginates can also exert a bioactive effect by activating macrophages within the chronic wound bed to generate pro-inflammatory signals, such as tumour necrosis factor (TNF)-alpha, interleukin (IL)-1, –6 and –12 [49]. This may then initiate a resolving inflammatory response characteristic of healing wounds. *In-vitro* studies have demonstrated that some dressings containing alginates can activate macrophages, as evidenced by their increased production of TNF-alpha [50].

Another example of an interactive dressing is Promogran, which is a sterile, freeze-dried matrix made up of collagen and oxidised regenerated cellulose. In the presence of wound exudate, the matrix absorbs liquid and forms a soft, conformable, totally biodegradable gel, which rebalances the wound environment. The gel binds and inactivates matrix metalloproteinases that, when present in excessive levels, have a detrimental effect on wound healing as they damage regenerating tissue [51]. The gel also binds growth factors secreted by macrophages and fibroblasts in the wound bed, protecting them from degradation by these proteases. As the gel is digested during the course of healing, the growth factors are released back into the wound bed in their active form, thereby promoting the healing process.

2.5.3 Tissue-engineered 'skin equivalents'

Surgical grafting of split-thickness autologous skin is the standard method for rapid closure of full-thickness burn wounds. Modern tissue engineering has now made possible grafts using either sheets of fibroblasts in a biodegradable matrix or cultured keratinocyte sheets [52, 53]. Superior results can be obtained when both dermal and epidermal components are combined in a bi-layer skin equivalent [54].

2.5.4 Cell-containing matrices

Artificial skins can be developed by combining cells with either synthetic matrices, such as polyglycolic acid mesh, or natural biological substrates such as collagen and glycosaminoglycans. For example, Dermagraft was developed by using a polyglactin-910 surgical mesh seeded with human dermal fibroblasts [55]. It has been found that this product can allow revascularisation and support human meshed split thickness skin grafts [56].

2.5.5 Cost versus effectiveness of new treatment regimens

As well as clinical efficacy and treatment effectiveness, cost is also an important issue in the development of new smart wound care materials. In considering the cost of new treatment regimens, it is important to evaluate the cost not only in terms of direct treatment costs, but also in terms of length of initial hospital stay, requirements for home care, additional bandaging regimens, and quality of the overall outcome. Whilst new smart wound care products are often more expensive than traditional products, in many cases this additional cost is justifiable. With respect to novel dressing types, it has been shown that not only are some of the new products cost effective, but they have also proven to be extremely beneficial in terms of their ability to reduce pain, odour and leakage from the wounds [57]. For example, the cost-effectiveness of tissue-engineered skin replacements, has been borne out by evidence from a number of studies. When treating venous leg ulcers, the annual estimated medical cost of patient management with a tissue-engineered skin replacement equated to $20,041, compared to $27,493 for traditional therapy using Unna's boots [58]. Despite the initial outlay being greater, the use of modern smart materials reduced the overall treatment cost considerably. In addition, patients' quality of life can also be improved.

2.6 Sources of further information and advice

For more information on wound care and wound management products, the readers can use the following publications.

A Prescriber's Guide to Dressings & Wound Management Materials, VFM Unit, Welsh Office Health Department, 1997.

G. Bennett and M. Moody, *Wound Care for Health Professionals*, Chapman and Hall, London, 1995.

C. Dealey, *The Care of Wounds*, Blackwell Science Ltd, Oxford, 1994.

D.J. Leaper and K.G. Harding (eds), *Wounds: Biology and Management*, Oxford University Press, 1998.

M. Morison, C. Moffatt, J. Bridel-Nixon and S. Bale (eds), *Nursing Management of Chronic Wounds*, Mosby, London, 1997.

S. Thomas, *Wound Management and Dressings*, The Pharmaceutical Press, London, 1990.

J. Wardrope and J.A.R. Smith, *The Management of Wounds and Burns*, Oxford University Press, Oxford, 1992.

2.7 References

1. S. Thomas, *Wound Management and Dressings*, The Pharmaceutical Press, London, 1990.
2. G.D. Winter, *Nature*, Vol. 193, 293–294, 1962.
3. C.D. Hinman and H. Maibach, *Nature*, Vol. 200, 377–378, 1963.
4. O.M. Alvarez, P.M. Mertz and W.H. Eaglstein, *J Surg Res*, Vol. 35, 142–148, 1983.
5. T.D. Turner, *Wounds: A Compendium of Clinical Research and Practice*, Vol. 1(3), 155–171, 1989.
6. S. Thomas, *J. Wound Care*, Vol. 6(10), 479–482, 1997.
7. C. Dealey, *The Care of Wounds*, Blackwell Science Ltd, Oxford, 1994.
8. P.G. Bowler, B.I. Duerden and D.G. Armstrong, *Clin Microbiol Rev*, Vol. 14(2), 244–269, 2001.
9. A.R. McLure and J. Gordon, *J Hosp Infect*, Vol. 21(4), 291–299, 1992.
10. H.J. Klasen, *Burns*, Vol. 26(2), 117–130, 2000.
11. H.J. Klasen, *Burns*, Vol. 26(2), 131–138, 2000.
12. S. Thomas and P. McCubbin, *J Wound Care*, Vol. 12(8), 305–308, 2003.
13. R. White, R. Cooper and A. Kingsley, *Br J Nurs*, Vol. 10(9), 563–78, 2001.
14. Y. Qin, *J Appl Polym Sci*, Vol. 91(3), 1641–1645, 2004.
15. Y. Qin and D.K. Gilding, *Medical Device Technology*, 19–22, November, 1996.
16. Y. Qin, *Textile Asia*, 25–27, November 2004.
17. K.J. Franklin and K. Bates, Brit. Pat. 1 375 572, 1974.
18. J.H.M. Miller, Brit. Pat. 1 328 088, 1973.
19. Y. Qin, *Textile Research Journal*, Vol. 75(2), 165–168, 2005.
20. Y. Qin, *J Appl Polym Sci*, Vol. 91(2), 953–957, 2004.
21. Y. Qin, original results.
22. L.L. Balassa and J.F. Prudden, in *Proceedings of the First International Conference on Chitin and Chitosan*, ed. R.A.A. Muzzarelli and E.R. Pariser, 1978.
23. G. Kunike, *J. Soc. Dyers Colourists*, Vol. 42, 318, 1926.
24. O.C. Agboh, PhD Thesis, University of Leeds, 1986.
25. Y. Qin, *Medical Device Technology*, 34–37, Jan/Feb 2004.
26. Y. Qin, PhD Thesis, University of Leeds, 1990.
27. G.C. East and Y. Qin, *J Appl Polym Sci*, Vol. 50, 1773–1778, 1993.
28. Y. Qin, *Textiles Magazine*, 12–14, Issue 1, 2005.
29. T. Krieg and K.G. Harding, in: T. Krieg and K.G. Harding (eds): *Aquacel Hydrofibre Dressing: The Next Step in Wound Dressing Technology*, Churchill Communications Europe Ltd, London, 1998.
30. F.R. Machado, in: T. Krieg and K.G. Harding (eds): *Aquacel Hydrofibre Dressing: The Next Step in Wound Dressing Technology*, Churchill Communications Europe Ltd, London, 1998.
31. S. Thomas, V. Banks and M. Fear, *J Wound Care*, Vol. 6, 333–336, 1997.
32. M.D. Sebern, *Arch Phys Med Rehabil*, Vol. 67, 726–729, 1986.
33. V. Banks, S. Bale and K.G. Harding, *J Wound Care*, Vol. 6, 266–269, 1997.
34. S. Bale, V. Banks, S. Haglestein and K.G. Harding, *J Wound Care*, Vol. 7, 65–68, 1998.
35. S. Thomas and P. Hay, *Ostomy Wound Man*, Vol. 41(3), 54–56, 1995.
36. S. Thomas, *J Wound Care*, Vol. 1(2), 27–30, 1992.
37. B. Gilchrist and C. Reed, *Br J Dermatol*, Vol. 121(3), 337–344, 1989.
38. S. Thomas and N.P. Hay, *Pharm. J*, Vol. 246, 264–266, 1991.

39. B. Griffiths, E.J. Jacques and S.A. Jones, in: *Proceedings of 7th European Conference on Advances in Wound Management*, Harrogate 1997, 1997.
40. V.M. Myles, B. Griffiths and S. Bishop, in: *Proceedings of 7th European Conference on Advances in Wound Management*, Harrogate 1997, 1997.
41. P.J. Terrill and G. Varughese, *J Wound Care*, Vol. 9(8), 359–363, 2000.
42. S. Thomas, *J Wound Care*, Vol. 3(1), 27–30, 1994.
43. P. Bugmann, S. Taylor, D. Gyger, A. Lironi, B. Genin, A. Vunda, G. La Scala, J. Birraux and C. Le Coultre, *Burns*, Vol. 24(7), 609–612, 1998.
44. J.C. Stockport, L. Groarke, D.A. Ellison and C. McCollum, *J Wound Care*, Vol. 66(10), 485–488, 1997.
45. H.Q. Yin, R. Langford and R.E. Burrell, *J Burn Care Rehabil*, Vol. 20(3), 195–200, 1999.
46. K. Dunn and V. Edwards-Jones, *Burns*, Vol. 30(Suppl 1), S1–9, 2004.
47. S. Thomas and P. McCubbin, *J Wound Care*, Vol. 12(3), 101–107, 2003.
48. S. Thomas and P. McCubbin, *J Wound Care*, Vol. 12(8), 305–08, 2003.
49. G. Skjak-Braek, T. Flo and O. Halaas, in: B.S. Paulsen (ed.), *Bioactive Carbohydrate Polymers*, Kluwer Academic Publishers, The Netherlands, 2000.
50. S. Thomas, *J Wound Care*, Vol. 9(2), 56–60, 2000.
51. A.B. Wysocki, L. Staiano-Coico and F. Grinnell, *J Invest Dermatol*, Vol. 101(1), 64–68, 1993.
52. V. Falanga, D. Margolis, O. Alvarez, M. Auletta, F. Maggiacomo, M. Altman, J. Jensen, M. Sabolinski and J. Hardin-Young, *Arch Dermatol*, Vol. 134(3), 293–300, 1998.
53. I.M. Leigh, P.E. Purkis, H.A. Navsaria and T.J. Phillips, *Br J Dermatol*, Vol. 117(5), 591–7, 1987.
54. V. Falanga and M. Sabolinski, *Wound Repair Regen*, Vol. 7(4), 201–207, 1999.
55. M.L. Cooper, J.F. Hansbrough, R.L. Spielvogel, R. Cohen, R.L. Bartel and G. Naughton, *Biomaterials*, Vol. 12(2), 243–248, 1991.
56. J.F. Hansbrough, M.L. Cooper, R. Cohen, R. Spielvogel, G. Greenleaf, R.L. Bartel and G. Naughton, *Surgery*, Vol. 111(4), 438–446, 1992.
57. K.G. Harding, V. Jones and P. Price, *Diabetes Metab Res Rev*, Vol. 16, Suppl 1, S47–50, 2000.
58. W.H. Schonfeld, K.F. Villa, J.M. Fastenau, P.D. Mazonson and V. Falanga, *Wound Repair Regen*, Vol. 8(4), 251–257, 2000.

3

Textile-based drug release systems

V A NIERSTRASZ, University of Twente,
The Netherlands

3.1 Introduction

Since the dawn of mankind textile materials have been produced and used to protect people from the surrounding environment. Over the years, textile properties like quality and wearing comfort have improved, and it is true to say that textile materials are an important aspect of our everyday lives. Logically, textile materials have found their way in the medical field as well, e.g., artificial aortas and bandages. However, advanced functional textile drug delivery systems were not developed until the end of the last millennium.

Why explore and develop textile materials in drug delivery systems? In many cases, drug delivery methods like pills and injections will give no problems, nevertheless, situations can be thought of where other systems would be more preferable. For example, in oral delivery systems like tablets, pills, capsules, the drug is absorbed in the stomach or intestinal tract. As some drugs are metabolised, they might lose their activity before being able to fulfil their purpose. Consequently, relatively high doses are necessary to achieve the desired effect (Fig. 3.1), which might give rise to adverse or toxic effects. Delivery through the skin bypasses the liver, making it possible to lower drug doses. Moreover, one can imagine situations where oral administration is less applicable or impractical, e.g., with children, people with swallowing difficulties or in the case of dementia. Transdermal and *in-vivo* drug delivery systems can be a good alternative in these situations. Furthermore, in cases of necessity for prolonged drug treatment, such a delivery system can possibly be preferred above daily injections or intake of pills. Advanced drug delivery systems can have many advantages in safety and effectiveness over conventional drug delivery systems by reducing dosage and frequency of dosing. However, when designing drug delivery systems one needs to be aware that not all drugs are applicable in prolonged drug dosage systems, and that such systems need to be developed taking into consideration drug properties, pharmacological demands and reliability.

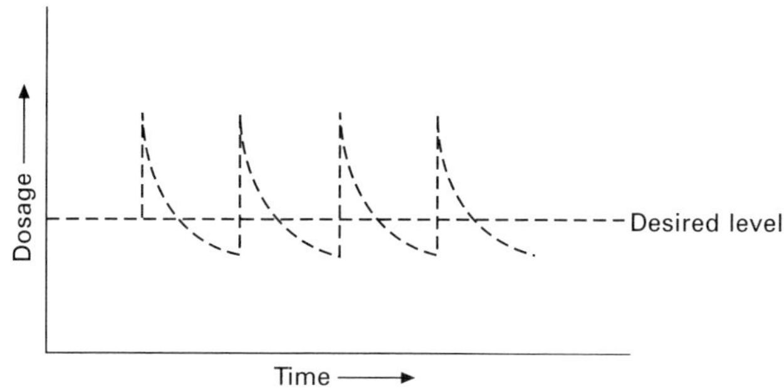

3.1 Drug dosage in time in a conventional drug delivery system.

Textile materials are extremely versatile materials, combining different materials and structures. Properties and functionalities of textiles are affected by chemical, physical and physical-chemical characteristics on micro-, nano-, meso- and macroscopic length scales (see Figs 3.2 and 3.3). On a macroscopic scale, although dependent on the actual fabrication process, textile materials are relatively 'open' and 'loose', permeable structures, with absorptive capacities as well. Especially the open permeable structure and large surface area makes textile materials a useful basis for *in-* and *ex-vivo* drug delivery applications. Moreover, people are used to wearing and using textile materials, making it a logical choice to use textile materials as a basis for *ex-vivo* drug delivery systems in professional and private situations. Textile drug delivery systems can thus contribute to a better quality of life.

Over the years, various delivery methods have been developed. A well-known category consists of so-called transdermal patches. They are mostly based upon multi-layer systems in which, besides an ointment or other drug-containing substance, a regulatory system like a membrane is used. In many cases the textile material in these transdermal patches is simply forming a support layer in the delivery system. Usually, no specific advanced treatments are required to gain useful patches. These kinds of slow release or delivery systems will not be the topic of this chapter. Owing to the enormous progress over the years in supramolecular chemistry, nanotechnology, nanobiotechnology, and polymer science and technology, high-performance textile drug delivery technologies have been developed (Breteler *et al.*, 2002). This chapter will essentially focus on aspects of more advanced and promising functional textile drug delivery systems or slow release systems like textile bearing cyclodextrins (e.g. Lee *et al.*, 2000; Lu *et al.*, 2001; Buschmann *et al.*, 2001; Martel *et al.*, 2002a,b; Szejtli, 2003; Voncina and Le Marechal, 2005), ion-exchange fibres (e.g. Jaskari *et al.*, 2000, 2001; Skundric *et al.*, 2002; Vuorio *et al.*, 2003, 2004), fibres containing (microencapsulated) drugs (e.g. Nelson, 2002; Liao *et al.*, 2005), microparticles (e.g. Gupta *et al.*, 2001; Berkland *et al.*, 2002) and (biodegradable) nano-fibres containing drugs

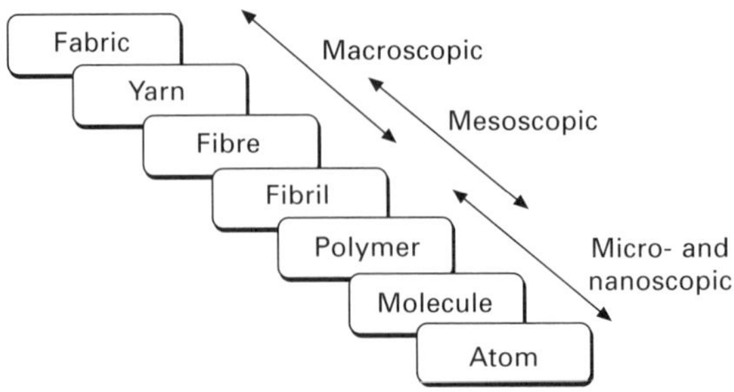

3.2 Different length scales.

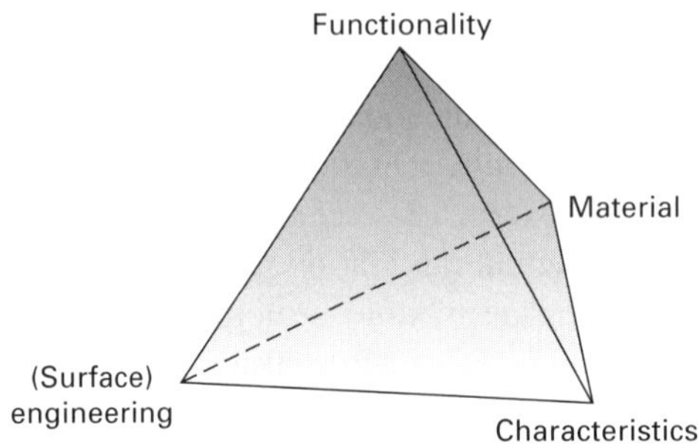

3.3 Functionality in textile materials.

produced by electrospinning (e.g. Kenawy *et al.*, 2002; Zeng *et al.*, 2003, 2005).

In the development and design of advanced textile drug deliverable systems various factors will affect performance of the release system apart from delivering the required amount of drug efficiently, precisely and for a defined period of time (controllability: dosage control, rate control and time control), like biocompatibility, biostability and biodegradability.

3.2 Mechanisms of drug release

For optimal performance textile drug release systems should be controlled in accordance with pharmaceutical requirements. As has been stated in the previous section, the objective of drug delivery systems is to deliver a defined amount of drug efficiently, precisely and for a defined period of time. By the selection of suitable carriers or host-molecules in textile drug release systems the rate and/or time of controlled release can be adjusted and regulated. Among other reasons this explains today's interest in advanced (textile) drug delivery systems.

3.2.1 Some typical release mechanisms

In general a few typical different types of release can be recognised relevant in textile drug delivery systems; immediate release, extended release and triggered or delayed release (e.g. Uekama *et al.*, 1998; Sansom, 1999). The different mechanisms are illustrated schematically in Fig. 3.4. Various, sometimes interchangeable, terms are used as well, and other delivery types do exist, like e.g. targeted drug delivery, site specific delivery, pulsed delivery, controlled delivery of multiple drug combinations (see Fig. 3.4), or modified delivery. Modified delivery is often a combination of other mechanisms in order to obtain more complicated dosage patterns (Uekama *et al.*, 1998). The release mechanisms mentioned will be illustrated using several examples.

Immediate release

In immediate release formulations, the drugs are available within a relatively short time. The rate is controlled by factors such as, for example, digestion in the stomach or intestinal tract, dissolution of the drugs and uptake of the drugs by the body. Initially the concentration increases rapidly, followed by a sharp decline as illustrated schematically in Fig. 3.5. Often a relatively high concentration is necessary to achieve the desired effect, dosing is quite often frequently. This type of release is required in situations where immediate action is essential. Other, often more conventional, formulations than textile drug delivery systems seem more appropriate and effective in immediate release of drugs.

Extended release

In extended release, sometimes called prolonged or sustained release, the availability of drugs is maintained at a lower concentration and for a prolonged

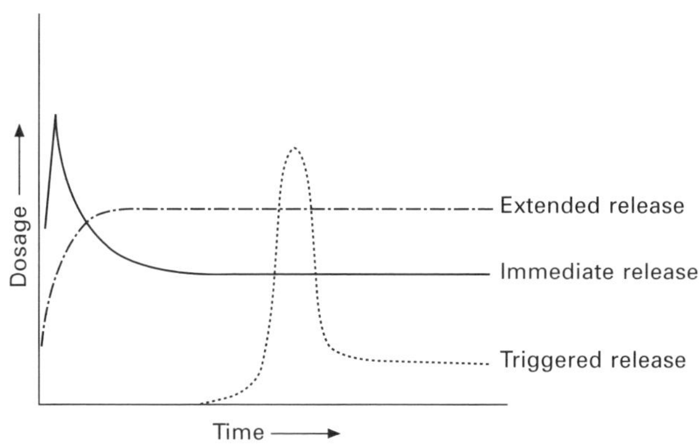

3.4 Different release mechanisms.

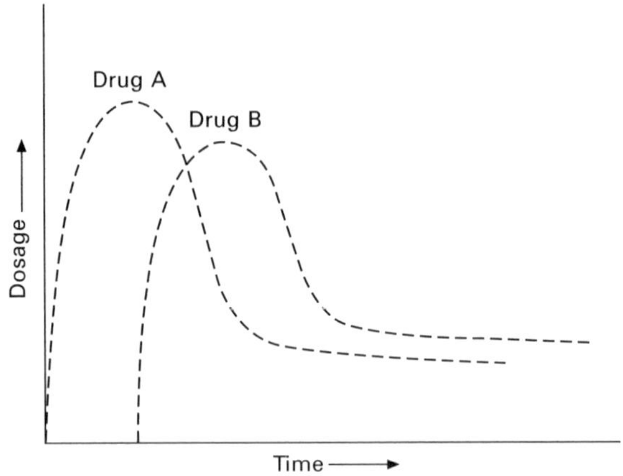

3.5 Controlled delivery of multiple drug combinations.

time compared to immediate release systems. In extended release systems the drug is delivered at a (very) slow rate and for a prolonged period of hours, days or even years, thereby usually reducing dosing frequency. The system can simply release the medication at a variable but slow rate, or release the medication at a constant rate over an extended period of time. Extended release systems are often slow release systems. Different principles are used to control the rate in extended release systems, such as diffusion, decomplexation, dissolution, ion exchange, erosion and degradation.

In diffusion controlled release systems the drugs are simply incorporated in the polymer matrix of the textile fibres, in hollow fibres or in fibres containing (micro-)encapsulated drugs. The concentration gradient and the diffusion coefficient of the drug in the polymer material determines the release rate. A typical example of a decomplexation controlled release system is textile materials bearing cyclodextrins (see Fig. 3.6). In decomplexation controlled systems, drugs can be incorporated in a host molecule bound to textile fibres. The complexation and decomplexation constants, k_c and k_d respectively, depend on the interactions between the drug, the guest molecule, and the cyclodextrin, the host molecule.

Fibres bearing encapsulated drugs are an example of a dissolution controlled release system (see Fig. 3.7). In dissolution controlled drug release systems, drugs are released by dissolution of the polymer. The release rate is thus determined by the dissolution rate of the polymer used to encapsulate the drug. This type of system can be relevant when designing triggered or delayed release systems as well (see below). Some drugs can be bound to ion-exchange materials. In ion-exchange textile drug release systems, the release rate of drugs bound to ion-exchange fibres is determined by ionic properties or the pH of the surrounding liquid and the choice of the ion-exchange material.

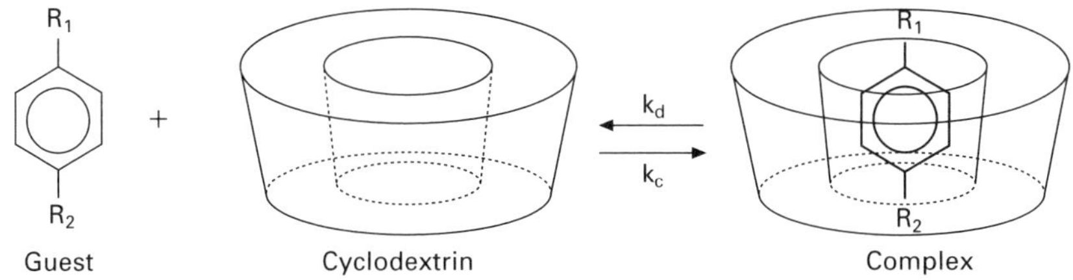

3.6 Schematic representation of cyclodextrin-guest complex formation.

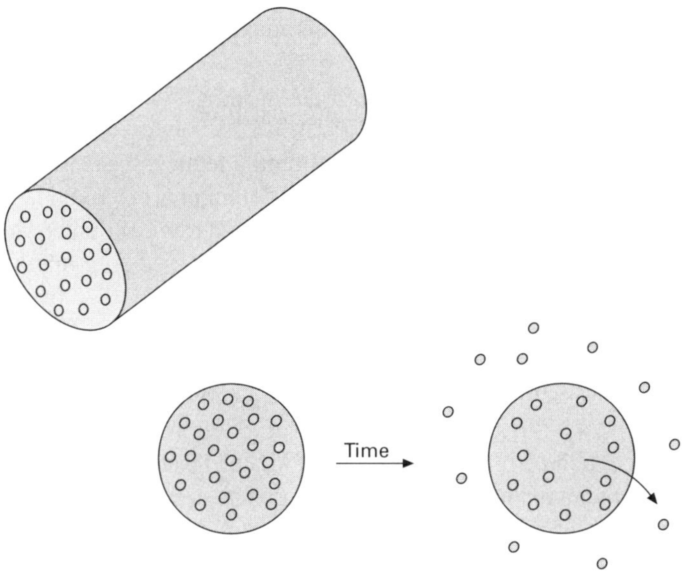

3.7 Release of drugs encapsulated in fibre.

This type of system can also be relevant when developing triggered or delayed release systems (see below).

Erosion and degradation controlled systems use a polymer matrix that is slowly eroded or degraded. As the polymer matrix is degraded or eroded the drugs are released. The erosion or degradation speed of the matrix carrying the drugs determines the release rate of the drugs. Like the previous two systems, this type of system can also be relevant when developing triggered or delayed release systems (see below). Biodegradable polymers and block copolymers (Kumar *et al*., 2001), for example, find their application in this type of release system.

Triggered or delayed release

The release of drugs from triggered or delayed release systems is determined by an (external) trigger/stimulus or time. The resulting release can be of the immediate type or slow-release type, depending on the design and the materials chosen. The degree and rate of erosion, degradation or dissolution are, apart from the matrix, a function of, e.g., pH, temperature, ionic strength, or even light and this determines time delay in delayed release systems. The release of the drug from the delivery system might also be triggered by a specific event, situation, or change in the environment such as a change in pH, temperature, ionic strength or even by an externally controllable trigger-like ultrasound for example (Bruinewoud *et al.*, 2004). Triggered release systems control drug dosage autonomously over an extended period of time, thus enabling precise dosage levels or more complicated dosage patterns.

3.2.2 Kinetics aspects of drug release

Textile drug delivery systems have the potential to meet the need for versatile delivery systems that are able to adapt to different pharmacological demands and to deliver drugs at a sufficiently well defined rate over a certain amount of time. A remarkably interesting feature of polymer-based drug-release systems is the potential of complex and novel release profiles, thereby increasing effectiveness and minimising toxic effects (Wise *et al.*, 1987; Berkland *et al.*, 2002), yet most developments in textile drug delivery systems emphasise slow release. Some pharmaceuticals require a constant but slow release rate for several hours, days or weeks. This seems relatively simple to achieve, nevertheless, such zero-order drug release kinetics is not that easily achieved. In zero-order release kinetics, the drug release rate is constant and independent of the drug concentration itself. Some textile drug release systems show pre-steady-state burst kinetics (see Fig. 3.8). In the initial phases a significant amount of the drug is already released (the 'burst'-phase) from the delivery system, followed by the desired period of zero-order kinetics. Burst release is undesirable because of potential toxic (side-)effects and drugs released in the initial phases are not available for slow release, thereby decreasing the efficiency of the delivery system. Release kinetics is strongly influenced by

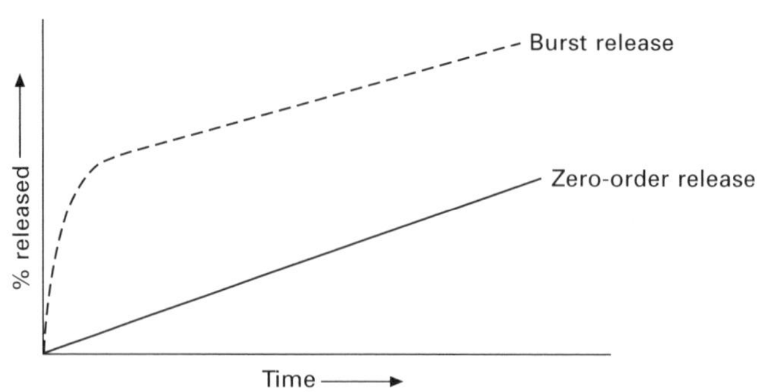

3.8 Burst- and zero-order release.

the surrounding environment and the choice of drug and carrier. There are numerous factors affecting kinetics and the amount of drug released from a carrier material, for example, molecular weight of the drug, concentration, diffusion coefficient, adsorption and desorption constants, charge (ion-exchange), degree of polymerisation, (bio)degradability, erosion of the carrier, ionic strength, temperature and pH.

Data of drug release from polymers or transdermal patches are generally analysed using a relatively simple model; the Korsmeyer equation (Korsmeyer *et al.*, 1983).

$$\frac{M_t}{M_\infty} = k_k t^n \qquad 3.1$$

where, M_t/M_∞ is the fractional release of the drug, M_t is the amount released at time t, M_∞ is the total amount of drug in the drug delivery system, k_k is a the Korsmeyer constant, a kinetic constant characteristic of the drug/polymer system, t is the release time and n is a diffusional exponent which characterises the mechanism of release. Zero-order drug release is characterised by $n = 1$, Fickian dominated diffusion is characterised by $n = 0.5$, and for non-Fickian diffusion $0.5 < n < 1$ (see Fig. 3.9). Models like the Korsmeyer equation are a very useful tool in analysing data of release systems, and can as such be used to improve delivery systems. Theoretical or predictive modelling of drug release kinetics of different delivery systems can of course act as a tool in the design and optimisation of such systems though that requires more advanced specific models. For example Vuorio *et al.* (2003) describes modelling of ion-exchange drug delivery systems, but such system-specific models are outside the scope of this chapter.

Transdermal textile drug delivery systems are often characterised and evaluated by determination of drug release into a certain liquid. In the design

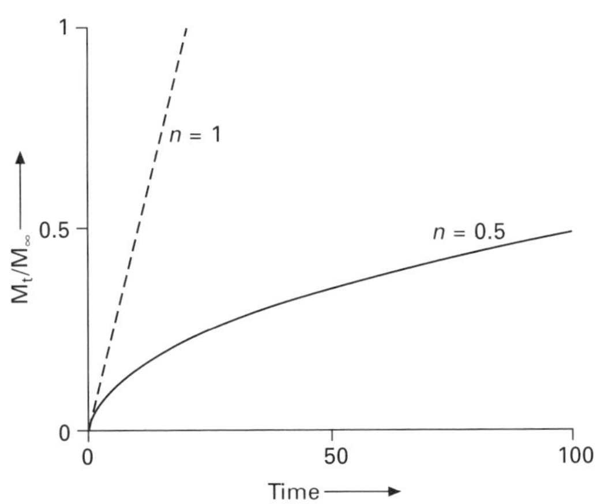

3.9 Zero-order and Fickian diffusion (Korsmeyer equation).

and development of transdermal textile drug delivery systems it is essential to quantify to which extent a system controls the overall drug delivery rate and pattern across the skin. Guy and Handgraft (1992) defined that in steady-state conditions the total resistance to transdermal drug delivery is:

$$R_{total} = R_{skin} + R_{delivery\ system} \qquad 3.2$$

where R_{total} is the total resistance to transdermal drug transport, R_{skin} is the resistance to drug transport across the skin and $R_{delivery\ system}$ is the resistance to drug release from the delivery system. Because the skin, and thus the resistance to drug transport across the skin, changes from person to person, age and anatomical site, drug delivery is preferably controlled by the delivery system.

3.3 Characteristics and application of drug release systems

In this section the potentials, constraints and characteristics of some specific textile slow release systems will be reviewed; cyclodextrins, ion-exchange fibres and drug-containing fibres (microencapsulated), microparticles and drug-containing nano-fibres produced by electrospinning.

3.3.1 Cyclodextrins

Cyclodextrins are considered as a relatively new class of molecules that have been widely investigated in the last three decades. They are the topic of an increasing amount of scientific papers on textile slow release systems as well. Despite their 'modern' image, cyclodextrins have been known for over 100 years and have already been described by Villiers in 1891 (Szejtli, 1998). The first patent on cylodextrin-inclusion complexes goes back to 1953 including the application of cyclodextrins in drug formulations (Freudenberg *et al.*, 1953), and the first application in textiles was already patented in 1982 (Szejtli *et al.*, 1980, 1982). In addition cyclodextrins have been used in complexation of dyes (Buschmann and Schollmeyer, 1997a). Cyclodextrins are able to form complexes with a variety of long-chain aliphatic or aromatic molecules like drugs, pesticides, hormones, detergents, fragrances and vitamin B. Other host-guest type systems exist, based on, for example dibenzo-crown ethers, aza-crown ethers or fullerenes (Buschmann, *et al.*, 1997b; Denter *et al.*, 1998a,b), but among all potential hosts, cyclodextrins seem to be the most attractive ones. The main reasons are:

- Cyclodextrins are semi-natural; they are enzymatically (amylase) produced from strarch, a renewable substrate.
- Since the end of the last century cyclodextrins are available in large quantities (over ten thousand tons/year). With the increase in production,

the price has been reduced considerably. Derivatives are industrially produced as well (e.g. methyl-, butyl-, 2-hydroxypropyl-, glucosyl-, maltosyl-, carboxymethyl-cyclodextrins) (Loftsson, T. and Brewster 1996; Szejtli, 1998).

- Cyclodextrins are from a toxicological point of view fairly safe, β-cyclodextrins are licensed as food additive.

Cyclodextrins are cyclic (α-1,4) linked D-glucopyranose residues. The most common cyclodextrins are α-, β-, and γ-cyclodextrin, which consist of six, seven or eight glucopyranose units respectively (see Fig. 3.10). Owing to the lack of free rotation of the units, cyclodextrins are not perfectly cylindrical but conical. Smaller cyclodextrins do not exist, as a result of sterical factors. Cyclodextrins of more units exist, but their cavity is not cylindrically shaped. The cavity is collapsed, therefore the actual space is smaller. For example, the cavity of δ-cyclodextrin (nine glucopyranose units) is smaller than that of γ-cyclodextrin. The approximate geometric of dimensions of α-, β-, and γ-cyclodextrins are schematically shown in Fig. 3.11 and some chemical and physical properties are listed in Table 3.1.

Most studies of the application of cyclodextrin-textile drug delivery systems focus on β-cyclodextrins. The cavity or the interior of the cyclodextrin molecule is rather hydrophobic, whereas the outer surface is hydrophilic. The hydrophobic interior is mainly responsible for complex formation. Despite the hydrophilic

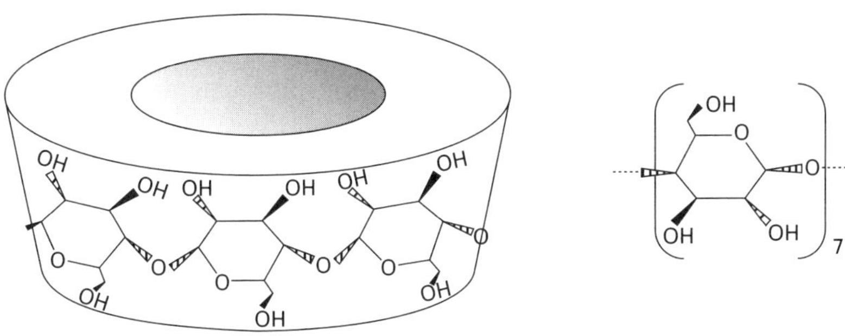

3.10 Schematic representation of β-cyclodextrin.

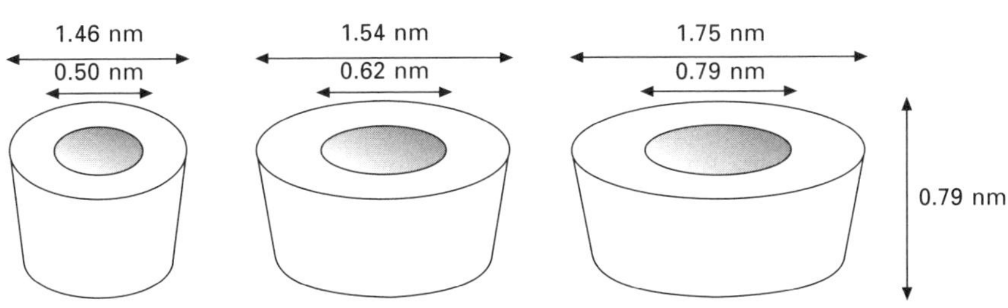

3.11 Dimensions of α-, β-, and γ-cyclodextrin.

Table 3.1 Some characteristics of cyclodextrins (Loftsson *et al.*, 1996; Szejtli, 1998)

	α	β	γ
Number of glucopyranose units	6	7	8
Molecular weight	972	1135	1297
Cavity diameter (nm)	0.47–0.53	0.60–0.65	0.75–0.83
Diameter (nm)	1.46±0.4	1.54±0.4	1.75±0.4
Height (nm)	0.79±0.1	0.79±0.1	0.79±0.1
Approximate cavity volume (Å^3)	174	262	427
Solubility in water at 25 °C (g/l)	145	185	232
Diffusion coefficient (m^2/s)	$3.4 \cdot 10^{-10}$	$3.2 \cdot 10^{-10}$	$3 \cdot 10^{-10}$
pK at 25 °C (potentiometry)	12.332	12.202	12.081

character of the outer surface the solubility of β-cyclodextrin is limited. Modification of the hydroxyl groups of the outer surface of the cyclodextrin can increase solubility, for example, by substitution of a hydroxypropyl or a carboxymethyl group, or decreasing solubility, for example, by substitution of an ethylhexyl glycidyl or an acetyl-group (Denter *et al.*, 1997; Hedges, 1998).

Complex formation is largely independent of chemical properties of the drug molecule as such, apart from the fact that the drug should fit in the cavity of the specific cyclodextrin, and thus the group of drugs compatible with a certain cyclodextrin is rather large (Loftsson and Brewster, 1996). This is underlined by the different types of drugs that have been investigated in drug-cyclodextrin complexes; varying from neutral to ionic, and from basic to acidic (Hirayama and Uekama 1999).Van der Waals forces are important in drug-cyclodextrin complex formation, complex formation is demonstrated to be enthalpy driven (Loftsson *et al.*, 1996). Drug-cyclodextrin complexation and decomplexation, i.e., the release of the guest from the host, is an equilibrium process. Assuming a host-guest ratio of 1:1, which is most frequently the case, we can write:

$$\text{CD} + \text{Drug} \underset{k_d}{\overset{k_c}{\rightleftarrows}} \text{CD-Drug}$$

$$K = \frac{k_c}{k_d} = \frac{[\text{CD} - \text{Drug}]}{[\text{CD}][\text{Drug}]} \qquad 3.3$$

where k_c and k_d are the complexation and decomplexation constants respectively and depend on the interactions between the drug, and the cyclodextrin. The enthalpy of complexation and decomplexation varies for different drug-cyclodextrin combinations, thus k_c and k_d differ as well for different drug-cyclodextrin combinations. Most scientific papers on cyclodextrin-drug complex formation deal with free cyclodextrins, like oral formulations, and not with cyclodextrins fixed to a substrate like textile materials. As fixation of cyclodextrins does not affect complexation power, it can be reasoned that the release pattern is not influenced by fixation either. For drugs with a weak interaction with the host, the drug release rate is controlled by dilution and degradation of the drugs as it shifts the equilibrium. For drugs with a stronger interaction with the host, competitive displacement affects the release rate too by decreasing the available amount of un-complexed cyclodextrin. Cyclodextrins can even be used to develop triggered or delayed release systems, for example, by a pH change or for water-insoluble drugs, changing the environment from aqueous to lipophilic will trigger drug release. Once the release has been triggered, the release is instantaneous and without delay. Currently, textile drug delivery systems based on cyclodextrins are mainly designed on the basis of experience and trial and error and not on the basis of specific design rules; the release pattern is to a large extent determined by the specific combination of drug and cyclodextrin.

Production of textile fibres bearing cyclodextrins

A variety of chemical and physical techniques exist for the production of textile fibres bearing cyclodextrins at their surfaces. An important feature is that attachment of cyclodextrin molecules is already achieved by conventional and well-developed as well as less conventional technologies (Denter and Schollmeyer 1996; Breteler *et al.*, 2002). Therefore textile drug delivery systems based on cyclodextrins have the potential to be produced by existing textile mills. Cyclodextrins can be fixed to the surface of textile fibres permanently or non-permanently; permanent fixation can be via covalent bonding (reaction of functional groups) as well as non-covalent bonding (cross-linking). Non-permanent techniques also exist, like anionically or cationically modified derivatives on, e.g., polyamide-6. In Fig. 3.12 various possibilities are schematically illustrated. The method preferred depends on application and on the fibre material itself (Denter and Schollmeyer, 1996).

Fixation of cyclodextrins by an anchor group is feasible when the anchor group or chain is capable of penetrating the textile fibres when the latter are in their amorphous state. Anchor groups are mainly hydrophobic ‘tails’, such as long alkyl chains that fit into the fibre’s hydrophobic inner environment, like PET. The hydrophilic outer surface of the cyclodextrin will prevent complete penetration into the fibre; hence, the functional cavity remains accessible on the fibre’s surface (Buschmann *et al.*, 2001). Upon lowering the temperature below the glass temperature, the mobility of the polymers is restricted thereby captivating anchor groups and fixating the cyclodextrins.

Grafting of cyclodextrins on textile materials seems most promising. α-, β- and γ-cyclodextrins have already been grafted on textile fibres like cotton, Tencell, wool, polyester, and polypropylene (for example, Denter and Schollmeyer 1996; Lee *et al.*, 2000; Le Thuaut *et al.*, 2000; Martel *et al.*,

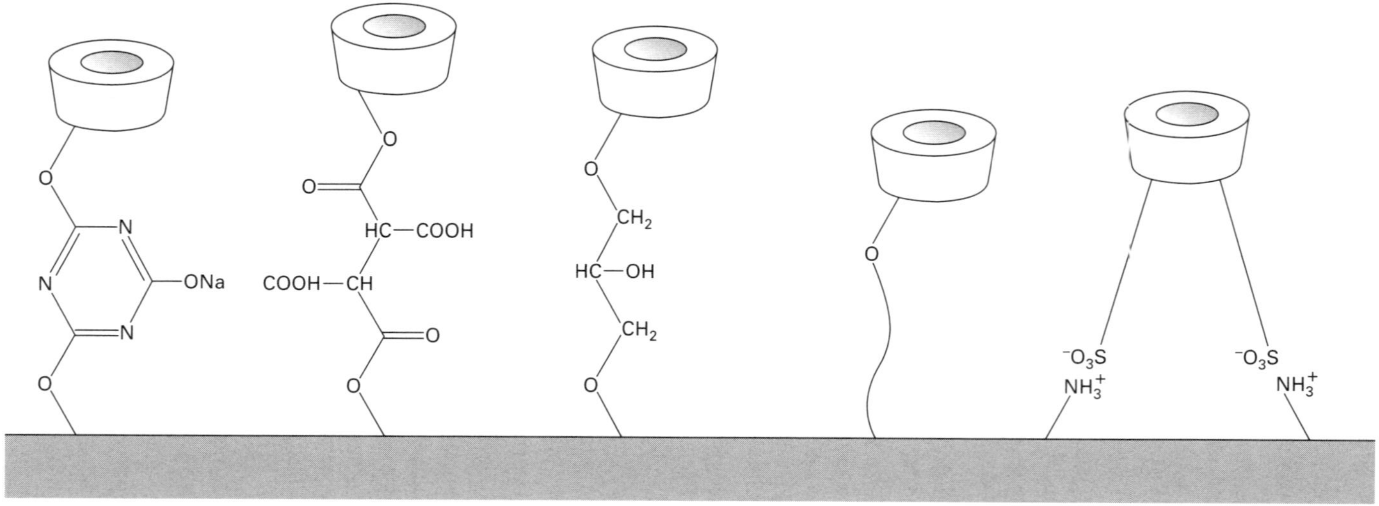

3.12 Schematic representation of cyclodextrin fixation: triazinyl, 1,2,3,4,-butanetetra-carboxylic acid, glyceryl ester, 'anchoring'of cyclodextrin with a long hydrophobic alkyl chain on, e.g., PET, anionically modified cyclodextrin (e.g. by sulfoalkylether on polyamide).

2000; Lu *et al.*, 2001; Breteler *et al.*, 2002; Lo Nostro *et al.*, 2002; Martel *et al.*, 2002a,b,c,d; Szejtli 2003; Voncina and Le Marechal 2005). Grafting of cyclodextrins on polypropylene to produce non-woven reactive filters was via activation of the polypropylene substrate by electrobeam, followed by grafting using glycidyl methacrylate (GMA). Three different approaches are often described in scientific literature: one approach is based on acryl-amido-methylated-β-cyclodextrin (CD-NMA), one on poly(carboxylic acids) and one on monochlorotriazynyl-β-cyclodextrin (MCT-CD).

Acryl-amido-methylated-β-cyclodextrin (CD-NMA)

In this grafting procedure cellulose is oxidised by cerium (IV), producing a free radical on the cellulose backbone. Due to consumption of cerium (IV) by CD-NMA as well it is beneficial to add the initiator, cerium (IV), before addition of the acryl-amido-methylated-β-cyclodextrin (Lee *et al.*, 2000). Grafting of CD-NMA was for one hour at 40 °C, and grafted β-cyclodextrins were mainly at the cellulose surface. The system studied was not evaluated for drug release properties, but for release of an antimicrobial component, benzoic acid, and a fragrance.

Polycarboxylic acids

Polycarboxylic acids have been used in production of cotton, wool and polyester fabrics carrying α-, β- and γ-cyclodextrins (e.g. Martel *et al.*, 2002a,b,c,d). 1,2,3,4,-butane-tetra-carboxylic acid (BTCA), polyacrylic acid and citric acid have been used as grafting agents. A cyclic anhydride is formed that reacts with hydroxyl groups of cellusose, forming an ester bond under the influence of heat and/or the presence of a catalyst, such as sodium dihydrogen hypophosphite. The remaining two carboxylic groups can again form a cyclic anhydride that can react with the cyclodextrin or with another cellulose chain. Process conditions vary with different textile substrates.

Monochlorotriazynyl-β-cyclodextrin (MCT-CD)

Monochlorotriazynyl-β-cyclodextrin (see Fig. 3.12) is a reactive cyclodextrin derivative that can be covalently linked to nucleophilic substrates, like cellulose, by a condensation reaction (Moldenhauer and Reuscher 1999, Lo Nostro *et al.*, 2002). Fixation of MCT-CD can be carried out in conventional textile finishing equipment. The fabric is simply dipped into the liquid containing the dissolved MCT-CD, followed by squeezing of the fabric. Fixation takes place at elevated temperature. Alkaline or acidic fixation are both possible. For alkaline fixation a fixation temperature of 150 °C results in a fixation yield of 80–85%. Fastness of the MCT-CD finish is reported to be very good

(Moldenhauer *et al.*, 1999). Apart from these methods, cyclodextrins can also be spun into the fibre. This can be achieved only with materials in which fibres are made using melt or solution spinning like polyamide-6. Cooling of the fibre leaving the spindle in a 'shock-wise' (or rapid) manner causes the cyclodextrins to migrate to the surface. Thereby the cyclodextrin molecules remain accessible as a host for drug molecules (Poukalis *et al.*, 1992).

Mass transport of cyclodextrins in textile materials

The time-determining step in a cyclodextrin impregnation process is often the transport of the molecules to the surfaces of the textile fibres in the yarn, especially in wet-to-wet applications. The porous textile structure will hinder free liquid flow, consequently diffusion of molecules through the pores to the fibre surfaces will be the main transport mechanism. This is a relatively slow process. The diffusion coefficient of un-complexed cyclodextrins is $3.2 \cdot 10^{-10}$ m^2/s, the diffusion coefficient of a cyclodextrin-guest complex will be lower (Szejtli 1998; De Azevedo *et al.*, 2000; Cameron and Fielding 2001). As an illustration, the time needed to remove 90% of various particles and cyclodextrin molecules from a yarn by diffusion as a function of the particle diameter has been calculated (see Fig. 3.13). For details on the calculation see Nierstrasz and Warmoeskerken 2003. The time needed before for cyclodextrins to adsorb at the fibre surfaces is consequently also much more than for regular textile chemicals.

Cyclodextrins are from a toxicological point of view considered to be safe; cyclodextrins are used as food additives and are considered harmful only in extremely high concentrations (Buschmann *et al.*, 2001). Toxicological properties of the groups used in fixation of cyclodextrins should, however,

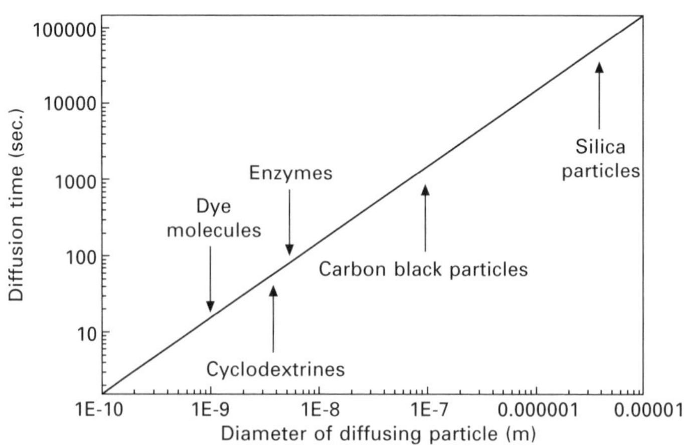

3.13 Time needed to remove 90% of particles from a yarn by diffusion as a function of the particle diameter.

not be neglected. Biodegradability and biocompatibility of textiles bearing cyclodextrins is mainly determined by the choice of the textile material itself. Therefore this is not considered to be a factor affecting application of cyclodextrins as a textile drug delivery system.

3.3.2 Ion-exchange fibres

Ion-exchange is a technique that has been known for quite some time and ion-exchange materials are widely used in various separation applications. Ion-exchange fibres have some advantages over other ion-exchange materials like a fast ion-exchange rate and a high separation capacity (Chen *et al.*, 1996). Ion-exchange fibres find their application in, for example, waste-water purification (Soldatov *et al.*, 1999), uranium enrichment from seawater (Chen *et al.*, 1996) and in textile drug delivery systems as well (Jaskari *et al.*, 2000, 2001; Skundric *et al.*, 2002; Vuorio *et al.*, 2003, 2004). Ion-exchange fibres have either a positive or a negative electric charge, which is compensated by mobile counter-ions of opposite charge. The overall charge depends on the pK-value of the functional groups, and is thus a function of the pH. In cationic fibres, ionic groups of ion-exchange fibres are formed by, for example, SO_3^-, COO^- or PO_3^-; anionic groups are, for example, $-NH_3^+$, $-NH_2^+$ or $-NH^+$. The principle of ion-exchange is based on the electroneutrality condition. Ion-exchange generally is a diffusional process, sensible to concentration gradients; the rate-determining step in ion exchange is diffusion either within the exchanger itself or in the so-called diffusion boundary layer. The amount of functional groups affects the loading capacity. Generally, the feature that ion-exchangers take up certain counter-ions in preference to others, influences specificity of the exchange process.

Many drugs are charged at physiological pH, therefore they can act as mobile counter-ions, and this allows them to be used in ion-exchange delivery systems. In addition drug stability during storage improves upon bonding them in ion-exchange fibres. Ion-exchange fibres suitable for drug delivery are already commercially available, examples are *Smopex*® fibres from SmopTech Co., consisting of a polyethylene backbone which is grafted with other polymers, e.g., poly(styrenesulphonic acid) (Smopex®-101) polyacrylic acid (Smopex®-102) or polyamide (Smopex®-108). Besides commercially available ion-exchange fibres, it is also possible to graft ion-exchange groups to textile fibres. Suitable fibres are cotton, flax, cellulose (derivatives) and wool, but also synthetic fibres like polyethylene, polystyrene, polyacrylonitril, polyamide and carbon fibres are possibilities (Järnström and Hirvonen 2001).

Both *in-* and *ex-vivo* ion-exchange drug delivery applications are developed. *In-vivo* the drugs can be released by ions present in bodily fluids, however, this might disturb homeostasis whereas in *ex-vivo* or transdermal applications the concentration of ions, like Na^+ and Cl^-, needed for the exchange process is determined by excretion through the skin. Consequently the release process might be difficult to control and will probably be relatively slow. To increase control, to reduce fluctuations and to increase drug permeation, ion-exchange is combined with iontophoresis (Jaskari *et al.*, 2000, 2001; Vuorio *et al.*, 2003, 2004). At physiological pH the human skin is negatively charged. As a result cationic drugs permeate the skin more easily than anionic drugs. Cationic drugs can associate with negative domains present in the skin, thereby neutralising the charge of the skin and hindering the iontophoretic process (Raiman *et al.*, 2003). Different ion-exchange fibres and drugs for transdermal iontophoretic drug delivery have been characterised, such as tacrin, propranolol, metoprol and nadolol with Smopex®-101 with strong ion-exchange groups and Smopex®-102 with weak ion-exchange groups (Jaskari *et al.*, 2000, 2001; Vuorio *et al.*, 2003, 2004). The ion-exchange material serves as a reservoir and a means to control delivery rate. In combination with iontophoresis drug release permeation across the skin may be controlled. Release kinetics are affected by the choice of the ion-exchange material and solution. Often, burst-release type is observed, however, when properly designed and controlled zero-order kinetics seems to be possible.

Skundric *et al.* (2002), studied ion-exchange fibres for *in-* and *ex-vivo* applications. Cation-exchange fibres based on polyacrylonitrile (PAN) were developed with –COOH as functional group. The potential of PAN fibres was evaluated because of good chemical stability and durability within living organisms, thereby avoiding problems that might result from biodegradation. Ion-exchange fibres with antibacterial properties (gentamicin sulphate, an antibiotic), or anaesthetic properties for, e.g., postoperative treatments (procaine hydrochloride) were successfully produced using PAN fibres with a functional carboxyl group. A very interesting development is the application of PAN ion-exchange fibres for the controlled delivery of insulin, to treat diabetes mellitus. The three different ion-exchange delivery systems, based on PAN fibres with functional carboxyl groups, exhibit burst-release type kinetics, however, satisfactory results were obtained with *in-vivo* experiments in rats with artificially provoked diabetes over a period of one month (Skundric *et al.*, 2002).

Toxicity, biocompatibility and biodegradability of ion-exchange materials are to a large extent determined by the choice of polymer. Toxicity could stem from ionic groups attached to the polymer backbones or degradation products of the polymers. In literature no specific comments were made on toxicity, biocompatibility and biodegradability as such, apart from the fact that PAN is chemically stable and durable within living organisms. In general it can be stated that in *ex-vivo* applications toxicity of ion-exchange materials is less critical, especially when compared to *in-vivo* applications.

3.3.3 Drug-containing fibres, microencapsulated drugs, microparticles and nano-fibres produced by electrospinning

Other often studied approaches in constructing textile drug delivery systems are based on polymeric systems in which the drugs are incorporated, e.g., hollow fibres, incorporating the drug during fibre preparation, polymer microcapsules containing the drug, and electrospinning. As in ion-exchange materials, toxicity, biocompatibility and biodegradability of ion-exchange materials are to a large extent determined by the choice of polymer. Hollow fibres drug delivery systems are small tubes filled with a drug (Ostad *et al.*, 1998). The fibre wall consists of a permeable membrane. The permeability of the membrane, chemical properties of the membrane and the radius controls drug release rate. Advantages of the hollow fibres are that they have a high surface area to volume ratio, and a high loading flexibility. Hollow fibre drug delivery systems comprise a hollow membrane filled with a liquid drug or a drug solution.

In hollow fibres, there still is a distinct separation in fibres and drug. Another method to incorporate drugs into fibres or particles is to suspend or dissolve a drug into a polymer solution used to produce the fibres. Selection of the polymer is based upon the solubility of the drug in the polymer solution. Drug loading efficiency is limited, and most often burst kinetics is observed. The resulting fibres can be further processed using regular techniques, like weaving.

Particles containing drugs can be fixed to other textile fibres by reaction or cross-links. The drug release rate is determined by the radius of the fibre or particle, the concentration gradient, the diffusion coefficient of the drug in the polymer material, erosion of the material, or electrostatic interactions in case of polyelectrolytes (Liao *et al.*, 2005). Burst kinetics is most often observed (Gupta *et al.*, 2001), however, when properly designed, zero-order kinetics seems possible in case of uniform micro-particles with controlled diameter (Berkland *et al.*, 2002). An interesting application is the application of biodegradable polymers such as poly(lactic acid). Upon degradation of the polymer, the drug is released. Drug release can thus be 'triggered', even by specific local conditions such as an infection for example (Woo *et al.*, 2000).

Another technology is to produce particles containing drugs is encapsulation (Nelson, 2002). Encapsulation can be achieved by a variety of methods, such as interfacial polymerisation, microemulsion polymerisation, precipitation polymerisation and diffusion. The drugs are brought into contact with monomers, oligomers or polymers. These assemble around the drugs and subsequent polymerisation produces the final particles. High drug loads are possible. Applications of encapsulated materials in textiles are not only in drug delivery systems, but in, for example, durable fragrances, skin softeners and insect repellents as well. Microencapsulated phase change materials are already applied in textile materials to reduce extreme temperature fluctuations.

A fairly new promising technology in the application of polymer based textile drug delivery systems is electrospinning (Kenawy *et al.*, 2002; Zeng *et al.*, 2003, 2005), even though the idea of electrospinning dates back to 1938 (Formhals, 1938). In electrospinning fibres are produced of nanoscopic dimensions. Depending on the experimental conditions, set-up and polymers fibre diameters are in the range of 16 nm up to 2 μm, which is orders of magnitude smaller than the diameter of fibres produced in conventional spinning processes (Jeager *et al.*, 1998; Bergshoef and Vancso 1999). Owing to their nanoscopic diameter, it is even possible to produce transparent composite materials (Bergshoef and Vancso, 1999). The technology for electrospinning is fairly straightforward (see Fig. 3.14). In electrospinning a strong electric field (5–45 kV) is applied to a polymer solution held in a capillary. At the critical field strength, depending on the polymer solution but typically around 10 kV, electrical forces overcome surface tension forces that keep the liquid in the capillary and a charged jet of the solution is ejected. The jet moves towards the collector. The solvent evaporates during spinning, and a non-woven mat is formed on the collector (Jeager *et al.*, 1998; Bergshoef and Vancso, 1999).

Kenawy *et al.* (2002) produced electrospun poly(L-lactic acid) (PLA) and poly(ethylene-covinyl acetate) (PEVA) fibres and blends thereof containing tetracycline, an antibiotic. The fibres were spun at 15 kV from chloroform solutions, containing a small amount of methanol to solubilise the tetracycline hydrochloride. Blends of electrospun PEVA and PLA fibres typically had a diameter of 1–3 μm, while electrospun PLA fibres had diameters of 3–6 μm.

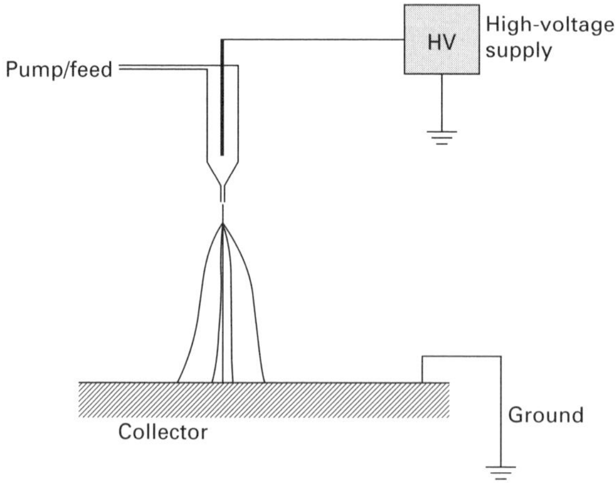

3.14 Schematic representation of set-up for electrospinning.

In initial drug release experiments burst release was observed, but smooth drug release has been described for a period of five days.

Zeng *et al.* (2003, 2005) tried to improve size distribution of the diameter of biodegradable electrospun PLA fibres to improve drug release characteristics. Fibres were spun at 30–45 kV from a chloroform-acetone solution. The influence of different surfactants (triethyl benzyl ammonium chloride, sodium dodecyl benzene sulphate and PPO-PEO ether) on fibre diameter and fibre uniformity was evaluated. The release kinetics of rifampin (an antibiotic), paclitaxel (an anti-tumour agent), doxorubicin and doxorubicin hydrochloride (a broad spectrum anti-tumour agent) was evaluated. Fibres spun at 23 kV in the absence of surfactant had diameters in the range of 0.3–4.2 μm, while fibres spun at 42 kV in the presence of triethyl benzyl ammonium chloride had diameters in the range of 0.3–0.5 μm. Fibres spun at 41 kV in the presence of sodium dodecyl benzene sulphate had diameters in the range of 0.68–1.35 μm, and fibres spun at 32 kV in the presence of PPO-PEO ether had diameters in the range of 0.34–1.35 μm. The release characteristics were determined in the presence of proteinase K, an enzyme capable of degrading the PLA fibres. In the absence of proteinase K no drug release was reported, release is triggered by degradation of the polymers. For the fibres produced in the presence of surfactants nearly zero-order kinetics was observed. This clearly demonstrates the potential of electrospun drug delivery systems compared to other polymeric drug delivery systems.

3.4 Future trends

As has been mentioned in paragraph 3.3, more often than not textile drug delivery systems based on, e.g., cyclodextrins are mainly designed on the basis of experience and trial and error, and not on the basis of specific design rules. Drug release rates and patterns are to a great extent determined by the combination of guest and the host or the carrier material. For *ex-vivo* applications this is not necessarily a problem hindering actual developments yet, but for *in-vivo* applications, where control of drug release rates is much more delicate and development costs are of another order of magnitude, this might block developments. This is a point of concern, that can possibly be addressed by, e.g., advanced computational techniques and more complicated release systems. Some polymer drug delivery systems suffer from burst-release kinetics. Novel techniques such as electrospinning clearly have the potential to combine triggered release with zero-order release kinetics. Today, most electrospinning processes are typically at lab-scale and not at industrial level though electrospinning is a technique strongly developing and up-scaling of the process is a matter of time.

A topic not being dealt with in this chapter is the potential of biotechnology in the development of textile drug delivery systems. However, it seems reasonable to expect that biotechnology will play a major role in textile drug delivery systems in the near future. Presently, strong efforts are being made to functionalise (bio-)polymer materials using enzymes, and enzymes have in principle the possibility to bind host- or drug-molecules to fibres. The development of innovative biodegradable materials can have a strong influence on the design of triggered drug release systems.

To meet pharmaceutical demands, industrial production of textile drug delivery systems require special production facilities apart from sufficient environmental and safety measures. The developments of suitable minimal application techniques, such as nozzles or digital finishing technology, have the potential to meet these demands and to increase efficiency, and competitiveness. This will allow actual implementation into the textile industry. Apart from applying these technologies in advanced drug textile delivery systems, new developments and applications of textiles or textile fibres bearing cyclodextrins are expected in the field of environmental protection, separation technology, and functional textile materials like sensoric, antibacterial and antifungal textiles (hygienic textile) or textiles releasing fragrances and adsorbing unwanted odours (Szejtli, 2003; Buschmann *et al.*, 2001).

3.5 Acknowledgements

The Textile Technology Group at the University of Twente acknowledges the financial support of the Foundation Technology of Structured Materials in the Netherlands and of the Dutch Ministry of Economic Affairs.

3.6 References and further reading

Bergshoef, M.M. and Vancso, G.J. (1999), Transparent nanocomposites with ultrathin electrospun nylon-4,6 fiber reinforcement, *Advanced Materials*, **11**(16), 1362–1365.

Berkland, C., King, M., Cox, A., Kim, K. and Pack, D.W. (2002), Precise control of PLG microsphere size provides enhanced control of drug release. *Journal of Controlled Release*, **82**, 137–147.

Breteler, M.R., Nierstrasz, V.A. and Warmoeskerken, M.M.C.G. (2002), Textile slow release systems with medical applications. *Autex Research Journal*, **2**(4), 175–189.

Bruinewoud, H., Kemmere, M.F. and Keurentjes, J.T.F. (2004), Drug delivery device comprising an active compound and method for releasing an active compound from a drug delivery device. Patent 113422.

Buschmann, H.J. and Schollmeyer, E. (1997a), Cucurbituril and β-cyclodextrin as hosts for the complexation of dyes. *Journal of Inclusion Phenomena and Molecular Recognition in Chemistry*, **26**, 167–174.

Buschmann, H.J., Cleve, E., Denter, U. and Schollmeyer, E. (1997b), Determination of complex stabilities with nearly insoluble host molecules. Part II. Complexation of alkali and alkaline earth metal cations with dibenzo crown ethers in aqueous solution. *Journal of Physical Organic Chemistry*, **10**, 781–785.

Buschmann, H.J., Knittel, D. and Schollmeyer, E. (2001), New textile applications of cyclodextrins. *Journal of Inclusion Phenomena and Macrocyclic Chemistry*, **40**, 169–172.

Cameron, K.S. and Fielding L. (2001), NMR diffusion spectroscopy as a measure of host-guest complex association constants and as a probe of complex size, *Journal of Organic Chemistry*, **66**, 6891–6895.

Chen, L.Q., Yang, G.L. and Zhang, J. (1996), A study on the exchange kinetics of ion-exchange fiber, *Reactive and functional polymers*, **29**(3), 139–144.

De Azevedo, M.B.M., Alderete, J.B., Lino, A.C.S., Faljoni-Alario, A. and Duran, N. (2000), Violacein/β-cyclodextrin inclusion complex formation studied by measurements of diffusion coefficient and circular dichroism, *Journal of Inclusion Phenomena and Macrocyclic Chemistry*, **37**, 67–74.

Denter, U. and Schollmeyer E. (1996), Surface modification of synthetic and natural fiber by fixation of cyclodextrin derivates. *Journal of Inclusion Phenomena and Molecular Recognition in Chemistry* **25**, 197 202.

Denter, U., Buschmann, H.J., Knittel, D. and Schollmeyer, E. (1997), Modifizierung von Faseroberflächen durch die permanente Fixierung supramolekularer Komponenten, Teil 2: Cyclodextrine, *Angewandte Makromolekulare Chemie*, **248**, 165–188.

Denter, U., Buschmann, H.J. and Schollmeyer, E. (1998a), Modifizierung von Faseroberflächen durch permanente Fixierung supramolekularer Komponenten, Teil 3: Azakrownether, *Angewandte Makromolekulare Chemie*, **258**, 75–81.

Denter, U., Buschmann, H.J. and Schollmeyer, E. (1998b), Modifizierung von Faseroberflächen durch die permanente Fixierung supramolekularer Komponenten, Teil 4: Fullerenen C60, *Angewandte Makromolekulare Chemie*, **258**, 87–91.

Formhals, A. (1938), Method and apparatus for the production of fibers. US Patent 2116942.

Freudenberg, K., Cramer, F. and Plieninger, H. (1953), Verfahren zur Herstellung von Einschlussverbindungen physiologisch wirksamer organischer Verbindungen. German Patent 895769.

Gupta, K.C., Majeti, N.V. and Kumar, R. (2001). pH dependent hydrolysis and drug release behavior of chitosan/poly(ethylene glycol) polymer network microspheres. *Journal of materials Science: Materials in Medicine*, **12**, 753–759.

Guy, R.H. and Handgraft, J. (1992), Rate control in transdermal drug delivery? *International Journal of Pharmaceutics*, **82**, R1–R6.

Hedges, A.R. (1998), Industrial applications of cyclodextrins. *Chemical Reviews*, **98**, 2035–2044.

Hirayama, F. and Uekama, K. (1999), Cyclodextrin-based controlled drug release system. *Advanced Drug Delivery Reviews*, **36**, 125–141.

Järnström, R. and Hirvonen, J. (2001), Composition for transdermal delivery of drugs. US Patent 6254883.

Jaskari, T., Vuorio, M., Kontturi, K., Urtti, A., Manzanares, J.A. and Hirvonen, J. (2000), Controlled transdermal iontophoresis by ion-exchange fiber. *Journal of Controlled Release*, **67**, 179–190.

Jaskari, T., Vuorio, M., Kontturi, K., Manzanares, J.A. and Hirvonen, J. (2001), Ion-exchange fibers and drugs: an equilibrium study. *Journal of Controlled Release*, **70**, 219–229.

Jeager, R., Bergshoef, M.M., Batlle, C.M.I., Schönherr, H. and Vancso, G.J. (1998), Electrospinning of ultra-thin polymer fibers, *Macromolecular Symposia*, **127**, 141–150.

Kenawy, E.R., Bowlin, G.L., Mansfield, K., Layman, J., Simpson, G., Sanders, E.H. and Wnek, G.E. (2002), Release of tetracycline hydrochloride from electrospun poly(ethylene-co-vinylacetate), poly(lactic acid), and a blend, *Journal of Controlled Release*, **81**, 57–64.

Korsmeyer, R.W., Gurny, R., Doelker, E., Buri, P. and Peppas, N.A. (1983), Mechanism of solute release from porous hydrophilic polymers. *International Journal of Pharmaceutics*, **15**, 25–35.

Kumar, N., Ravikumar, M.N.V. and Domb, A.J. (2001), Biodegradable block copolymers. *Advanced Drug Delivery Reviews*, **53**, 23–44.

Le Thuaut, P., Martel, B., Crini, G., Maschke, U., Coqueret, X. and Morcellet, M. (2000), Grafting of cyclodextrins onto polypropylene nonwoven fabrics for the manufacture of reactive filters. I Synthesis parameters, *Journal of applied Polymer Science*, **77**, 2118–2125.

Lee, M.H., Yoon, K.J. and Ko, S.W. (2000), Grafting onto cotton fiber with acrylamidomethylated β-cyclodextrin and its application. *Journal of Applied Polymer Science*, **78**, 1986–1991.

Liao, I.C., Wan, A.C.A, Yim, E.K.F. and Leong, K.W. (2005), Controlled release from fibers of polyelectrolyte complexes. *Journal of Controlled Release*, **104**, 347–358.

Lo Nostro, P., Fratoni, L. and Baglioni, P. (2002), Modification of a fabric with β-cyclodextrin for textile finishing applications. *Journal of Inclusion Phenomena and Macrocyclic Chemistry*, **44**, 423–427.

Loftsson, T. and Brewster, M.E. (1996), Pharmaceutical applications of cyclodextrins. 1 Drug solubilization and stabilization. *Journal of Pharmaceutical Sciences*, **85**(10), 1017–1025.

Lu, J., Hill, M.A., Hood, M., Greeson, jr., D.F., Horton, J.R., Orndorff, P.E., Herndon, A.S. and Tonelli, A.E. (2001), Formation of antibiotic, biodegradable polymers by processing with Irgasan DP300R (Triclosan) and its inclusion compound with β-cyclodextrin. *Journal of Applied Polymer Science*, **82**, 300–309.

Martel, B., Le Thuaut, P., Crini, G., Morcellet, M., Naggi, A.M., Maschke, U., Bertini, S., Vecchi, C., Coqueret, X. and Torri, G. (2000), Grafting of cyclodextrins onto polypropylene nonwoven fabrics for the manufacture of reactive filters. II Characterization, *Journal of applied Polymer Science*, **78**, 2166–2173.

Martel, B., Weltrowski, M., Ruffin, D. and Morcellet, M. (2002a), Polycarboxylic acids as crosslinking agents for grafting cyclodextrins onto cotton and wool fabrics: study of the process parameters. *Journal of Applied Polymer Science*, **83**, 1449–1456.

Martel, B., Morcellet, M., Ruffin, D., Ducoroy, L. and Weltrowski, M. (2002b), Finishing of polyester fabrics with cyclodextrins and polycarboxylic acids as crosslinking agents. *Journal of Inclusion Phenomena and Macrocyclic Chemistry*, **44**, 443–446.

Martel, B., Morcellet, M., Ruffin, D., Vinet, F. and Weltrowski, M. (2002c), Capture and controlled release of fragrances by CD finished textiles. *Journal of Inclusion Phenomena and Macrocyclic Chemistry*, **44**, 439–442.

Martel, B., Le Thuaut, P., Bertini, S., Crini, G., Bacquet, M., Torri, G. and Morcellet, M. (2002d), Grafting of cyclodextrins onto polypropylene nonwoven fabrics for the manufacture of reactive filters. III Study of sorption properties, *Journal of applied Polymer Science*, **85**, 1771–1778.

Moldenhauer, J.P. and Reuscher, H. (1999), Textile finishing with MCT-β-cyclodextrin. In *Proceedings of the 9th International Symposium on Cyclodextrins*. Torres Labandeira, J. and Vila-Jato, J.L., eds., Kluwer Academic Publishers, Dordrecht, 161–165.

Nelson, G. (2002), Application of microencapsulation in textiles. *International Journal of Pharmaceutics*, **242**, 55–62.

Nierstrasz, V.A. and Warmoeskerken, M.M.C.G. (2003), Chapter 4: Process Engineering and industrial enzyme applications. In Cavaco-Paulo A. and G.M. Gübitz, *Textile Processing with Enzymes*, Cambridge, Woodhead Publishing Ltd.

Ostad, S.N., Malhi, J.S. and Gard, P.R. (1998), *In-vitro* cytotoxicity and teratogenicity of norethisterone and levonorgestrel released from hollow nylon monofilaments, *Journal of Controlled Release*, **50**, 179–186.

Poulakis, K., Buschmann, H.J. and Schollmeyer, E. (1992), Antiperspirant finish for polyester textiles – comprises cyclodextrin and/or derivs., chemically and/or physically bonded by cellulose polymer. German Patent 4035378 A1.

Raiman, J., Hänninen, K., Kontturi, K., Murtomäki, L. and Hirvonen, J. (2003), Drug adsorption in human skin: a streaming potential study, *Journal of Pharmaceutical Sciences*, **92**(12), 2366–2372.

Sansom, L.N. (1999), Oral extended-release products. *Australian Prescriber*, **22** (4), 88–90.

Skundric, P., Medovic, A. and Kostic, M. (2002), Fibrous systems with programmed biological-activity and their application in medical practice. *Autex Research Journal*, **2**(2), 78–84.

Soldatov, V.S., Shunkevich, A.A., Elinson, I.S., Johann J. and Iraushek, H. (1999), Chemically active textile materials as efficient means for water purification, *Desalination*, **124**(1–3), 181–192.

Szejtli, J. (1998), Introduction and general overview of cyclodextrin chemistry. *Chemical Reviews*, **98**, 1743–1753.

Szejtli, J. (2003), Cyclodextrins in the textile industry. *Starch/Stärke*, **55**, 191–196.

Szejtli, J., Zsadon, B., Fenyvesi, É., Otta, H. and Tüdös, F. (1980 and 1982), Sorbents of cellulose basis capable of forming inclusion complexes and a process for the preparation thereof. Hungarian Patent 181733 (1980) and US Patent 4357468 (1982).

Uekama, K., Hirayama, F. and Irie, T. (1998), Cyclodextrin drug delivery systems. *Chemical Reviews*, **98**, 2045–2076.

Voncina, B. and Majcen Le Marechal, A. (2005), Grafting of cotton with β-cyclodextrin via poly(carboxylic acid). *Journal of Applied Polymer Science*, **96**, 1323–1328.

Vuorio, M., Manzanares, J.A., Murtomäki, L., Hirvonen, J., Kankkunen, T. and Kontturi, K. (2003), Ion-exchange fibers and drugs: a transient study. *Journal of Controlled Release*, **91**, 439–448.

Vuorio, M., Murtomäki, L., Hirvonen, J. and Kontturi, K. (2004), Ion-exchange fibers and drugs: a novel device for the screening of iontophoretic systems. *Journal of Controlled Release*, **97**, 485–492.

Wise, D.L., Trantolo, D.J., Marino, R.T. and Kitchell, J.P. (1987), Opportunities and challenges in the design of implantable biodegradable polymeric systems for the delivery of antimicrobial agents and vaccines. *Advanced Drug Delivery Reviews*, **1**, 19–39.

Woo, G.L.Y., Mittelman, M.W. and Santerre, J.P. (2000), Synthesis and characterization of a novel biodegradable antimicrobial polymer, *Biomaterials*, **21**, 1235–1246.

Zeng, J., Xu, X., Chen, X., Liang, Q., Bian, X., Yang, L. and Jing, X. (2003), Biodegradable electrospun fibers for drug delivery. *Journal of Controlled Release*, **92**, 227–231.

Zeng, J., Yang, L., Liang, Q., Zhang, X., Guan, H., Xu, X., Chen, X. and Jing, X. (2005), Influence of the drug compatibility with polymer solution on the release kinetics of electrospun fiber formulation. *Journal of Controlled Release*, **105**, 43–51.

4

Application of phase change and shape memory materials in medical textiles

B PAUSE, Textile Testing and Innovation, USA

4.1 Introduction

Shape memory materials and phase change materials are fascinating materials with unique properties which differentiate them significantly from other materials. However, the shape memory technology and the phase change material technology are relatively new technologies which are currently in the stage of being established in different textile applications. Medical textiles are one of the most important areas in which both technologies will be used in the future. The application of the two technologies will add substantial benefits to textile products used for all kinds of medical applications. Despite the variety of differences between the two technologies, such as materials, properties, functionality and product manufacturing – one major similarity exists; their physical effects are triggered by changes in their material temperatures. That means both technologies are based on thermally generated effects. Because of this connection, the two technologies, their effects and their applications in medical textiles will be introduced and discussed together in this chapter.

The first observation of the transformation that yields the shape memory effect was made by Chang and Read in 1951 on a sample of a Gold-Cadmium alloy.[1] In 1962, scientists at the Naval Ordinance Laboratory (USA) found the shape memory effect in alloys of Nickel and Titanium.[2] The Nickel-Titanium alloys became the number one commercially used metallic alloys in the following years under the trade name NiTiNOL. With the discovery of NiTiNOL, the level of product development using shape memory alloys began to accelerate. But it took another seven years until the Raychem Corp. launched a hydraulic pipe coupling with a NiTiNOL actuator. Nowadays, there are a variety of medical and consumer products using shape memory alloys. NiTiNOL is used, for instance, for medical implants and for minimal invasive surgical devices.[4]

Starting in 1987, Mitsubishi Heavy Industries developed the first shape memory polymer.[5] Additional shape memory polymers were later discovered by other researchers.[7] Shape memory polymers are specifically suitable for textile applications.[6] They are currently used in medical, healthcare, and aerospace products.

The technology for incorporating phase change materials into textile structures was developed in the early 1980s as part of a research program funded by the US National Aeronautics and Space Administration (NASA). The program's aim was to improve the thermal performance of space suits to provide astronauts with protection against the extreme temperature fluctuations they encounter in outer space. The concept never led to any practically applicable materials for use in the space program, but the basics of the technology were further developed into 'terrestrial' applications. Today, textiles with phase change material treatment are widely used in garments and home furnishing products.

Currently, there are no specific applications of this technology in the medical field. However, this area has tremendous potential. In the near future, the field of medicine is sure to be affected significantly by the application of the phase change material technology.

4.2 Physical effects

4.2.1 Physical effects obtained by shape memory material

Shape memory materials possess the ability to 'remember' a shape, as triggered by heat through a strain recovery. In addition, they show a highly elastic behaviour in a certain temperature range. The shape memory effect is mainly observed in metallic alloys and polymers.

Shape memory effect

The shape memory effect is the result of a phase transition. The phase transition occurs during a heating process at a certain temperature.[10] Forced by mechanical work, which follows the phase transition, the shape memory alloy or the shape memory polymer reverts to a previously held shape. During this phase transition, the metallic alloys undergo a change in their crystalline structure. The previous less-stable martensitic crystalline structure is transformed into a very stable austenitic crystalline structure. The shape memory polymers change at their glass transition temperatures from a glassy state into a rubbery state. The original hard polymer material becomes soft. In addition to its thermal activation, the shape memory effect of shape memory polymers can also be triggered by light or a chemical reaction in some circumstances.[12]

Elastic memory effect

An elastic behavior takes place in the austenitic stage of shape memory alloys above the transition temperature. For shape memory alloys, this elasticity is 20 times the elasticity of conventional materials and, therefore, called 'superelasticity'. The impressive amount of 'elastic' strain observed in shape memory alloys forces the material to spring back immediately to its original shape if an applied stress is removed. Shape memory polymers possess this property of high elasticity if they are in the rubbery stage above the glass transition temperature.

Martensitic transformation

Martensitic transformation of shape memory alloys is a shear-like mechanism which takes place below the transition temperature. The martensitic transformation can be induced by mechanical forces or by temperature changes in a cooling process. While a substantial martensitic shape transformation of shape memory alloys can be obtained by mechanical forces, the shape transformation induced by temperature changes is comparatively small. Shape memory polymers are usually deformed under stress at a temperature below the glass transition temperature. The deformed shape is fixed in a cooling process. The memory effects which shape memory alloys go through are shown in Fig. 4.1. Figure 4.2 shows the memory effects which are received by the application of shape memory polymers.

4.2.2 Physical effects obtained by phase change material

Phase change material possesses the ability to change its physical state within a certain temperature range. When the melting temperature is obtained in a

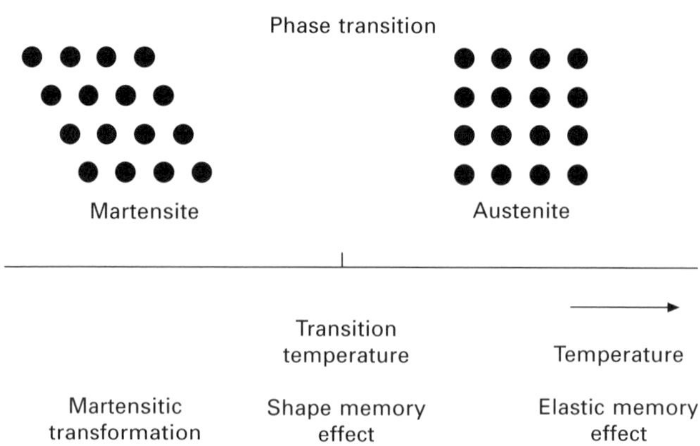

4.1 Memory effects of shape memory alloys.

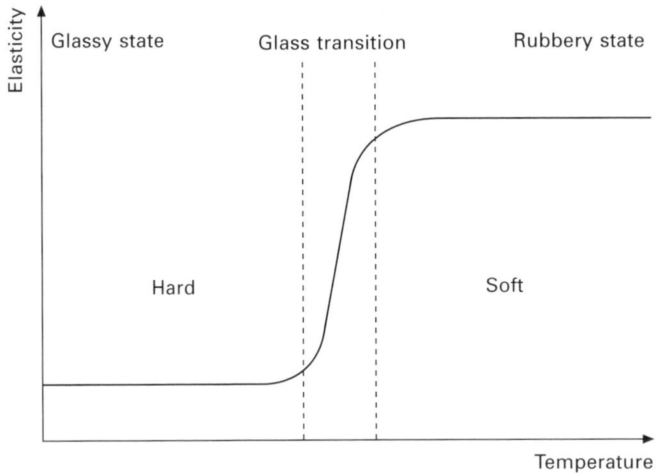

4.2 Memory effects of shape memory polymers.

heating process, the phase change from the solid to the liquid state occurs. During this melting process the phase change material absorbs and stores a large amount of latent heat. The temperature of the phase change material and its surroundings remains nearly constant throughout the entire process. In a cooling process of the phase change material, the stored latent heat is released into the environment in a certain temperature range, and a reverse phase change from the liquid to the solid state takes place. During this crystallization process, the temperature of the phase change material and its surroundings remains also nearly constant. After the phase change is complete, a continued heating/cooling process results in a further temperature increase/decrease. The absorption or release of high amounts of latent heat without any temperature changes, is responsible for the appeal of the phase change material as a suitable heat storage medium.[16]

In order to compare the amount of latent heat absorbed by a phase change material during the actual phase change with the amount of sensible heat absorbed in an ordinary heating process, the ice-water phase change process will be used for comparison. When ice melts, it absorbs an amount of latent heat of about 335 J/g. When the water is further heated, it absorbs a sensible heat of only 4 J/g while its temperature rises by one degree Celsius. Thus, water needs to be heated from about 1 °C up to about 84 °C in order to absorb the same amount of heat which is absorbed during the melting process of ice.[18]

In treating textile structures with phase change material the following thermal benefits are obtained:

- a cooling effect, caused by heat absorption of the phase change material
- a heating effect, caused by heat release of the phase change material

- a thermo-regulating effect, resulting from either heat absorption or heat release of the phase change material.

The efficiency of each of these effects and their duration are mainly dependent on the thermal capacity of the phase change material and, hence, the applied phase change material quantity. Furthermore, phase change temperature range and application temperature range need to correspond in order to realize the desired thermal benefits. In addition, the structure of the carrier system also influences the efficiency of the phase change effect. For instance, dense and thin carrier systems readily support the cooling process.[17]

4.3 Materials

4.3.1 Shape memory materials

Shape memory properties are observed in metallic alloys, polymers, ceramics and gels. Among these materials shape memory alloys and shape memory polymers are most suitable for textile applications.

Shape memory alloys

Shape memory alloys are made of compositions of different metals such as Nickel, Titanium, Copper, or Aluminum. Currently, the Nickel-Titanium alloys are the most commonly used shape memory alloys, possessing transition temperatures ranging from –50 °C up to 110 °C. There are several reasons for the preference of the Nickel-Titanium alloys in comparison to other alloys. The Nickel-Titanium alloys are comparatively inexpensive. They can be fabricated with common metalworking techniques. The transition temperature of the shape memory effect can be tailored to specific needs by simply changing the ratio between Nickel and Titanium. Nickel-Titanium alloys are biocompatible. Furthermore, they possess a high shape memory strain of up to 8%.

In a primary heat treatment process, the transition temperature is adjusted, the mechanical properties are established, and the shape memory alloy is formed into its final shape which will be 'remembered'. In use, the shape memory alloy can be deformed at will (martensitic transformation). However, if the shape memory alloy is then heated up to the point where the transition temperature is reached, the shape of the shape memory alloy will be transformed immediately into the shape given during the production process (final shape).

Fabrication forms include clamps, springs, wires, films and foils. Wires or foils of shape memory alloys, for instance, can be incorporated into a textile matrix. At the University of Aachen in Germany, fine NiTiNOL wires have been successfully processed on conventional textile machinery using warp knitting, braiding and weaving technologies.[13]

Shape memory polymers

Shape memory polymers are usually block copolymers that have hard and soft segments. The hard segments form a continuous crystalline phase which is needed to create the points of physical cross-linking. These segments determine the permanent shape. For instance, hard segments are made of polyurethane. The soft segments create the glassy phase which is responsible for the shape memory behavior of the material. These segments also possess the function to fix the temporary shape of the shape memory polymer at temperatures below the transition temperature. Polyether or polyester diol are used, for instance, for the soft segments.

The shape memory polymers are available, e.g., in the form of pellets. They can easily be compounded and formed by extrusion or injection molding. The processing temperature in this first step of the production process needs to be high enough, so that both segments are molded during this process. Cooling the formed object to a temperature at which both phases are solid again creates the permanent shape. Heating the shape memory polymer for a second time to only soften the glassy phase allows the shape memory polymer to be deformed under load. In the following cooling process, the shape memory polymer obtains its temporary shape. During a further heating process where the phase transition from the glassy state into the rubber state takes place, the recovery of the shape memory polymer's temporary shape into the shape memory polymer's permanent shape will occur. By a calendaring procedure, which follows the extrusion or the injection molding process, the shape memory polymer can be compressed into a thin film and laminated to a textile substrate.

There are shape memory polymers available with variable ranges of hardness and softness as well as different transition temperatures between –30 °C and 70 °C. Beside the shape memory effect, where the shape memory polymer transforms from its temporary into its permanent shape, there are other effects which have been determined in a variety of tests. For instance, cooling the shape memory polymer down to its glassy state leads to length shrinkage of about 3% and shrinkage of the material's volume of about 9%. On the other side, heating the thin film made of the shape memory polymer leads to an increase in the material's breathability. Furthermore, the described shape memory polymer possesses a sufficient chemical resistance.

There are several advantages of shape memory polymers compared to shape memory alloys, such as:

- substantial higher deformability
- ease of manufacture
- comparatively low production costs
- biocompatibility
- substantially easier shaping procedure
- sufficient shape stability.

A disadvantage of shape memory polymers in comparison to shape memory alloys is the much lower stiffness which leads to a relatively small recovery force under constraint. However, when incorporated into a fiberglass-reinforced composite, the stiffness and, hence, the recovery force of the shape memory polymer can be improved substantially.[8,9]

4.3.2 Phase change materials

In addition to ice (water) which has been discussed in 4.2.1, more than 500 natural and synthetic phase change materials are known. These materials differ from one another in their phase change temperature ranges and their latent heat storage capacities. The most common phase change materials presently used in a variety of applications are paraffins, summarized in Table 4.1.

Compared to other phase change materials, paraffins possess very high latent heat storage capacities. Furthermore, paraffins can be mixed in order to realize desired temperature ranges in which the phase change takes place. Paraffins are non-toxic, non-corrosive, and non-hygroscopic. The thermal behavior of the paraffins remains stable also under permanent use. Paraffins are byproducts of petroleum refining and therefore inexpensive.

Before applying a phase change material to a textile matrix, it needs to be integrated in a durable containment structure in order to prevent dissolution while in its liquid stage. In one part of the phase change material technology the phase change materials are encapsulated in very small spheres.[14,15] These microcapsules possess approximate diameters of between 1 μm and 20 μm. The microcapsules are resistant to mechanical actions (e.g. abrasion, shear and pressure), heat and most types of chemicals.

Textiles are treated with phase change material microcapsules in the following ways:

- inside fibers
- as a coating
- as a foam dispersion
- dispersed in the fiber matrix of a non-woven.

Table 4.1 Phase change materials

Phase change material	Melting temperature (°C)	Crystallization temperature (°C)	Latent heat storage capacity (J/g)
Hexadecane	18.5	16.2	237
Heptadecane	22.5	21.5	213
Octadecane	28.2	25.4	244
Nonadecane	32.1	26.4	222
Eicosane	36.1	30.6	247

At present the in-fiber technology is applied only to acrylic fibers. A wet spinning process is used in manufacturing such fibers whereby the phase change material microcapsules are totally surrounded by the fiber material. Therefore, the encapsulated phase change material is permanently locked within the fibers. The fibers are further spun into yarns from which fabrics or knits are then made. Microencapsulated phase change material is also integrated in the polymeric binder which is used to bond the fiber web in order to create nonwoven textiles. For coating applications, the phase change material microcapsules are embedded in a coating compound (e.g. Acrylic, Polyurethane or Rubber Latex coating compounds) and topically applied to a fabric or foam.

Finally, applied as a dispersion into a foam, the phase change material microcapsules are mixed into a water-blown polyurethane foam matrix. The foam with incorporated phase change material microcapsules is then formed in a drying process where the water is taken out of the system. These foams are often topically applied to a fabric in a lamination process. In contrast to the micro-encapsulation, the phase change material is directly integrated in a polymer matrix and is durable contained therein. The polymer matrix with the incorporated phase change material is either coated onto a textile structure or is made in the form of a film which is then laminated onto a textile. The macro-encapsulation of phase change material possesses some advantages in comparison to the micro-encapsulation of phase change material. The macro-encapsulation technology is comparatively cheaper. Furthermore, using the macro-encapsulating technology, a substantially higher latent heat storage capacity is obtained due to the larger amount of phase change material which is contained within a comparative volume.

4.4 Application in medical textiles

4.4.1 Application of shape memory materials in medical textiles

Shape memory materials are already used in medical applications such as implants and surgical devices. Two examples of these applications are stents and wound closures.

Stents

Stents are used to hold up a lumen such as a blood vessel. Stents are made, for instance, of NiTiNOL wires knitted together and formed into a tubular shape. The comparatively large stent is first folded into a small sheet to fit into a catheter. The catheter with the stent is then pushed into the vessel. Inside the blood vessel the stent deploys under body temperature utilizing the shape memory effect of the NiTiNOL wires. When positioned inside the artery, the superelasticity of the material is used to provide a force which keeps the vessel open.[3]

Wound closure

In endoscopic surgery there is a need to close an incision or an open lumen effectively. It is especially difficult to press the wound lips together under the right stress. When the force which fixes the knot is too strong necrosis of the surrounding tissue is likely to occur. On the other side, a too weak force of the knot can lead to the formation of hernias. The solution is the use of a yarn made of a shape memory polymer. The suture is made when the shape memory polymer is in its temporary shape. Under the body temperature the suture shrinks and tightens the knot. In this way, the right force is applied to the knot.[7]

Medical products made with shape memory materials which are currently under development include, for example, surgical protective garments and emergency care products.

Surgical protective garments

The newly designed medical textiles which can be used for gowns, caps and gloves are composites consisting of a shape memory polymer film laminated to non-woven or woven fabric.[11] The shape memory polymer film provides a barrier function against the permeation of blood and other fluids. However, in addition, the shape memory polymer film possesses a temperature dependent water vapor transfer. The water vapor transfer through the shape memory polymer film increases with an increase in the temperature. Figure 4.3 shows test results received for the composite's water vapor permeability depending on temperature.

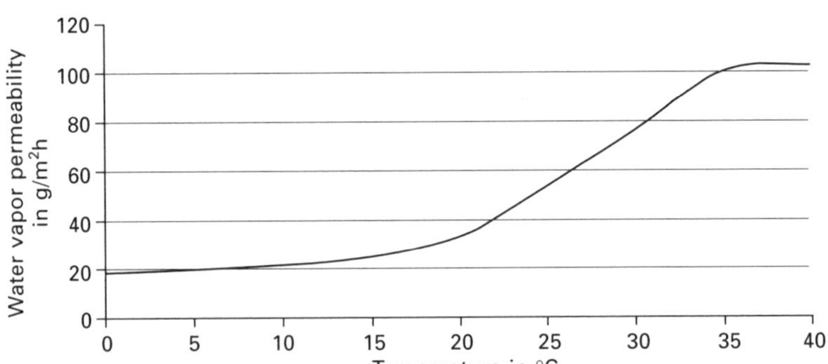

4.3 Temperature dependence of water vapour transfer through a shape memory polymer film/fabric composite.

The test results indicate that at a temperature below 15 °C, the water vapor transfer through the fabric is only small. But after the phase transition of the shape memory polymer at about 15 °C, the water vapor transfer increases steadily. At a temperature of 35 °C, the water vapor transfer totals about four times the water vapor transfer received at a temperature of about 15° C.

In addition to the other features, the shape memory polymer film/fabric composite is flexible, thin and lightweight. By using such shape memory polymer composites for surgical garments, their thermo-physiological comfort can be enhanced substantially without a decrease in the garment's protective function.[12]

Emergency care product

The shape memory effect of shape memory alloys is also used in a new type of emergency blanket. A shape memory alloy foil is used as an inner liner between two thin cover fabrics. In its basic configuration, the blanket is very thin and can be stored in a small pocket. For rescue operations under cold weather conditions the blanket will be inflated as a result of the shape memory effect initiated by the body heat of the injured person or someone from the rescue team.

4.4.2 Application of phase change materials in medical textiles

Microencapsulated phase change material is already applied to bedding products which could be used in hospital setups.

Bedding products

Microencapsulated phase change material integrated in the textile matrix of non-woven fabrics or topically applied to a non-woven fabric in the form of a coating is currently used in a variety of bedding products such as comforters, pillows, or mattress covers. Integrated in these bedding products, the microencapsulated phase change material provides a thermo-regulating feature to them by either absorbing or releasing heat. The thermo-regulating effect keeps the microclimate temperature in the comfort range and, therefore, prevents sweat from being produced by the body. Used in a hospital, the thermo-regulating feature of such bedding products would specifically support the healing process of the patients.

Currently, a variety of medical products are under development where macro-encapsulated phase change material is used. Such products include heating and cooling patches, warming blankets as well as surgical protective garments.

Heating and cooling pads

Heating and cooling patches consist of a polymer matrix in which phase change material is integrated. The patches are embedded in a textile cover in order to meet health care requirements. The heating patch is used for thermal therapy provided in different parts of the body. Before the therapy can take place, the patch needs to be put into a microwave or oven and heated until the temperature desired for the specific therapy is reached. Then the patch is brought in contact with the part of the body which has been selected for the thermal therapy. The heat stored in the phase change material is slowly released into the patient's body.

In contrast, cooling patches can be directly applied to the body part which is injured by an inflammation. The phase change material contained in the patch absorbs the heat generated by the body and provides a cooling effect in the area where the inflammation takes place. In comparison to ice packs, which are used for the same purpose, the cooling effect provided by the cooling patches is much gentler because of a higher surface temperature. Furthermore, in contrast to the ice packs, the cooling patches do not need to be stored in a refrigerator in order to regenerate. The recharge of the phase change material applied to the cooling patches takes place under room temperature.

Warming blankets

Warming blankets are suitable for use in the operating theatre or in intensive care in order to prevent hypothermia of the patient's body during surgery and thereafter. The blanket consists of a polymer pad in which a phase change material is integrated. The polymer pad is contained in a cover which can be cleaned with disinfectants. Before the application, the warming blanket is heated up by a heating circuit. The power supply to the blanket can be disconnected after a short period of time. The heat stored in the phase change material as a result of the initial heating effect is slowly released into the patient's body during the course of surgery. Hypothermia can thus be prevented. No additional power supply is normally necessary during long-lasting surgery. By using the phase change material for the heating process, the heat is evenly divided over the whole area of the blanket and overheating can be prevented.

Surgical protective garments

Surgical protective garments such as gowns, caps and gloves are often worn by surgeons for several hours at a time in the operating room. Because these materials are designed primarily to prevent permeation of particles and liquids which carry bacteria, the thermo-physical wearing comfort of such garments is usually very poor. The thermo-physical comfort of these garments can be improved substantially by coating the inside of the garments with a polymeric film which contains phase change material.

In the application of surgical protective garments, the main function of the phase change material will be the absorption of excessive heat generated by the body during surgical procedures. Heat absorption by the phase change material will keep the microclimate temperature in the comfort range over an extended period of time preventing a greater amount of sweat from being produced by the skin. As a result, the thermo-physiological wearing comfort of surgical protective garments will be enhanced substantially which will also help the surgeons and nurses to better perform their duties.[19] The polymer film with the incorporated phase change material is impermeable to blood, other liquids and even bacteria, which provides an additional benefit to the surgical garments.

4.5 Future trends

There is no doubt that textiles with a shape memory function or a phase change material treatment can provide a significant contribution in order to enhance the performance of various kinds of medical products. Medical devices with a shape memory function already support the surgeon in carrying out complicated surgeries successfully. More of these useful devices will be developed in the future. Patches and blankets with thermal storage properties based on the application of phase change material are currently under development. They are suitable for thermal therapy and the prevention of hypothermia in the operating theatre and in intensive care. Both products will be on the market in the near future. Medical textiles with both shape memory function and phase change material treatment can be used to improve significantly the thermo-physiological comfort of existing surgical garments, such as surgical gowns or gloves. However, a substantial amount of effort will be necessary to further develop these products and bring them to the marketplace.

4.6 Sources of further information and advice

4.6.1 Research on shape memory materials

Reseach on shape memory materials is carried out, for instance, by the following reseach institutes:

- Textile Testing & Innovation, LLC, 7161 Christopher Court, Longmont, CO 80503, USA,

- GKSS-Research Center Geestacht GmbH, Institute for Chemistry, Kantstr. 35, D-14513 Teltow, Germany,
- RTWH Aachen, Institut für Textiltechnik, Eilfschornsteinstrasse. 18, D-52062 Aachen, Germany.

4.6.2 Sources of information on shape memory products

The following companies are suitable sources of information pertaining to shape memory products:

- Diaplex Co., Ltd., 3-1 Marunouchi 2-Chrome, Chiyoda-Ku, Tokyo 100-0005, Japan.
- Shape Memory Applications, Inc., 1070 Commercial Street, Suite No. 110, San Jose, CA 95112, USA.

4.6.3 Research on medical textiles with incorporated phase change materials

The company Textile Testing & Innovation, LLC, located at 7161 Christopher Court, Longmont, CO 80503, USA is specialized in the development and the test of medical and other end-use products.

4.6.4 Sources of information on textiles treated with microencapsulated phase change material

The following companies are suitable sources of information pertaining to textiles with microencapsulated phase change material:

- Outlast Technologies, Inc., The Valmont Building, 5480 Valmont Street Suite 200, Boulder, CO 80301, USA.
- Freudenberg Vliesstoffe KG, D-69456 Weinheim, Germany.
- Schoeller Textil AG, Bahnhofstr., CH-9475 Sevelen, Switzerland.

4.7 References

4.7.1 References related to shape memory material

1. Chang L C, Read T A (1951), *Trans. AIME*, 189, 47.
2. Buehler W J, Gilfrich R C, Wiley J (1963), *Journal Applied Physics*, 34, 1475.
3. Duerig T W (1995), 'Present and future applications of shape memory and superelastic materials, *Materials Research Society Symposium Proceedings*, 360.
4. Otsuka K, Wayman C M (1999), *Shape memory materials*, Cambridge, Cambridge University Press.
5. Russell D A, Hayashi S (1999) 'Potential use of shape memory film in clothing, *Technical Textiles International*, 10, 17–19.

6. Pause B, 'Textile application of shape memory material', 11th International Conference on *Textile Coating and Laminating*, Atlanta, USA, 2001.
7. Lendlein A, Langer R (2002), 'Biodegradable, elastic shape-memory polymers for potential biomedical applications, *Science*, 296, 1673–1676.
8. Gall K, Dunn M L, Liu Y, Finch, D, Lake M, Munshi N A (2002), 'Shape memory polymer nanocomposites', *Acta Materialia*, 50, 5115–5126.
9. Abrahamson E R, Lake M S, Munshi N A, Gall K (2003), 'Shape memory mechanics of an elastic memory composite resin, *Journal of intelligent material systems and structures*, 14, 623–632.
10. Lendlein A, Kelch St (2002), 'Shape memory polymers', *Angewandte Chemie, Int. edn*, 41, 2034–2057.
11. Pause B, 'Application of shape memory material in medical textiles, 12th International *Techtextil Symposium*, Frankfurt, Germany, 2003.
12. Lendlein A, Jlang H, Juenger O, Langer R (2005), 'Light-induced shape-memory polymers, *Nature*, 434, 879–882.
13. Budillon F, Sri Harwoko M, Gries T, 'Nitinol textiles for medical application, 13th International *Techtextil Symposium*, Frankfurt, Germany, 2005.

4.7.2 References related to phase change material

14. Bryant Y G, Colvin D P, 'Fibers with enhanced, reversible thermal energy storage properties, 4th International *Techtextil Symposium*, Frankfurt, Germany, 1992.
15. Pause B, 'Phase Change Materials – the technology and incorporation into textiles, 5th International Conference on *Textile Coating and Laminating*, Williamsburg, USA, 1995.
16. Pause B, 'New possibles in medicine: Textiles treated with PCM microcapsules, 10th International *Techtextil Symposium*, Frankfurt, Germany, 1999.
17. Pause B (2001), 'Textiles with improved thermal capabilities through the application of Phase Change Material (PCM) micro-capsules, *Melliands Textilberichte*, 9, 753–754.
18. Pause B (2003), 'Nonwoven protective garments with thermo-regulating properties, *Journal of Industrial Textiles*, 33, 93–99.
19. Pause B (1999), 'Phase change materials show potential for medical applications, *Technical Textiles International*, 9, 23–26.

5 The use of electronics in medical textiles

M CATRYSSE, F PIROTTE, Centexbel, Belgium and R PUERS Katholieke Universiteit Leuven, Belgium

5.1 Introduction

5.1.1 Electronics of the future: ambient intelligence

Based on the ever increasing performance of microelectronics (as predicted by Moore's Law), a new paradigm, that might drastically change our environment in the next decades, is emerging: ambient intelligence [Boek 02, Mar 03, Aarts 03]. Ambient intelligence, pervasive or ubiquitous computing, the smart environment: these are all synonyms, referring to the same principle: electronics everywhere and always. A distributed network with small, low-power and high performance circuits, wireless communications, new sensors and actuators, autonomous power sources and user-friendly interfaces will make electronic systems disappear by integration into clothing and the environment (e.g. carpet and walls). In the ambient intelligence era, each consumer will have its own, adaptive personal area network (PAN) offering multimedia functions, such as GPS, internet connection, mobile phone, music (MP3) player, and health care monitoring by different (implantable and wearable) sensors. Clothes with integrated electronics may become key elements in the ambient intelligence era. Recent developments already illustrate the promising character of these 'smart clothes'. It is clear, however, that the era of ambient intelligence is not tomorrow's reality yet. First, both psychological (e.g. privacy concerns) and technological barriers should be overcome for its introduction. In this chapter, research efforts, overcoming the technological barriers are discussed.

5.1.2 Medical applications: ambulatory monitoring and telemedicine

The concept of ambient intelligence has fostered a dramatic growth of interest for wearable medical technology, resulting in the development of ambulatory monitoring systems and telemedicine, as parts of the smart environment

[Bona 03, Dan 03]. The image of an Australian farmer aided by the Flying Doctors, is being replaced by the image of that same farmer with a wearable ECG monitoring unit and sending the measured data via a mobile phone or internet connection to the physician 500 km away. This interest for wearable medical technology is both socially driven (the rising cost of medical assistance, the ageing of the population, the need for chronic follow up of patients and the need to improve early illness detection and intervention) and technologically driven, by the advances in sensor technology, data communication and processing [Para 03]. The ideal ambulatory monitoring system should be non-obtrusive and provide continuous and long-term monitoring of patient vital signs, resulting in an improved autonomy and quality of life of the patient/wearer. Moreover, by providing direct feedback to its wearer, it should improve the patient's awareness and potentially allow better control of his own condition.

Despite the sociological aspect, technology is the key factor in these developments and in the enhancement of the quality of life for everyone in the continuum of life from newborns to senior citizens – whether it is the safe delivery and care of undernourished premature babies or extending the life of a senior citizen through monitoring and treatment. Technology is indeed the catalyst that can rapidly transform health care and the practice of medicine. So, any technology to minimize the loss of human life and/or enhance the quality of life has a value that is priceless [Park 03].

5.1.3 What are 'Textronics'?

Depending on the degree of integration, the combination of electronics and textiles can be divided into three categories: embedded electronics, textronics and fibertronics, as is shown in Fig. 5.1.

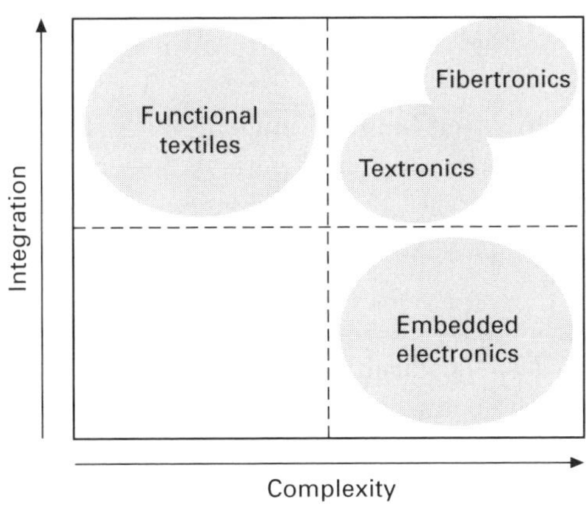

5.1 Integration and complexity level of different textile–electronics combination methods (adapted from [Mech 04]).

Embedded electronics

These are referred to as the building-in of existing (commercially available) electronic components in a textile. Examples are ICD+ suit, developed by Philips and Levi's [Aarts 03] and the Lifeshirt from Vivometrics [Wil 02, Vivo]. In the ICD+ suit, a mobile phone and an MP3 player are integrated in a jacket. The level of integration of the electronics of this suit is low, as an existing mobile phone and an existing MP3 player are used and the connection between the different parts (player, headphone, ...) is made by regular electrical wire. Moreover, the whole system can easily be disconnected from the suit, as the electronics and the interconnections cannot endure a washing machine. The Lifeshirt is intended for sports and health care applications. Respiration, ECG, blood pressure, position and movement can be monitored by attaching existing, removable sensors to a shirt. The data is stored on a PDA also attached to the shirt, and can be read out by, e.g., a physician. As is illustrated by the examples, the major advantage of the embedding of existing electronics in textiles is the ease of combining electronics and textiles. As a consequence, embedded electronics are already available on the market. The disadvantages of this method are the lack of flexibility and washability of the embedded electronics circuitry, and the large dimensions of the circuitry, which may cause discomfort to the wearer (in the case of embedding electronics in clothing).

Textronics

This refers to the manufacturing of electronic components by textile production techniques and textile materials. Examples are the developments at the University of Pisa where suits for monitoring of rehabilitation, studying of ergonomics, virtual reality and ambulatory monitoring were developed by integrating fabric based sensors [Mazz 02, Rossi 03]. Two technologies are used for the fabrication of the sensors, resulting in electrodes for the measurement of ECG and strain gauges for the measurement of posture, movement and respiration. In a first fabrication method PolyPyrrol (PPy) is used as a conducting polymer and coated onto Lycra, the second one produces electrodes and strain gauges made of carbon filled rubber. The carbon-rubber mixture can be either directly printed on the fabric or carbon filled rubber coated fibers can be woven.

The major advantage of textronics technology is the ease of integration of the electronics in the textiles, the disadvantage is the limited amount of components that can be built in this way. The design and application of textronics will be discussed throughout the remainder of this chapter.

Fibertronics are referred to as the building-in of electronic building blocks such as transistors into yarns. Fibertronics will be dealt with in section 5.6 of this chapter.

5.2 Challenges when integrating electronics in textiles

Figure 5.2 depicts the basic components of an electronic system. It consists of a processor and memory, sensors and actuators and wired or wireless connections to other electronic systems. The whole system is powered by a power source and packaged. When integrating this kind of electronic system into textiles, three major challenges should be overcome:

- realisation of the electronic components (section 5.3)
- ensuring constant power delivery to the system (section 5.4)
- providing a washable and flexible packaging, which does not cause any discomfort to the wearer (section 5.5).

5.3 Textile-based electronic components

As mentioned above, the major disadvantage of textronics technology is the limited amount of components that can be built with it: the technology allows only the building of electronic components on a macro scale, such as sensors (and input devices), antennas and wired interconnections. The importance of textronics technology is the possibility for textile manufacturers to create an added value for their products. Whereas in the case of embedded electronics, essentially anybody can build in the existing electronic components in a textile material, for the textronics technology, knowledge of and access to textile production is necessary. Several textile production techniques can be used to build electronic components:

- weaving conductive yarns in weft and/or in warp direction, combined with a specific weaving pattern and specific weaving techniques (jacquard, loop weaving) for the realisation of contacts

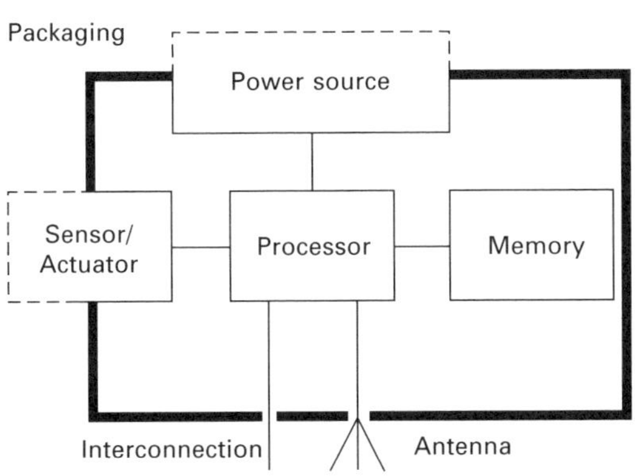

5.2 Schematic overview of an electronic system.

- knitting conductive yarns using either plain knitting, circular knitting, warp knitting or crocheting
- during the textile finishing process, e.g., coating or screenprinting. Recently, some first experiments of screenprinting with conductive inks were successfully carried out by the author.
- during the textile confection process, e.g., by the embroidering of conductive yarns on textile.

The application of the different techniques for the building of sensors, input devices, interconnections and antennas will be illustrated with some examples.

5.3.1 Woven RFID antenna

Figure 5.3 shows a woven RFID antenna developed by TITV [Gimp 04]. For the realization of this antenna, a three-layered Jacquard weaving technique was used. In the bottom layer, conductive yarns were used in the warp direction, in the top layer, conductive yarns were used in the weft direction. The conductive yarns in both layers are separated by the insulating intermediate layer. By a specific Jacquard weaving technique only at certain selected locations, the conductive yarns in the top layer and in the bottom layer are connected, in order to form the functional coil structure for the RFID antenna. This RFID antenna can be used in combination with a microchip to which it should be connected as a tag, e.g., to sort out clothing in a laundry.

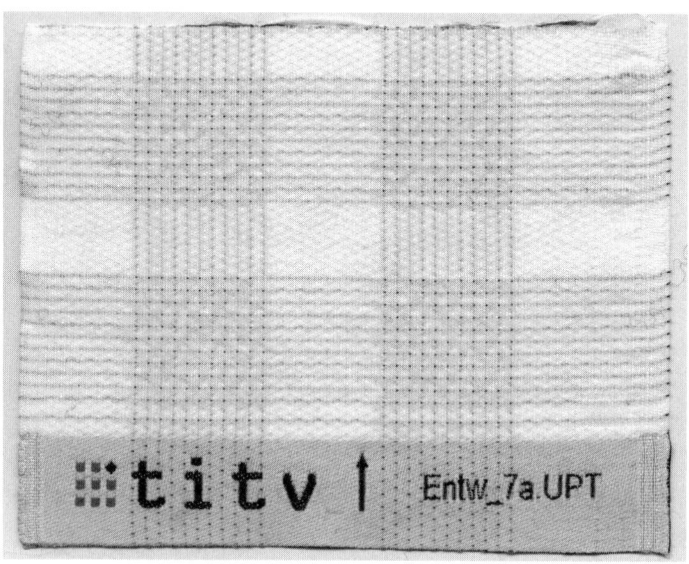

5.3 Woven RFID antenna [Gimp 04].

5.3.2 Knitted sensors for the measurement of physiological parameters

A lot of research in the field of smart textiles has been conducted on medical applications. The measurement of physiological parameters such as heart rate or ECG and respiration rate by sensors integrated into clothing is studied by several research groups and attracts a lot of attention due to several reasons, as already discussed in section 5.1.

As an alternative to conventional gel electrodes, knitted stainless steel electrodes, called 'Textrodes', as shown in Fig. 5.4, were developed for the measurement of ECG [Cat 04]. The advantage of the Textrodes is their non-irritating character (in contrast to the conventional gel electrodes, which may cause skin irritation or allergic reactions) and the possibility of integration in a shirt or a suit. The major drawback however of the Textrodes is their inherent high skin–electrode impedance.

Next to the Textrode, a fabric sensor, the 'Respibelt' was developed by the author, as an alternative to the conventional respiration measurement methods. The Respibelt is made of a stainless steel yarn, knitted in a Lycra-containing belt, providing an adjustable stretch. Figure 5.5 shows the Respibelt knitting structure. By placing the Respibelt as a coil around the abdomen or thorax, circumference and length changes of the Respibelt, caused by breathing, result both in an inductance and resistance variation. In this way, both changes in the perimeter and cross-section are measured.

The two sensors described above were successfully applied in several measurement conditions and integrated in two prototype suits. A first suit was built for the wireless monitoring of children during a hospital stay or,

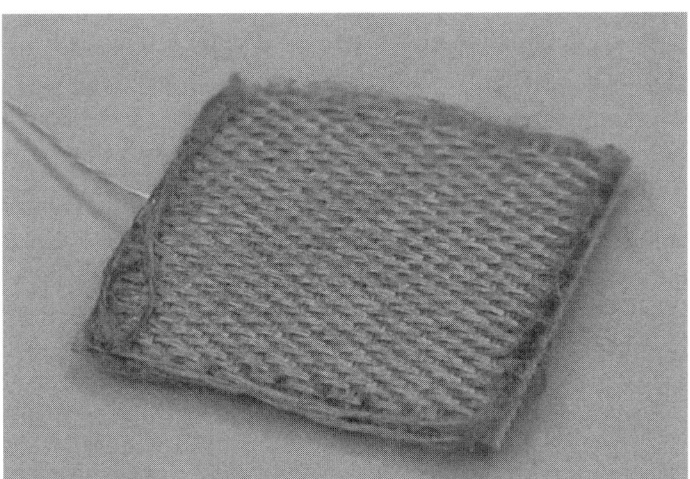

5.4 Knitted ECG electrode.

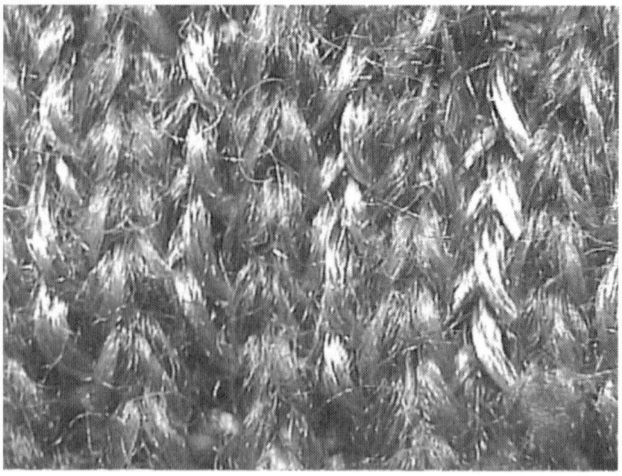

(a)

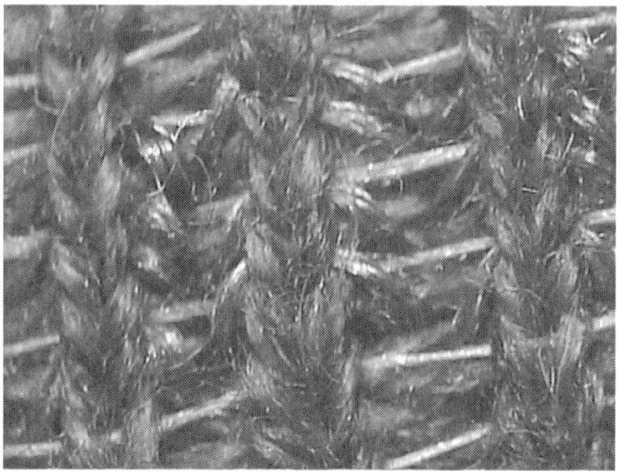

(b)

5.5 Detail of the Respibelt respiration sensor (a) rest position; (b) stretched.

e.g., to prevent cot death. A second prototype suit was built for the follow up of adults and is shown in Fig. 5.6 [Piro 05].

5.3.3 Embroidered and knitted keyboards

One of the first developments in the field of smart textiles was done at MIT. A capacitive numerical keyboard, made of embroidered silk screened with copper and integrated in fabric, was conceived as an interface for, e.g., mobile phones or portable music players [Post 97]. Figure 5.7 shows a knitted keyboard [BE20050269]. As in many other examples presented here, conductive yarns made of stainless steel are used. Due to the knitting technique, the obtained keyboard has a flexible structure, which can easily follow the body curves, without a decrease in functionality. The major advantage of using this knitting technology for the realization of a keyboard is that the keyboard can be introduced in, e.g., pieces of clothing during the knitting process; no additional production or confection step is needed.

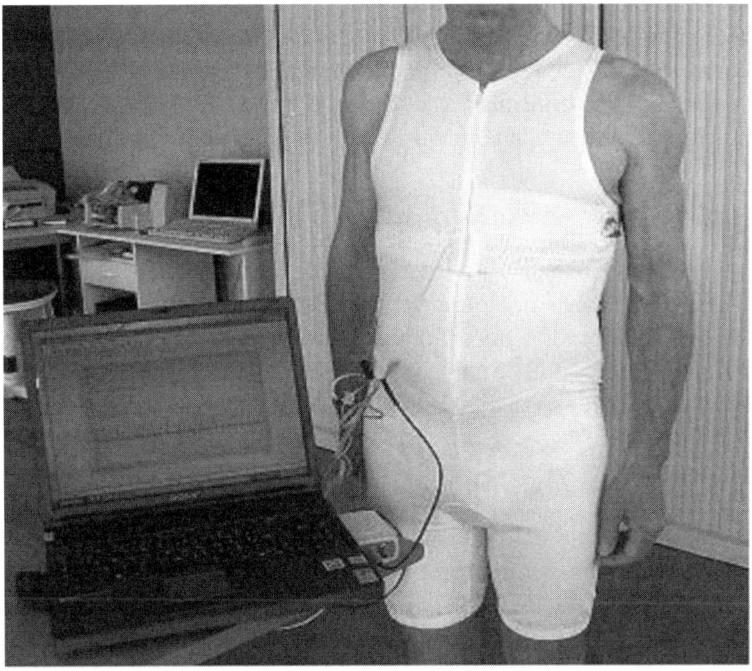

5.6 Prototype suit with integrated sensors for heart rate and respiration rate.

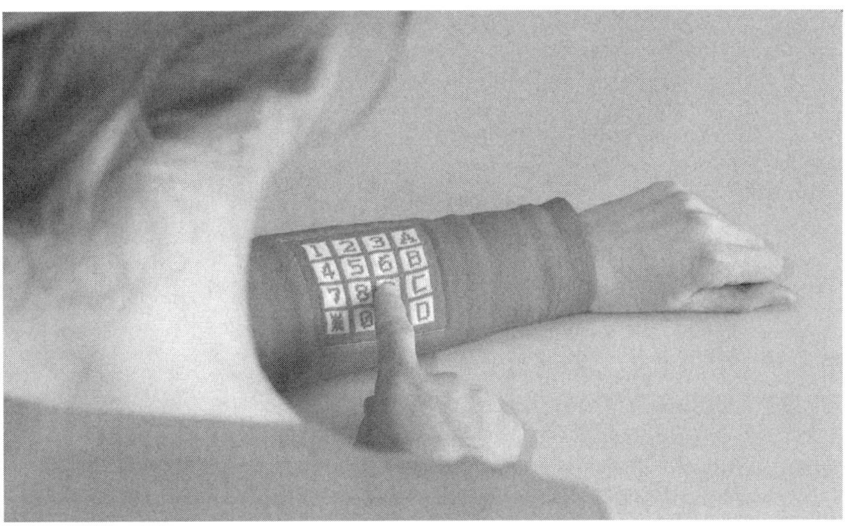

5.7 Knitted textile keyboard.

5.3.4 Embroidered antenna

Figure 5.8 depicts an embroidered spiral antenna which can be used for power and data transmission at the same time [Cat 04]. More details on the functionality of the antenna are given in paragraph 5.4.

5.4 Power management

Several methods can be used to provide energy to autonomous electronic systems integrated in clothing. In this section an overview will be given of the combination of different power sources and power storage systems. The different options will be compared to each other regarding both power density and integration aspects. Finally some design examples will be given.

5.4.1 Overview of the different possibilities

It should be clear that the connection of clothes to the mains (220 or 110 V) is not an option, as in this way the mobility of the wearer is drastically reduced. A more straightforward method is the use of primary (non-rechargeable) or secondary (rechargeable) batteries. Furthermore, power can be harvested from a source which is in the first place not intended to deliver

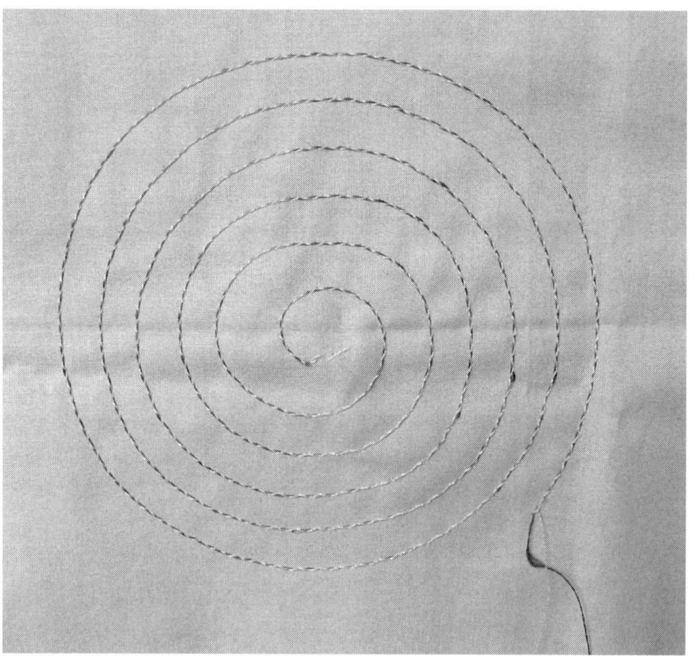

5.8 Embroidered secondary coil of an inductive power link.

power. Examples are power harvested from the temperature difference between the wearer and the environment and power harvested from the movement of the wearer. This parasitic power harvesting imposes an extra load on the source from which the power is harvested; power harvesting from the movement of a wearer, e.g., will cause an attenuation of this movement. Table 5.1 gives an overview of the different possibilities for the powering of electronics embedded in clothes. The use of primary and secondary batteries will be discussed in the next section. The other techniques from Table 5.1 – power harvesting techniques – will be discussed in brief here.

Solar cells

A first possibility for power harvesting is by using sunlight. Apart from visible light, solar radiation contains among others ultraviolet and infra-red light. In (amorphous or crystalline) silicon solar cells, the photonic energy from solar radiation is converted into an electric current. Recently, flexible solar cells became available on the market [VHF]. Typical maximal power output is currently 20 W/m^2, which means that for a state-of-the-art mobile phone (e.g. Nokia 8310) an area of 20 cm × 20 cm is needed. The price of state-of-the-art flexible solar cells varies between 1000 and 2000 €/m^2.

In recent years, organic semiconductors have been developed that allow polymer (also called 'plastic' or 'organic') electronics products to be fabricated. These are lightweight, flexible, and low-cost. An additional benefit is that their production requires a great deal less energy than the production of conventional (mostly silicon) electronics because by definition only low-temperature processes are used. Polymer solar cells are one of the electronic products that have successfully been demonstrated. They are an ideal candidate

Table 5.1 Overview of the different possibilities for the powering of electronics embedded in clothes

Energy source	Available amount of energy	Remarks
Primary batteries (Li)	400 Wh/kg, 800 Wh/l	–
Secondary batteries (Li-Ion)	75 Wh/kg, 200 Wh/l	Lifetime: 2000 cycles
Si solar cells	20 W/m^2	Illumination or sunlight needed
Recovery of body heat	0.01 W/m^2	@ DT = 5 °C
Power harvesting from breathing	0.4 W	Uncomfortable for wearer
Power harvesting from walking	0.25 W	Continuous walking necessary
Microcombustion	10–50 W/cm^3	Fuel needed

for a lightweight, extremely flat and flexible, autonomous electrical power source that can be integrated into clothing, baggage or accessories (backpacks, etc.) for powering wearable electronics – either directly or via rechargeable batteries.

Recovery of body heat

Recovery of body heat to power embedded electronics is done by using thermopiles. The working principle of a thermopile is based on the Seebeck effect. An elementary thermopile or a thermocouple consists of two different conductive materials (usually metals), which form a junction at one side. If a temperature difference occurs between this junction and the other sides of both metals, an electric voltage will be generated across the two sides of the materials which do not form a junction. When a resistance is placed between these two sides, a current will flow through this resistance. The output voltage and power can be increased by joining different thermocouples, forming a thermopile. An example of such a system, integrated in an IC is given by Laut [02]. This IC was integrated in textiles and able of delivering 1 $\mu W/cm^2$ at a temperature difference of 5 °C. The limited amount of power that is available in this way can currently be used only by passive systems with a low power consumption.

Power harvesting from movement

By using electromechanical systems or piezoelectric materials, (mechanical) energy from movement can be converted into electric energy [Star 96]. The energy can be obtained from the movement of several body parts: thorax (respiration), arms, legs, feet (walking). Although electromechanical systems, using pistons and flywheels, have a higher efficiency (e.g. 0.25 W versus 2 mW for walking), piezoelectric materials produced in flexible films are preferred due to the more straightforward integration into textiles and the less nuisance caused to the wearer. If a pressure is applied to a piezoelectric material, an electric voltage is generated. Several crystals (e.g. PZT or lead zirconate titanate) show piezoelectric behavior as well as some industrially produced polymers (e.g. PVDF or PolyVinyliDenFluoride).

Micro fuel cells

The use of micro fuel cells is very promising, due to the high power density that can be obtained [Mehr 00]. However, these power densities are currently obtained in laboratory experiments. The technology lacks sufficient maturity to be used in powering smart clothes.

5.4.2 Possible configurations

In this section the possible system configurations of powering embedded electronics are discussed.

Use of primary batteries

Figure 5.9 shows the evolution of several technologies that are used for wearable electronics. It is clear that during the last 15 years, battery power has not evolved in the same way as, e.g., disk capacity or CPU speed. Technological evolutions like the increase in CPU speed or disk capacity, however, result in an increase of the overall power consumption. New types of batteries (e.g. Li-based) have an increased power capacity [Tak 96] but are insufficient to bridge the gap with the other technological evolutions.

Primary batteries should be used only if the embedded electronics do not consume a lot of power or if it concerns disposable clothing. Applications that require no large memory space or high speed, and in which the electronics are designed and optimised towards minimal power consumption, can benefit from the use of primary batteries. Generally, it concerns applications that are limited to the (passive) measurement of a certain parameter (e.g. heart rate) and do not permit interactions with the wearer. Recently, research has been conducted on the development of textile batteries [Inn 02]. Until now, the specifications of these textile batteries are far below the specifications of

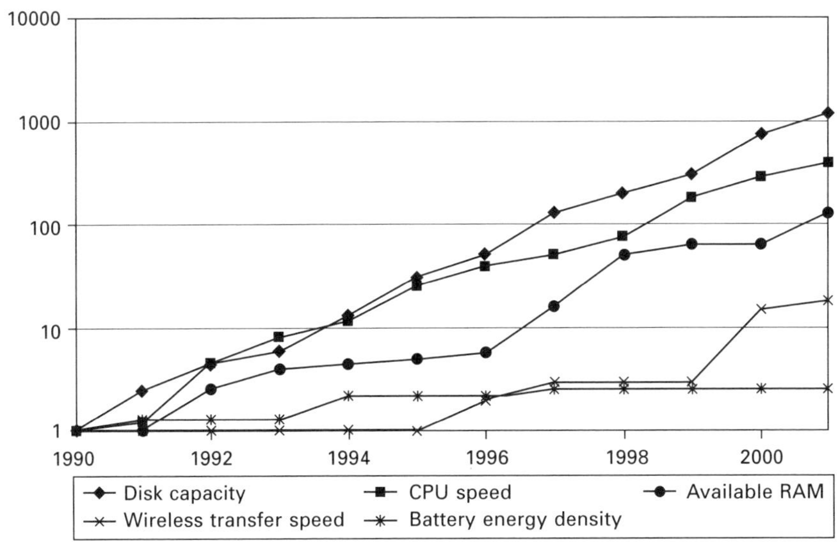

5.9 Evolution of the different technologies for wearable electronics [Star 02].

classic primary batteries. In future applications, however, this type of batteries, and more generally flexible batteries, should be envisaged.

It is clear from Fig. 5.9 that to make the vision of ambient intelligence and smart textiles become reality, the presently available hardware must be further reduced in size and power consumption. On the other hand, the users of these wearable devices want to be more independent of power supply systems. Development of low power electronics and of new power supply systems should go hand in hand and 'meet in the middle'.

Use of secondary batteries

Secondary batteries can be used in two ways:

- wearer-controlled recharging of the batteries, i.e., the wearer takes action to recharge the batteries
- non-wearer-controlled recharging of the batteries.

An example of the first method is the recharging of heating ski shoes. The recharging of the batteries occurs at a given moment (e.g. at night) and care should be taken that the power density of the batteries is sufficient to bridge the period between two recharging moments. In the second case, parasitic power harvesting (as discussed above) can be used for the recharging of the batteries. This configuration is useful if periods in which power harvesting can occur are alternated with periods in which no power harvesting can occur. During the power harvesting period, the battery can be recharged and the embedded electronics can be powered directly through the harvesting; during the non-power-harvesting period, the embedded electronics should be powered through the battery. Design parameters for this configuration are the available amount of power of the parasitic source, the power density of the battery and the alternation between the harvesting period and the non-harvesting period, as a function of the needed power for the embedded electronics.

Direct parasitic power harvesting

A last option is direct parasitic power harvesting without the use of a battery. In this configuration, the parasitic power source should always be available.

5.4.3 Examples

Inductive powering

A first example is shown in Fig. 5.8. It concerns the use of an inductive link for the recharging of a battery, embedded in a suit for the measurement of physiological parameters [Cat 04]. The inductive link is composed of two coils: the primary coil that is integrated in a mattress generates an alternating magnetic field, the secondary coil, shown in the picture, is embroidered on the suit. In this way, a battery can be recharged while the wearer lies on the bed. The system is able to transmit the required 25 mW over a distance of 10 cm with an efficiency of 32%.

Solar cells

Within the Belgian research consortium 'Soltex', the feasibility of integrating flexible solar cells in textiles is demonstrated. On the one hand, the project starts from proven plastic solar cell technology that is adapted to achieve a solar-cell sheet that is suitable for lamination on textiles. On the other hand, certain parts of the solar cell are selectively replaced in order to improve its performance in the desired environment. From the several possible approaches to producing textiles with integrated flexible solar cells, lamination has been selected as the preferred means of integration. Lamination is a procedure well established and largely adopted by textile manufacturers. It allows a maximum freedom of the type of textile. It is compatible with the production of large areas and provides genuine integration of the solar cell with the textile. It allows the textile manufacturer to be minimally involved in the production of the electronics part, in this case the solar cell. To demonstrate the potential of this technology a demonstrator was built, as shown in Fig. 5.10. An LCD display powered by solar cells was integrated into a suitcase. The LCD display could have various functions, e.g., digital ID-tag with contact details of the owner as well as destination and flight information.

From the overview in this section, it should be clear that there are different options for the powering of embedded electronics and textronics in textiles. To choose the right technology and system configuration for a given application in the first place, the following questions should be answered:

- How much power is needed?
- What kind of application is envisaged?
- How mobile is the wearer?

5.5 Packaging issues

One of the major challenges to be tackled in the development of smart textiles is the packaging of the electronics. As already mentioned above, the textronics technology can be used to build a limited amount of components such as sensors, antennas and interconnections. Until now, more complex electronic components such as microprocessors and memory cannot be built with this technology and therefore available electronics need to be embedded in the clothing.

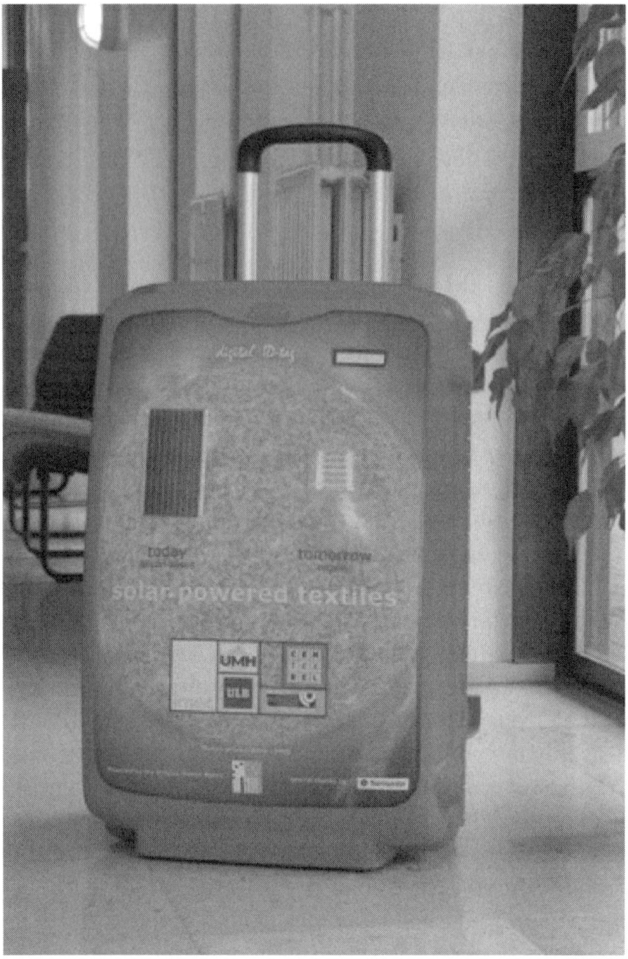

5.10 Suitcase with integrated solar cells.

There are several factors to consider when embedding electronics in textiles:

- mechanical stress, circuit bending and cracking
- chemical stress, corrosion by washing, rain and sweat
- thermal stress, heating in the sun or ironing.

The packaging of the electronics should provide a hermetic encapsulation of the electronics and should be sufficiently strong. At present, a packaging technology is not finalized, not only for the developments presented here. It remains the bottleneck in every wearable electronics or intelligent textiles development [Lukow 00, Burch 01] and, as already mentioned above, most applications require removal of the electronics before starting the cleaning or washing process. Moreover, discomfort, dimensions, ease of integration –

through confection, laminating or another textile production technique – should be considered. A first step towards a solution could be by adapting packaging techniques for implantable systems.

Within the Bioflex research project, [Bioflex] http://www.elis.ugent.be/ELISgroups/tfcg/project/bioflex/Welcome.html e.g., research is being conducted to develop an electronics substrate that is flexible and stretchable. To be applicable both in implants and in clothing, biocompatibility and washability are also envisaged. In the case of clothing, the mixture with fashion, however, poses some extra requirements to the packaging as well. While in the case of implantable systems esthetics are a minor issue, they are an important prerequisite for the successful market introduction of smart clothes. To arrive at a commercial end product, a multidisciplinary approach, including material science, electronics, textiles and design is needed.

5.6 Future trends

As is shown in Fig. 5.1, complete integration of electronics in textiles will be achieved only by fibertronics technology. Textronics technology offers the possibility of integrating some specific components such as sensors and antennas in textiles, but other more complex electronic components, such as microprocessors, cannot be realized in this way and should still be embedded in textiles.

Research on the integration of basic electronic building blocks in yarns – the so-called fibertronics technology – is already ongoing [Clem 03, WO02095839] however. This technology is based on semiconductor processing techniques and will allow the full integration of microprocessors in textiles in the future. A fiber computer, however, should not be expected within the next fifteen years.

5.7 Sources of further information and advice

Further information on the topics discussed in this chapter can be found in the references. Recent developments of research groups active in the field of smart textiles can be found on their respective websites:

- Georgia Tech School of Polymer, Textile & Fiber Engineering: http://www.ptfe.gatech.edu
- Virginia Tech E-Textiles Laboratory: http://www.ccm.ece.vt.edu/etextitles
- Wearable Computing Lab, ETH Zürich: http://www.wearable.ethz.ch
- Research Center E. Piaggio, University of Pisa: http://www.piaggio.ccii.unipi.it

An interesting introduction to the materials that can be used to build smart textiles is given by the Intelligent Textiles project of the Tampere

University of Technology: http://www.tut.fi/units/ms/teva/projects/intelligenttextiles

5.8 Acknowledgements

Our gratitude goes to our colleagues for the advice and help during the developments which are presented in this chapter: Tom Meyvis, Daniël Verstraete, Jan Laperre, Bart Hermans, Johan Coosemans, Carla Hertleer and Lieva Van Langenhove.

5.9 References

[Aarts 03] E. Aarts and S. Marzano, *The New Everyday – Visions on Ambient Intelligence*, 101 Publishers, Rotterdam, The Netherlands, 2003.

[BE20050269] Belgian patent application number BE2005/0269.

[Boek 02] F. Boekhorst, 'Ambient Intelligence, the Next Paradigm for Consumer Electronics: How will it Affect Silicon?', in *Proceedings of the IEEE International Solid-State Circuits Conference*, San Francisco (CA), USA, Feb. 2002, pp. 28–31.

[Bona 03] P. Bonato, 'Wearable Sensors/Systems and Their Impact on Biomedical Engineering', *IEEE Engineering in Medicine & Biology*, vol. 22, no. 3, pp. 18–20, May 2003.

[Burch 01] B. Burchard, S. Jung, A. Ullsperger and W. D. Hartmann, 'Devices, Software, their Applications and Requirements for Wearable Electronics', in *Proceedings of the IEEE International Conference on Consumer Electronics*, Los Angeles (CA), USA, June 2001, pp. 224–225.

[Cat 04] M. Catrysse, 'Wireless power and data transmission for implantable and wearable monitoring systems', PhD Thesis, K.U. Leuven, 2004.

[Clem 03] F. Clemens *et al.*, 'Computing Fibers: A Novel Fiber for Intelligent Fabrics?', *Advanced Engineering Materials*, vol. 5, no. 9, pp. 692–687, 2003.

[Dan 03] J. P. Dan and J. Luprano, 'Homecare: A Telemedical Application', *Medical Device Technology*, pp. 25–29, Dec. 2003.

[Inn 02] P. C. Innis *et al.*, 'Inherently Conducting Polymers for Wearable Energy Conversion (Actuator) and Storage Systems', *Proc. International Interactive Textiles for the Warrior Conference*, Cambridge (MA), USA, July 2002.

[Gimp 04] S. Gimpel *et al.*, 'Textile-based Electronic Substrate Technology', *Journal of Industrial Textiles*, vol. 33, no. 3, pp. 179–189, Jan. 2004.

[Laut 02] C. Lauterbach, M. Strasser, S. Jung and W. Weber, '"Smart Clothes" Self-Powered by Body Heat', *Proceedings Avantex*, 2002.

[Lukow 00] P. Lukowicz and G. Troster, 'Packaging Issues in Wearable Computing', in *Proceedings of the International Workshop on Chip Package Codesign*, Zürich, Switzerland, Mar. 2000, pp. 19–22.

[Mar 03] K. Marent, J. Wauters and J. Van Helleputte, 'De intelligente omgeving: de noodzaak van convergerende technologie en een nieuw businessmodel', *IWT Studies 44*, Mar. 2003.

[Mazz 02] A. Mazzoldi, D. De Rossi, F. Lorussi, E. P. Scilingo and R. Paradiso, 'Smart Textiles for Wearable Motion Capture Systems', *AUTEX Research Journal*, vol. 2, no. 4, pp. 199–203, Dec. 2002.

[Mech 04] S. Mecheels, 'Smart Clothes, The stony way from the vision to the marketable product', *Proceedings of the International Dornbirn Conference on Chemical Fibres, Dorbirn, Austria*, Sept. 2004.

[Mehr 00] A. Mehra, X. Zang, A. A. Ayon, I. A. Waitz, M. A. Schmidt and C. M. Spadaccini, 'A Six-Wafer Combustion System for a Silicon Micro Gas Turbine', *Journal of Microelectromechanical Systems*, vol. 9, no. 4, Dec. 2000, pp. 517–527.

[Para 03] R. Paradiso, 'Wearable Health Care System for Vital Signs Monitoring', in *Proceedings of the Information Technology Applications in Biomedicine Conference*, Birmingham, UK, Apr. 2003.

[Park 03] S. Park and S. Jayaraman, 'Enhancing the Quality of Life Through Wearable Technology', *IEEE Engineering in Medicine & Biology*, vol. 22, no. 3, pp. 41–48, May 2003.

[Piro 05] F. Pirotte *et al.*, 'MERMOTH: Medical Remote Monitoring of Clothes', *Proc. Ambience 05*, Tampere, Finland, Sept. 2005.

[Post 97] E. R. Post and M. Orth, 'Smart Fabric, or Washable Computing', in *Proceedings of the IEEE International Symposium on Wearable Computers*, Cambridge (MA), USA, Oct. 1997, pp. 167–168.

[Ross 03] D. De Rossi, F. Carpi, F. Lorussi, A. Mazzoldi, R. Paradiso, E. P. Scilingo, and A. Tognetti, 'Electroactive Fabrics and Wearable Biomonitoring Devices', *AUTEX Research Journal*, vol. 3, no. 4, pp. 180–185, Dec. 2003.

[Star 96] T. Starner, 'Human-powered wearable computing', *IBM Systems Journal*, vol. 35, pp. 618–629, 1996.

[Star 02] T. Starner, 'Thick Clients for Personal Wireless Devices', *IEEE Computer*, vol. 35, no. 1, pp. 133–135, Jan. 2002.

[Tak 96] E. S. Takeuchi, 'Developments In Battery Technology', in *Biotelemetry XIII*, C. Cristalli, C. J. Amlaner Jr. and M. R. Neuman, Eds., Wageningen, The Netherlands, 1996, pp. 49–55, International Society on Biotelemetry.

[VHF] http://www.vhf-technologies.com

[Vivo] http://www.vivometrics.com

[Wil 02] F.H. Wilhelm, E. Handke and W.T. Roth, 'Measurement of respiratory and cardiac function by the Lifeshirt: initial assessment of usability and reliability during ambulatory sleep monitoring', *Biological Psychology*, vol. 59, pp. 250–251, 2002.

[WO02095893] International patent application number WO02/095839.

6
Textile sensors for healthcare

L VAN LANGENHOVE, C HERTLEER and P WESTBROEK, Ghent University, Belgium and J PRINIOTAKIS, TEI Pireaus, Greece

6.1 Introduction

The term 'smart textiles' is derived from intelligent or smart materials. The concept 'smart material' was defined for the first time in Japan in 1989. The first textile material that, in retroaction, was labelled as a 'smart textile' was silk thread having a shape memory effect (by analogy with the better known 'shape memory alloys'). The discovery of shape memory materials in the 1960s and intelligent polymeric gels in the 1970s were, however, generally accepted as the birth of real smart materials. It was not before the late 1990s that intelligent materials were introduced in textiles. It is a new type of product that offers the same potential and interest as technical textiles.

Smart textiles can be described as textiles that are able *to sense* stimuli from the environment, *to react* to them and *adapt* to them by integration of functionalities in the textile structure. The stimulus as well as the response can have an electrical, thermal, chemical, magnetic or other origin. The extent of intelligence can be divided in three subgroups [Zhang, 2001]:

- passive smart textiles can only sense the environment, they are *sensors*
- active smart textiles can sense the stimuli from the environment and also react to them, besides the sensor function, they also have an *actuator* function
- finally, very smart textiles take a step further, having the gift to adapt their behaviour to the circumstances.

So two components need to be present in the textile structure in order to bear the full mark of smart textiles; a sensor and an actuator, possibly completed with a processing unit which drives the actuator on the basis of the signals from the sensor.

6.2 Smart textiles

6.2.1 Why textiles?

Intelligence is currently embedded in daily objects like watches. However, textiles show several advantages as clothes and are unique in several aspects. They are extremely versatile in products as well as processes. The building stones of the textile material are *fibres* or *filaments*. Innumerable combinations of these source materials result in a whole range of textile materials. Fibres are available in a very broad range of materials, single or combined: natural or synthetic, strong, elastic, biocompatible, biodegradable, solid or porous, optical or electro-conductive. They can have varying lengths, fineness, cross-sectional shape, surface roughness, etc. Fibres of various types can be arranged at random or in a strictly organized way in yarns or fabric structures. From this, even three-dimensional structures can be constructed. After treatments allow the creation of very special properties such as a hydrophilic/hydrophobic nature, antimicrobial, selective permeability etc. Textile materials are able to combine advanced multifunctionality with traditional textile properties.

Clothes are our own personal house. They can be made to measure, with a perfect fit and high level of comfort. Clothes make contact with a considerable part of the body. They are a common material to all of us, in nearly all of our activities. They look nice and attractive, the design and look being adapted to the actual consumer group. We all know how to use them. Maintaining textiles is a daily practice; house as well as industrial laundry are well developed. Last but not least, textiles and clothes can be produced on fast and productive machinery at reasonable cost. These characteristics open up a number of applications that were not possible before, especially in the area of monitoring and treatment, such as:

- long-term or permanent contact without skin irritation
- home applications
- applications for children in a discrete and carefree way
- applications for the elderly; discretion, comfort and aesthetics are important.

It is clear that the intelligent character of the textile material can be introduced at different levels. It can occur at fibre level, a coating can be applied, other threads can be added to the textile material, it is even possible to closely connect completely independent appliances with the textile. Full success however will be achieved only when the sensors and all related components are entirely converted into 100% textile materials. This is a big challenge because, apart from technical considerations, concepts, materials, structures and treatments must focus on the appropriateness for use in or as a textile material. This includes criteria like flexibility, water (laundry) resistance, durability against deformation, radiation, etc.

As for real devices, ultimately most signals are being transformed into electric ones. Electroconductive materials are consequently of utmost importance with respect to intelligent textiles.

6.2.2 Functions of smart textiles

The functionalities of smart textiles can be classified in five groups: sensoring, data processing, actuation, communication and energy. At the moment, most progress has been achieved in the area of sensoring. Many parameters can be measured:

- temperature
- biopotentials: cardiogram, myographs, encephalographs
- acoustic: heart, lungs, digestion, joints
- ultrasound: blood flow
- biological, chemical
- motion: respiration, motion
- pressure: blood
- radiation: IR, spectroscopy
- odour, sweat
- mechanical skin parameters
- electric (skin) parameters.

Some of these parameters are well known, like cardiogram and temperature. Nevertheless, permanent monitoring also opens up new perspectives for these traditional parameters too. Indeed, today evaluation is usually based on standards for global population groups. Permanent monitoring supported by self-learning devices will allow the set up of personal profiles for each individual, so that conditions deviating from normal can be traced an soon as possible. Also diagnosis can be a lot more accurate.

Apart from the actual measuring devices data processing is a key feature in this respect. These types of data are new. They are numerous with multiple complex interrelationships and are time dependent. New self-learning techniques will be required. The introduction of such an approach will be slow, because no evidence of the benefits are available at this moment. 'We don't measure because we don't know the meaning, we don't know the meaning because we don't measure.'

Actuation is another aspect. Identification of problems makes sense only when followed by an adequate reaction. This reaction can consist of reporting or calling for help, but also drug supply and physical treatment. A huge challenge in this respect is the development of high-performance muscle-like materials.

Mechanisms of actuation are:

- chemical: drug supply, skin care
- mechanical: artificial muscles, massage, pressure bandages
- optical: UV irradiation
- thermal: heating/cooling
- electrical: electrotherapy.

Some materials are available today, many need to be developed.

Data processing is a limiting factor as well. The optimal reaction needed strongly depends on the individual. Here again self-learning dynamic steering and control algorithms are required. A smart suit should be a stand-alone unit, not requiring any wired connections for communication and energy supply. These are the topics of other chapters in this book. The textile systems should also resist the normal conditions of use: multiple deformation (extension, bending, compression, etc.) as well as laundry (water, elevated temperatures, detergents, enzymes). This will be discussed in the sections that follow.

6.3 Conductive fibres and fibrous materials

Sensors can be divided into active and passive sensors [Carpi, 2005]. Passive sensors require an external power source, while active sensors are able to convert the input energy (elastic, thermal, etc.) into a measurable difference of potential. Conductive fibres and structures made from them are passive sensors according to this definition. Active sensors are, for instance, based on piezo-electric effects. Electro-conductive fibres are used on a large scale for a variety of functions: antistatic applications, electromagnetic shielding (EMI), electronic applications, infra-red absorption, protective clothing in explosive areas, etc. Their use as a sensor, however, is a rather new field of application.

6.3.1 Fibrous sensors

Heart signals are one of the basic parameters in health care. The heart is basically a muscle that is controlled by the brain though electric impulses. The body being a vessel filled with an electrolyte solution, these signals can be detected in all of its parts. Small metal plates are commonly used to capture these signals while instruments analyse the results, extracting the required parameters such as frequency, phases, etc. Conductive fibres are being used as passive sensors for monitoring biopotential, mainly heart rate. Several research projects have been carried out on this topic (Table 6.1) [Van Langenhove 2003, Smartex, Medes, Georgia Tech]. The feasibility has clearly been demonstrated, although the sensor needs to be optimized and practical problems need to be solved.

Table 6.1 Textile electrodes for measuring heart rate

Name	Application	Level of transformation
Smartex	Health care	Woven/knitted textile sensors
Intellitex	Children's health care	Knitted textile structures, textile antenna
VTAM	Health care	Partly textile structures
Wearable motherboard	Health care, military	Partly textile structures

As will be explained in the following sections, several mechanisms cause the resistance to go up or down due to extension of the material. This is called a piezo-resistive effect. The global effect of these combined mechanisms depends on the type of material and its structures. The piezo-resistive effect makes the textile a versatile tool for a broad range of sensor applications where extension is a crucial parameter. This is the case, for instance, for respiration measurements (expansion/contraction of the chest), all kinds of movements (dance, sports, etc.) as well as volumetric changes like volume of inhaled air. For applications as a passive sensor like electrocardiogram electrodes, the conductivity of the textile materials should be as consistent as possible, the piezo-resistive effect being a source of error. This can be achieved by careful selection of fibre type and proper design of the textile structure. The resistance of such a structure is constant when, for instance, a cyclic extension is applied as a simulation of the breathing movement (Fig. 6.1).

6.3.2 Textile strain sensors

Conductive fibres show piezo-resistive effects. By extending the fibres, fibre cross-section is reduced causing the electrical resistance to go up. Secondly the fibre length increases again causing resistance to increase. As a result resistance becomes an indicator of its extension. However, the level of this type of piezo-electric effect is insufficient to allow accurate readings. Additional piezo-electric effects have to be achieved using other principles. Such principles, for instance, exploit mechanisms of conductivity as described by Mattes [2003]. Later, the inclusion of conductive nanoparticles can generate piezo-electric effects, as conductivity will depend on the distance between the nanoparticles [Devaux 2005]. This distance will change due to fibre extension.

Arranging conductive fibres in a structure like textiles generates a material with a complex behaviour in terms of conductivity. Fibre length being limited, the electron flow has to be transferred from one fibre to the other, from one yarn to the other. Contact resistance between fibres plays a determining role here. Contact resistance usually is quite high as compared to the intrinsic

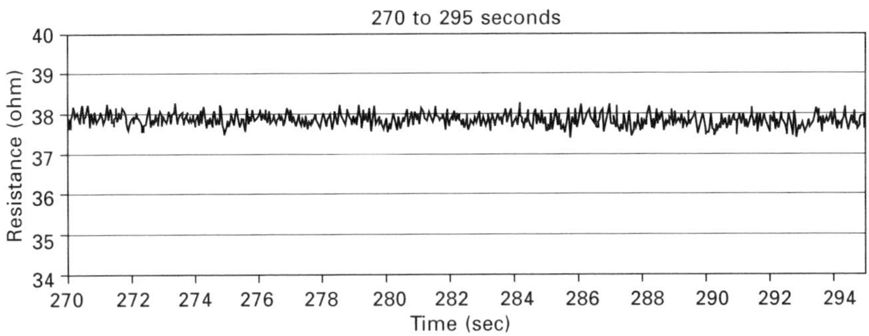

6.1 Textile structure without piezo-resistive effect.

conductivity of the material. Any rearrangement of the fibres in a textile may affect the global conductivity of the structure. It changes the contact resistance, number of contact points, path followed by the current and hence the piezo-resistive effect. Consequently, any process that alters fibre arrangement also has an impact on the sensor properties. It makes the long-term behaviour of such sensors not obvious.

6.3.3 Smart textile structures

The applications mentioned in the previous sections are rather straightforward. Careful design of the textile structure enables more advanced sensing properties. The basic mechanisms are related to conductivity, changes in conductivity, currents or change in currents and so on. Any mechanism that affects such parameters is useful. Electrochemistry is an extremely important discipline in this respect.

A set of fibres, yarns or fabrics separated one way or another can be considered as a double electrode system. Such a system can be used to detect water. The presence of water will be reflected in an increase of conductivity between the two electrodes. This increase will be bigger when the water contains salt. The reaction of such a textile sensor (i.e. resistance as a function of time), consisting of two conductive yarns, on wetting with water with different salt concentrations is given in Fig. 6.2 [Priniotakis 2005].

Impedance spectroscopy has been used to optimize the test set up

A double set of such a two-electrode system of which one is coated with a coating that is impermeable to the salt but permeable to water allows separation of the quantity of water and the quantity of salt. Coatings with selective permeability can be the base for a huge number of specific sensors, for instance, for a qualitative as well as quantitative analysis of sweat. This basic method is suited for a huge range of applications, provided the right

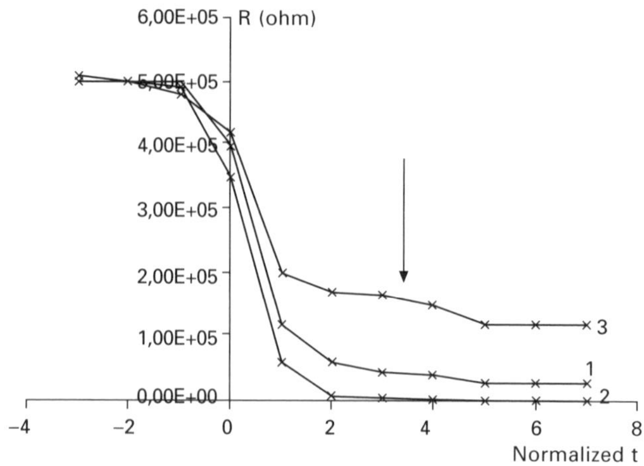

6.2 Decrease of electrical resistance due to wetting of the sensor (1 and 2 high salt content, 3 low salt content).

electrode configuration, measuring conditions and textile configuration are selected. Electrode configuration, for instance, includes diameter of the fibres or yarn electrodes and distance between the electrodes.

Another approach to designing conductive fibre based sensors is based on the piezo-resistive effect, whereby the separation of conductive (nano)particles is not achieved by fibre extension, but by fibre swelling. In this case also one basic technology is capable of generating an enormous range of sensing capabilities. Selection of adequate polymeric materials for the fibres or inclusion of swelling components like gels must be adapted to the triggering agent. In addition coatings with selective permeability can be applied to increase selectivity and specificity of the sensor system. These are just two examples of relatively simple systems with an enormous range of applicability.

6.4 Testing of ECG electrodes

Textile sensors to be used for medical purposes are usually in contact with the skin. This is particularly the case for electrodes used for monitoring heart signals (cardiogram). In order to test the performance of textile structures for this application an actual cardiogram can be recorded. All studies show textile electrodes are basically inferior to classical electrodes and need special treatment for achieving good readings. Skin contact is a first key issue. Electro-conductive gels are commonly used to improve skin contact. Such gels, however, cause skin irritation when used for longer than 24 hours. One of the reasons for choosing textile electrodes is that they can be worn permanently without affecting comfort. One of the main problems here is the extreme variability of the skin properties. Skin conductivity changes between persons and for one person in time and with activity making objective testing very difficult. In addition, any movement changes the textile to skin contact and this is another major source of artifacts. Therefore a phantom test set up has been developed [Westbroek 2006]. In this method an electrolyte is used to simulate body fluids, separated from the textile electrodes by polymeric membranes mimicking the skin. (Fig. 6.3)

Signal transfer is analysed using impedance spectroscopy. This method allows the separation of the impedance of the separate components of the system. By varying different parameters, their influence on resistance can be studied quite easily in an accurate and reproducible way. In this section the overall resistance has been measured. It is composed of the following resistances:

- the textile
- the contact textile/membrane
- the electrolyte solution.

The two first resistances are far bigger that the third. Size and shape of the electrodes has to be optimized as well as distance between the electrodes on the body. The effect of distance between the electrodes can be simulated by varying the length of the PVC tube. The skin properties can be varied by using different membranes (thickness and pore size).

The textile structure itself has a major impact too of course. The following values of the overall resistance have been measured:

- reference material: 310 kΩ
- woven structure: 29 kΩ
- knitted structure: 3.2 kΩ
- non-woven structure: 0.315 kΩ

The textile structures have been made from stainless steel fibres, palladium has been chosen as a reference material. The effect of the size of the electrodes on the resistance of the cell is presented in Fig. 6.4. The four lines represent

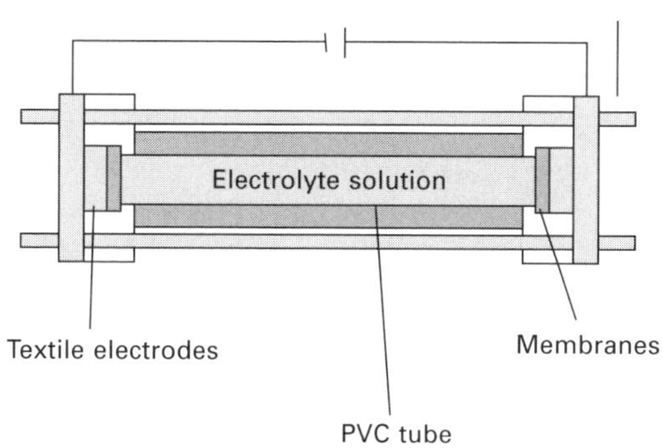

6.3 Impedance spectroscopy for characterizing textile electrodes.

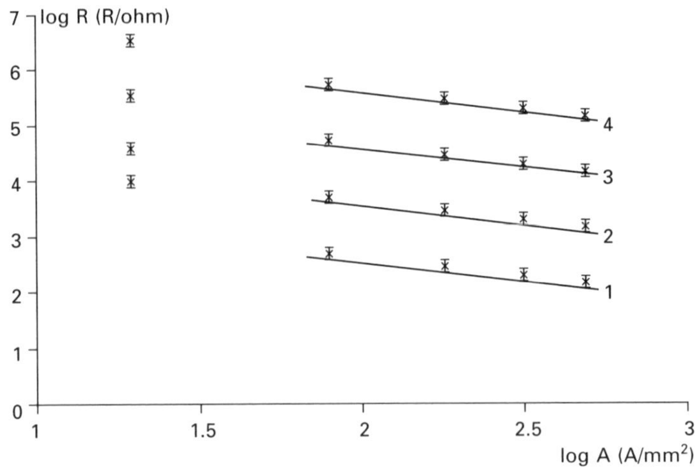

6.4 Effect of electrode size on the resistance of the cell.

different salt concentrations of the electrolyte. As would be expected, the resistance decreases linearly with the logarithm of the electrode surface, except for small areas. This can be explained by edge effects that play a bigger role in smaller electrodes. As resistance should be minimal, electrodes should be large. On the other hand, bigger electrodes are more sensitive to deformation and motion artifacts, so an optimal size should be chosen.

The distance between the positions of the electrodes is another parameter that has to be defined. The effect of this parameter can be seen in Fig. 6.5. The four lines have been measured at different salt concentrations. The resistance increases relative to the logarithm of distance. At short distances the results deviate. This is due to the surface roughness of the textile; the exact distance between the texile is not defined because of this parameter, and this error has an impact when the distance is small.

When permanently worn on the body the textile electrodes will become wet due to sweating. In order to simulate this effect, a porous membrane has been used. The electrolyte migrates through the pores and wets the textile. As can be seen from following graph (Fig. 6.6), sweating considerably reduces the resistance leading to improved measurements (curves 2–4). When wetted with clear water (curve 1), this effect is negligible.

Apart from the positive effect of sweating, corrosion has to be considered as well. Although stainless steel fibres resist corrosion due to, for instance, NaCl, at the skin a voltage also occurs, causing electrochemical attack. As a consequence the electric resistance increases in time when the material is in contact with artificial sweat (measured using the set up described above) [Westbroek 2006] (Fig. 6.7). This graph clearly demonstrates that corrosion has a significant impact on the conductivity of the sensor: the resistance

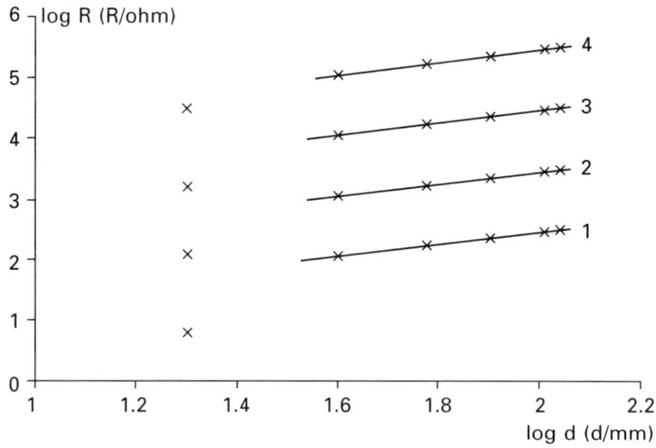

6.5 Effect of distance between the electrodes on the resistance of the cell.

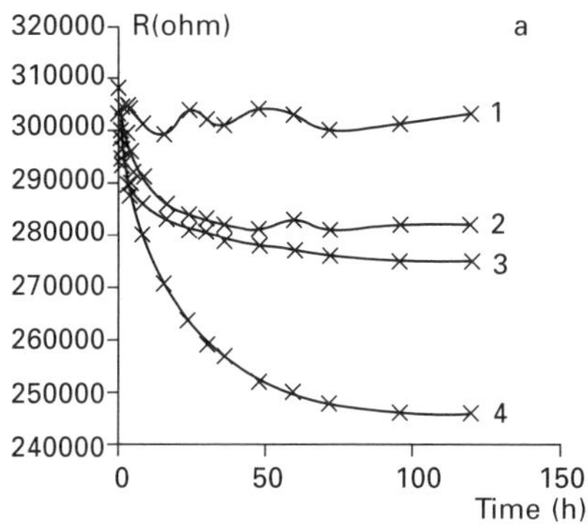

6.6 Effect of sweating on cell resistance.

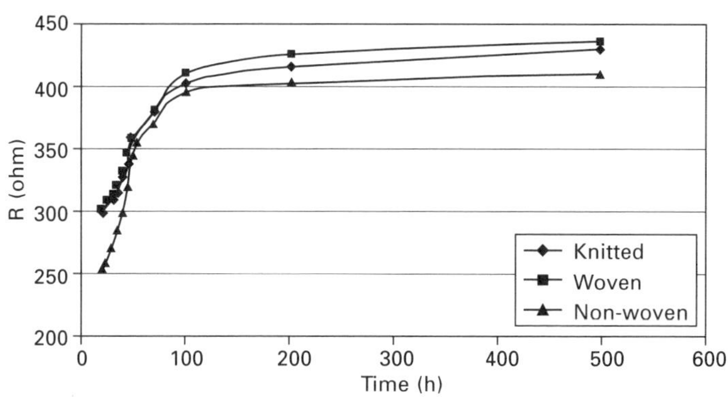

6.7 Effect of corrosion of stainless steel fabrics on electrical conductivity.

nearly doubles in a couple of weeks. This means that the accuracy of the sensor will be reduced significantly.

6.5 Testing of strain sensors

6.5.1 Physical effects

Conductive fibres often have mechanical properties that are quite different from those of 'regular' textile fibres. This causes them to react differently to deformation, bending, extension. As a result a slow but consistent migration of those fibres occurs. This eventually leads to separation of both components and this effect may become clearly visible after long-term use as, for instance, a breathing sensor (Fig. 6.8.) This effect is obviously not welcome for several reasons:

- it negatively affects the aesthetic aspect of the fabric
- it may affect the sensor function
- contacts may occur with the skin or the environment, leading to false signals, increased noise, etc.
- fabric feel may be affected.

6.5.2 Fibre breakage

Apart from the quite obvious macroscopic effect described in a previous paragraph more complex phenomena influence the sensor function of textile

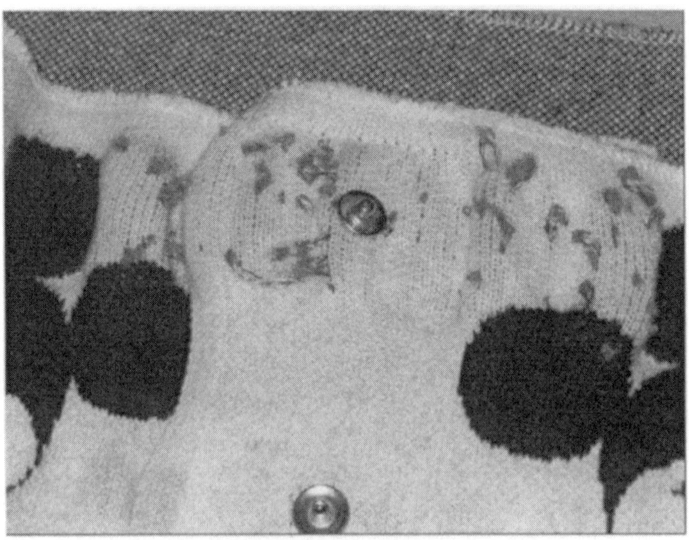

6.8 External loops formed by stainless steel yarns due to repeated extension.

sensors. Stainless steel fibres, for instance, are rather brittle, so repeated extension and bending causes them to break. Consequently, the number of fibre to fibre switches will increase with each fibre breakage and contact resistance being the biggest resistance by far, overall resistance of the textile structure will drastically increase. Particularly during laundry, deformation is quite intensive and laundry is of course a very relevant operation so it is a good way to test the impact of deformation. Measuring changes in length of fibres in an actual textile structure is very difficult because the fibres are embedded in the textile structure and its unravelling may cause more fibres to break. Fibres may also be crimped considerably so the length measurement in itself becomes difficult. An indirect method to evaluate fibre length is yarn strength as this relationship has been demonstrated in numerous studies (Fig. 6.9).

Mechanical damage of fibres has also been reported by Tao [2004]. This work describes the appearance of cracks at the surface of PANi and PPY coated fibres at extensions from 6% onwards. It is quite clear that all factors that affect the conductivity of the material also affect its proper functioning in the intelligent textile (Fig. 6.10). Mechanical damage due to multiple deformation in general is an important problem for all kinds of conductive textile materials. Also interconnections between different components (sensors, actuators, electronics, battery, wires) have been reported in many studies as

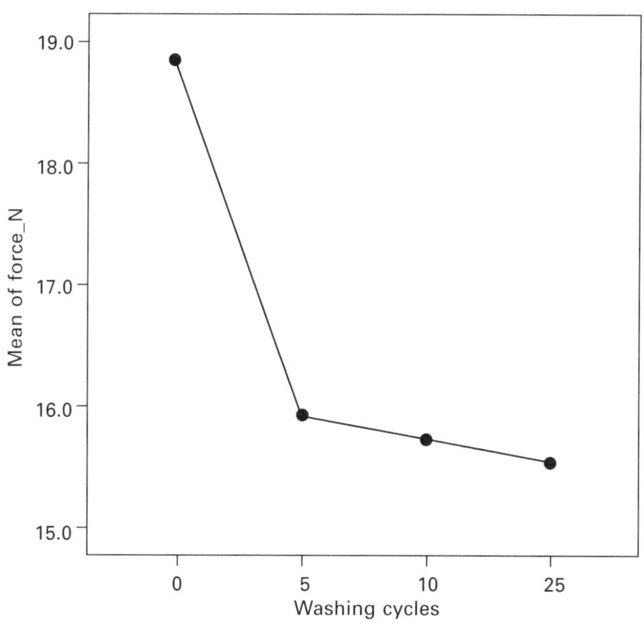

6.9 Influence of repeated extension during washing on yarn strength as a measure of fibre breakage.

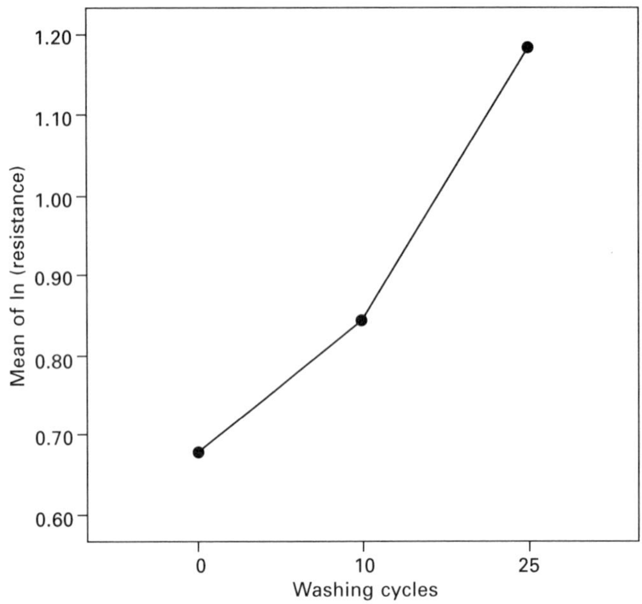

6.10 Effect of fibre breakage due to multiple deformation on yarn resistance.

weak spots, in particular at places where soft (textile) and hard (electronics) elements are connected.

6.5.3 Resulting long-term behaviour of textile strain sensors

As explained earlier, several factors may affect the proper sensor function of textile strain sensors. To test this a cyclic loading was applied whilst measuring the resistance of the textile structure [Lanfer 2005]. This resistance should go up and down with extension and the amplitude should be high enough for an accurate sensor (Fig. 6.11). The strain gauges were used for the characterization of the sensors and for accurate and precise measurement of strain [Heriott Watt 2004]. It is a very simple and handy system applied for sensors with the linear dependence of resistance changes on strain (or elongation) [Puers 1973]. All the developed formulas are true for the homogeneous materials and products. In general, the gauge factor (GF) is given by the following formula:

$$GF = \frac{\Delta R}{R_0} \Big/ \frac{\Delta L}{L_0}$$

where:

ΔR – an increase of resistance and $\Delta R = R_i - R_0$;

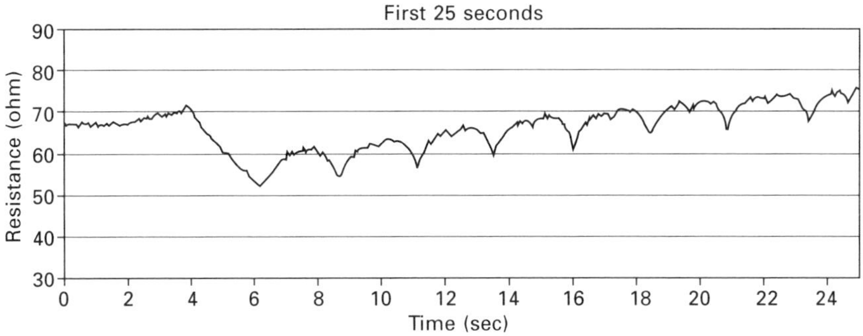

6.11 Variation of resistance due to cyclic loading of the textile strain sensor.

R_0 – initial resistance value;
ΔL – an increase of length and $\Delta L = L_i - L_0$
$\Delta L/L_0$ – the formula describes strain.

Rearrangement of the fibres happens mostly in the initial phase of use. As a result, resistance of a fabric will experience its fastest changes at the beginning of deformation tests; later on it will stabilize more or less (Fig. 6.12). From this figure it can be seen that the gauge factor is maximum at the start of the experiment and stabilizes after about 1.5 minutes. For many textile structures this gauge factor slowly goes down turning the textile material into an unreliable sensor (Fig. 6.13).

Washing is another important process of use that needs to be considered. Surprisingly the amplitude temporarily increases after washing. This is probably due to a rearrangement of the fibres in the textile structure after washing following the considerable fibre rearrangement during washing (Fig. 6.14). The sensor sensitivity of some textile structures actually improves due to washing. This is reflected in the gauge factor (Fig. 6.15). The gauge factor clearly goes up after washing. The more washing cycles that have been completed, the greater the increase and the better the sensitivity of the sensor. The effect partly disappears again during use, but partly it is permanent. It can be concluded that textile structures behave in a very complex way as sensors. Depending on the actual fibre type and the fabric structure a wide range of responses can be found.

6.6 Future applications of smart textiles

As stated earlier, the potential of smart textiles for health care is still largely unexploited. Apart from individual health, smart textiles can also play a role in public health. Epidemia, and more particularly pandemia, are one of the major threats of the future [Yayaraman 2006]. In the past particular types of flu have caused enormous casualties. With our very mobile society pandemic

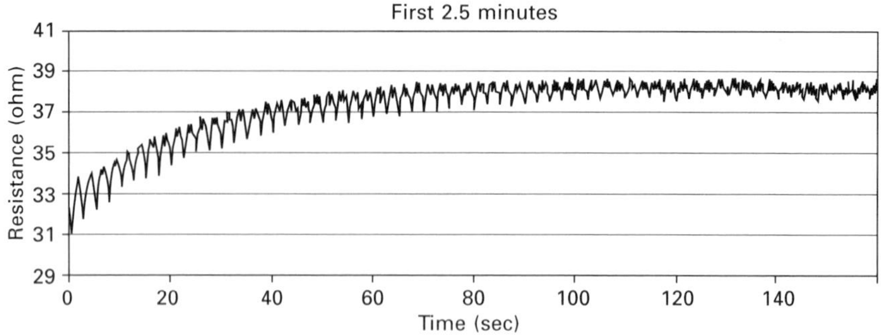

6.12 Change of resistance of a conductive yarn during initial phase of use.

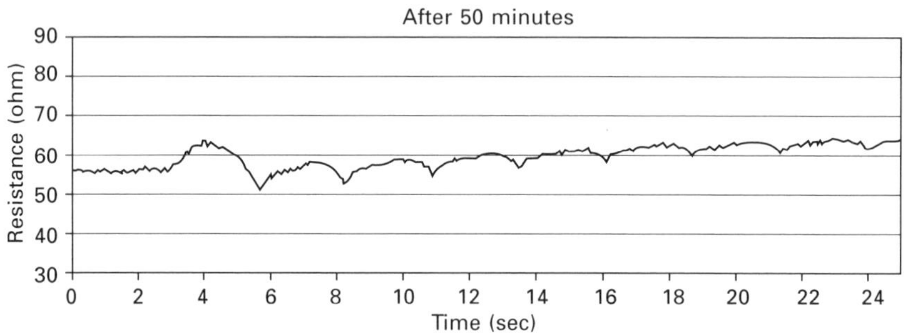

6.13 Loss of sensor capacity due to multiple deformation.

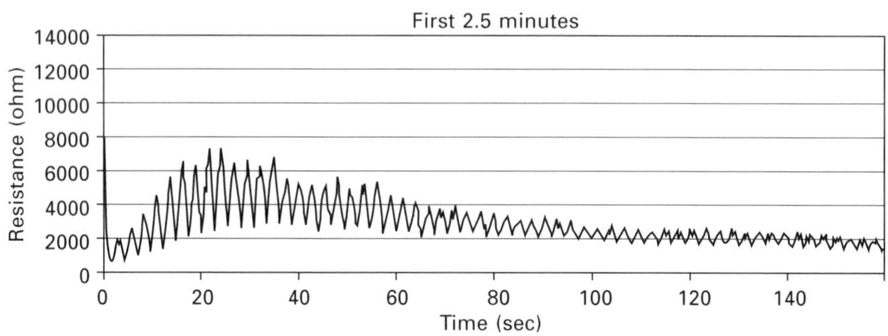

6.14 Effect of washing on sensor capacity of a textile material.

diseases will spread far quicker than ever before. Smart textile suits can play a role in remote monitoring, diagnosis and advanced protection. In an ageing society, falling becomes an increasing risk. Let us look at what smart textiles can offer in this respect. The suit will help to avoid risky situations. It communicates with the house in order to switch on the light when entering a room. It informs about objects lying on the ground. The suit detects when a person has an increased risk of falling, for instance, by detecting a drop in blood pressure or frequent instabilities. It sends out a warning in order to

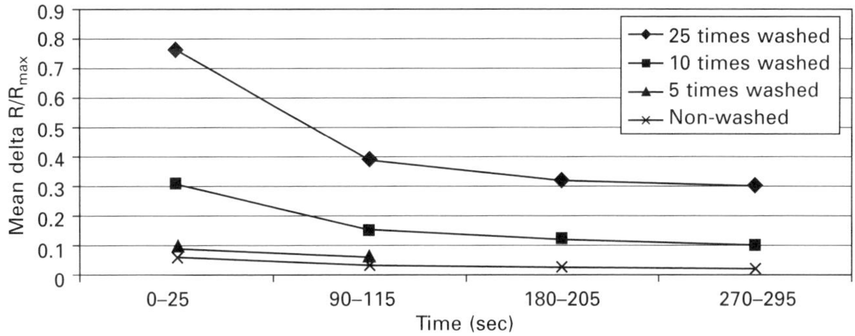

6.15 Impact of washing on textile strain sensor sensitivity.

inform the person and his relatives. The suit can supply drugs should this be necessary.

Integrated artificial muscles help to maintain equilibrium. When detecting an actual fall, in spite of the integrated muscles, the suit instantaneously turns into an impact-absorbing material. Air bags or mechanical actuators could be used to this end. After a fall, the smart suit assesses whether help is needed. If so, it calls for help and sends out information on the situation. It treats wounds and provides a splint should this be necessary. The suit also provides help in rehabilitation, for instance, by stimulating the healing process or by keeping the body in shape during immobilization. And all this in a discreet way, without any special care or loss of comfort. Of course the components, systems and materials for such a suit are far from being available today but it sets our mind on what could be possible tomorrow.

6.7 Conclusions

Smart textile structures are here to stay. They have demonstrated their feasibility both from the point of view of technical specifications as well as their textile character. The enormous versatility of textiles in terms of (combinations of) fibre types to be used, processing technologies and textile structure is at the same time an opportunity to be exploited but also a confusing space of possibilities. Different textile materials may show different, even opposite behaviour. It is a huge challenge to find the right set of materials for each particular application. Properties that are beneficial for one application may be disruptive for another one. Technical features may be in contrast to textile characteristics so a balance may have to be looked for. Objective testing is another field of research. No evaluation is possible without an accurate and reliable test method but the result will be worthwhile; it will definitely lead to a better quality of life.

6.8 References

Carpi, F., De Rossi D. Electroactive polymer based devices for e-textiles in biomedicine, *IEEE transations on information technology in biomedicine*, vol 9 (3), September 2005.

Devaux E., Saiha, D., Campagne, C., Roux, C., Kim, B., Rochery, M., Koncar, V. *Nanocomposite fibres for the processing of intelligent textile structures,* 5th World textile conference AUTEX, (2005), 2–8.

Georgia Tech: www.gtwm.gatech.edu

Heriott Watt www.hw.ac.uk/mecWWW/courses/d_towers/233Ld1/233LD1_Strain_Gauges_NOTES.doc (April 2004).

Lanfer, B. Master thesis: *The development and investigation of electroconductive textile strain sensors for use in smart clothing*, Ghent University, June 2005.

Mattes, B. R. Electronic textiles based on intrinsically conducting polymer fibre, *New generation of wearable for e-health: towards a revolution of citizens' health and lifestyle*, December 11–14 Lucca, Italy (2003).

Medes: http://www.medes.fr/VTAMN.html

Priniotakis J., PhD thesis: *Study of Conductive Textile Electrodes as Analytical Tool for Detection of Parameters related to human body by (EIS) Electrochemical Impedance Spectroscopy*, Ghent University, (September 2005)

Puers, R. Converting Stress Into Strain: Basic Techniques, chapter in the book: *Monitoring of Orthopedic Implants – A Biomaterials-microelectronic Challenge*; F. Burny, R. Puers, European Materials Research Society monographs, Volume 7, 1993 Elsevier Science Publishers B.V.

Smartex: http://www. smartex.it/ uk/projects/physensor.htm

Tao, X. *Fibre based interactive textiles and nanotechnology*, International Conference on Intelligent Textiles, Gent 25 June, 2004.

Van Langenhove, L., Hertleer, C. *Smart textiles for medical purposes*, MEDTEX 03, International Conference and Exhibition on Healthcare and Medical Textiles, July 7–9th, Bolton UK (2003).

Westbroek, P., Priniotakis, G., Palovuori, E., De Clerck, K., Van Langenhove L. and Kiekens, P. Method for quality control of textile electrodes used in intelligent textiles by means of (EIS) Electrochemical Impedance Spectroscopy, *Textile Research Journal* (76) 2 pp. 152–159 (2006).

Yayaraman, S., Kiekens, P., Grancaric, A. M. *Intelligent textiles for personal protection and safety*, Nato Security through Science series, IOS Press, ISBN 1-58603-599-1 (2006).

Zhang, 2001: Zhang, X., Tao, X. *Smart textiles: Passive smart*, June 2001 p 45–49, *Smart textiles: Active smart*, July 2001 pp. 49–52, *Smart textiles: Very smart*, August 2001, pp. 35–37, Textile Asia.

7

Smart dyes for medical and other textiles

T RIJAVEC and S BRAČKO,
University of Ljubljana, Slovenia

7.1 Introduction

Due to various physical and chemical changes in molecules, dyes can change their colour in the presence of acids, alkalis or when exposed to sunlight, water, mechanical loading, electric power, etc. Such changes are temporary or permanent. In this chapter we describe dyes that respond to changes of temperature, irradiation (ultraviolet rays in particular), solvents, electric power and other factors by changing their colour and which revert to the original colour after the establishment of normal conditions. They have become recognized as smart dyes. A very important natural smart dye with a reversible colour capacity is rhodopsin, a photosensitive compound, which is present in the retina of the eye. The rhodopsin activated by light induces nerve stimuli, which are transmitted to the brain where they provide visual perception. Rhodopsin has been also discovered in a primitive bacterium, *Halobacterium halobium*, where it transforms sunlight into energy, which is required for metabolism. The activity of photochromic Bacteriorhodopsin in simple archaebacteria is less complex than the activity in highly developed organisms. Due to its extraordinary resistance to photodegradation, rhodopsin is a photoswitchable biomaterial that is suitable for various applications such as optical data storage and security applications (Hampp, 2005a,b).

Scientific research into the phenomenon of reversible colour change dates back to the 19th century. The first noticed photochromic effect under the influence of ultraviolet (UV) rays was by J. Fritzsche on a solution of tetracene and later by E. ter Meer on a solid potassium salt of dinitromethane. (Bouas-Laurent, 2001) Until now, several smart dyes have been discovered, natural and synthetic. Among them very few smart dyes are suitable for dyeing textile materials with adequate resistance to external influences such as washing agents, sunlight and higher ironing temperatures, and very few smart dyes have an adequate fatigue resistance, i.e., an ability to develop colour after several reversible molecular transformations. Smart dyes have significant potential in the development of smart textile materials, especially for fashion, decorating, toys (Shibahashi, 2004), camouflage clothing, thermoregulation, flexible smart sensors, etc.

The following section deals with the phenomenon of smart dyes in connection with their application on textile materials. The basic colour change mechanisms are explained and the advantages and disadvantages of the potential use of smart dyes on textiles are discussed. As the research in this field and the commercial applications of smart dyes have shown a steady increase in the past few years, examples of uses on textiles as well as on other materials and the future trends are given consideration.

7.2 Colour change mechanisms

The phenomenon of reversible colour change is known as chromism. It is based on the phenomena that generate the change of the electron density of substances, especially π- or d-electron state, or the change in the arrangement of the substance supramolecular structure. Independently of the factors that trigger reversible colour change, several kinds of chromism are known:

- photochromism (induced by sunlight or UV rays)
- thermochromism (induced by changes in temperature)
- solvatochromism (polarity of the solvent)
- hygrochromism (moisture)
- ionochromism (ions)
- halochromism (pH value)
- acidochromism (acids)
- chemochromism (specific chemical agents like dangerous gases, warfare agents, etc.)
- electrochromism (electricity)
- piezochromism (pressure)
- mechanochromism (deformation of substances).

In this chapter we present the mechanisms of those phenomena that are applicable in the textile sector or are included in ongoing investigations.

7.2.1 Photochromic compounds

Photochromism is a reversible photochemical process during which a photochromic material temporarily changes its chemical structure and, consequently, also its electromagnetic waves absorption spectrum under the influence of irradiation involving UV rays. The reaction can be presented in eqn 7.1:

$$\text{A (colourless)} + h\nu_1 \rightarrow \text{B (coloured)} \qquad 7.1$$

The colourless photochromic material A does not absorb visible light. It can only be activated by high-energy photons ($h\nu_1$) from the near UV range of the electromagnetic spectrum. Due to the changes in the electron density, the material B is capable of absorbing low-energy photons ($h\nu_2$) from the visible part of the electromagnetic spectrum, which results in colouration of the material B. The absorption spectrum of the material A (in the absence of UV rays) is different from that of the material B (in the presence of UV rays) (Fig. 7.1).

A reverse reaction (eqn 7.2) takes place when the excited molecule B absorbs visible light ($h\nu_2$) with the frequency near absorption maximum and returns to the non-excited colourless state A. This reaction is also called decolourization.

$$\text{B (coloured)} + h\nu_2 \rightarrow \text{A (colourless)} \qquad 7.2$$

A reverse reaction in thermosensitive materials can be induced also by heat absorption. In the open air in the presence of UV rays and visible light, both reactions are going on; the reaction 7.1 is very quick, the reaction 7.2 is usually slower. Decolourization of a photochromic dye under the influence of UV rays is called negative photochromism.

At present, many inorganic and organic photochromic substances are known. Most inorganic substances, such as various metal oxides, alkaline earth metal sulphides, titanates, copper compounds, mercury compounds, certain minerals, transitional metal compounds and others, are not suitable for dyeing textile and leather materials. Organic photochromic dyes, on the other hand, are

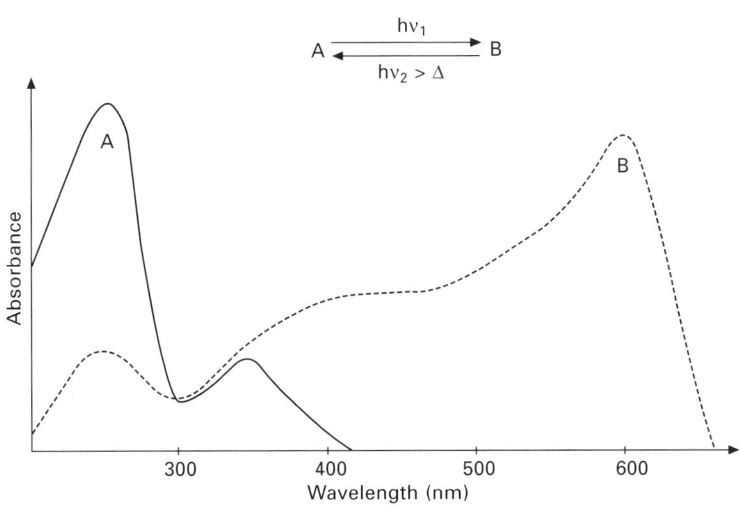

7.1 Absorption spectra of photochromic compounds: spectrum A changes under UV rays (hv1) into spectrum B. Reversible reaction occurs photochemically (hv2) or thermally (ν).

much more effective and environmentally friendly. The most important organic photochromic dyes are those belonging to the families of spiropyrans, spirooxazines, chromenes, fulgides, fulgimides and diarylethenes. Spiropyrans, spirooxazines and chromenes are sensitive to thermal effects and return to the colourless state under heat or visible light. Fulgides and diarylethenes are thermally stable. They decolourize by visible light. The mechanism of spiro compounds, particularly spiropyrans, is the most researched mechanism of organic photochromic substances. Slightly less researched is the mechanism of spirooxazines. (Bamfield, 2001)

Spiro compounds (Fig. 7.2(a)) consist of a pyran ring linked to another heterocyclic ring via a spiro group. Spirooxazines are nitrogen-containing analogues of spiropyrans. A colourless molecule of spiropyrans or spirooxazines has a non-planar molecular structure which prevents delocalization of π electrons and colouration. The absorption of UV rays ($h\nu_1$) induces heterolytic cleavage of a relatively weak C(spiro)-O bond within the pyran ring of spiro compound, which in turn enables the formation of a planar ring-opened molecular structure with the enlarged system of double conjugated bonds. Such a structure enables delocalization of electrons and colouration. This excited form is the zwitterionic merocyanine, a *cis* isomer, which transforms to a *trans* isomer. The reverse open-to-close process takes place under the influence of visible light and/or heat. Due to thermal instability, merocyanine reverts to the uncoloured spiro form after a certain period of time. In general, spiropyrans are instable in the excited form and, when exposed to sun rays and heat, they fade very quickly. Usually, colours are weaker at higher temperatures than at room temperature. The slow-down of the reverse reaction in solutions can be improved by using polar solvents, which stabilize the zwitterionic merocyanine form.

The reaction of spiro compounds colouration takes place when the photochromic dye is in solution or embedded in various matrices or polymers but, usually, it does not start when this dye is in crystalline state. The photochromic mechanism of chromenes is similar to the mechanism of spiro compounds. By introducing various substituents into the basic molecular structure, it is possible to tune the colour.

Fulgides (Fig. 7.2(b)) can exist in two isomeric forms, E or Z, which are produced by rotation around a double bond. Under the influence of UV rays, Z-form, which is colourless, may isomerize into E-form, and with cyclization of this form, an intensively coloured form called P-state may be produced. When exposed to visible light, the coloured compound can revert to E-form, however, it does not react to heat.

7.2.2 Thermochromic compounds

Thermochromism is a reversible change of molecular or supramolecular structure induced by heat and closely connected with the changes within the

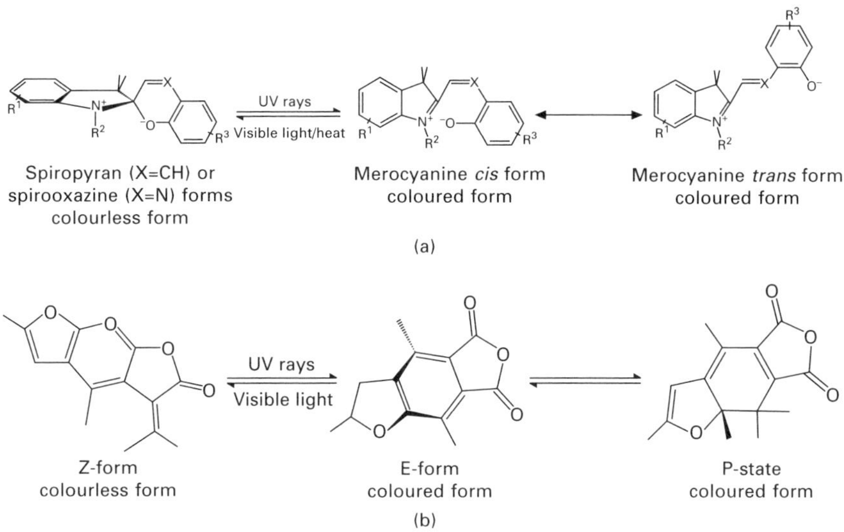

7.2 (a) Photochromic reaction of colourless spiropyrans or spirooxazines into coloured merocyanine form (b) photochromic reaction of fulgides.

absorption spectrum of a thermochromic molecule, usually in the visible light range. Thermochromic substances can be of inorganic or organic origin. Among inorganic thermochromic substances, few examples of metal oxides are known: indium oxide (In_2O_3) is yellow at lower temperatures and becomes yellowish brown with heating, zinc bloom (ZnO) is white at room temperature and turns to yellow at higher temperatures, a system chromium hemitrioxide-alum earth (Cr_2O_3-Al_2O_3) is red at 20 °C and changes to grey at 400 °C, etc. Reversible colour change takes place with the change of aggregate state or with the change of the geometry of ligands in metal complexes. The usage of inorganic thermochromic systems in the textile sector is restricted because reversible colour changes occur at very high temperatures and because the colour change usually takes place in solution. For usage on textiles, it would be ideal if colour changes were to occur between the ambient and body temperatures.

Organic thermochromic substances can reversibly change colour by different direct (intrinsic) or indirect mechanisms (Burkinshaw, 1998; Towns, 1999). For a direct mechanism relatively high energy is needed, which induces molecular changes such as the cleavage of a covalent bond or the change of molecular conformation. Heat triggers the change of molecular structure and the change of colour but after elimination of the source of heat, the system reverts to the thermally more stable form. The change of colour may be also the result of different structural changes, such as in crystalline liquid crystals.

Rearrangement of molecules

The cleavage of covalent bonds and the opening of cyclic structures may lead to the enlargement of the conjugated bonds system and to the formation of new chromophoric groups. The result is a coloured compound. The example is *bis*-spiropyran, which converts through heating in n-propanol at 60 °C into red coloured mono-merocyanine, and at 70 °C into blue *bis*-merocyanine.

Stereoisomerism

Heating may cause transition between two stereoisomers, which leads to changed light absorption. Such behaviour can be noticed with certain compounds, such as biantrons, dixanthylenes and xanthilidenantrons. Since a very high temperature, even above the melting point, is usually required for such transition, these systems are not suitable for textile products (Aitken, 1996).

Macromolecular systems

It is characteristic for some polymer systems (e.g. poly (3-alkylthyophene)) that their colour undergoes change under the influence of heat and that such colour change is usually reversible. The change is the result of hypsochromic shift of the absorption maximum which occurs due the fact that the structure of a polymer is planar at lower temperatures but at higher temperatures, the arrangement decreases and the structure ceases to be planar.

Changes in crystalline structures

Cholesteric liquid crystals (CLCs) represent the intermediate state between the crystalline phase, which is formed at low temperatures, and the liquid phase, which is formed at a sufficiently high temperature. In this state, rigid molecules are moving similarly to liquid but at the same time they retain a certain degree of arrangement, which is characteristic for the solid crystalline state. Molecules are orientated in a certain direction, which periodically changes the crystal lengthwise. The repeat distance along the direction of periodicity is a pitch. The pitch length is the distance along which the orientation of molecules changes for 360° (Fig. 7.3) (White, 1999). It is related to the wavelength of the reflected light λ and the average refractive index n of the crystal, according to eqn 7.3:

$$p = \lambda/n \tag{7.3}$$

If CLCs are optically birefringent, they typically do not reflect a single wavelength. In this case, the pitch is defined according to eqn 7.4:

$$p = \Delta\lambda/\Delta n \tag{7.4}$$

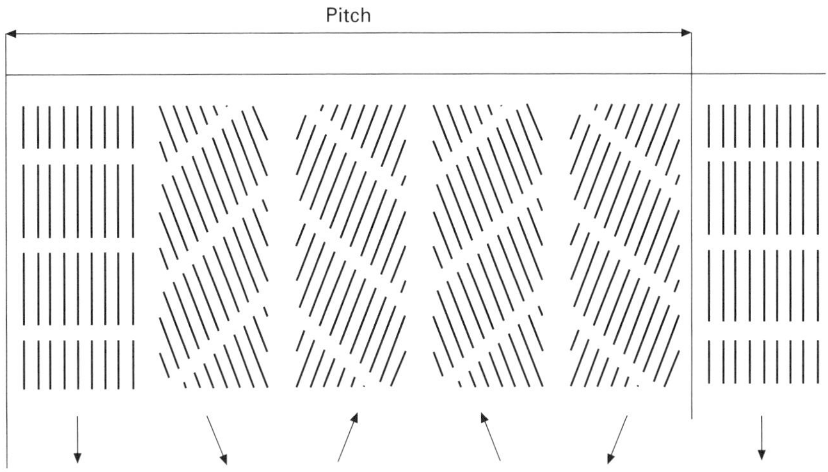

7.3 A scheme of a cholesteric structure of liquid crystalline compound with a survey of progressively changing orientation of rigid-rod molecules in neighbouring layers. A pitch defines the repeat distance along the direction of periodicity.

Such arrangement leads to colouration and its dependence on temperature. On individual layers of such orientated molecules, light reflection and interference occur, therefore, the perception of colour depends on the mean crystal refractive index and the pitch length. Several layers, which are separated with the pitch or integer multiple of the pitch, have the same orientation. The change of temperature generates the changes of distances between individual layers and the change of the pitch length. Since the pitch changes with temperature, the colour changes accordingly; with the increase of pitch the wavelength of the reflected light increases and vice versa. Thermochromic liquid crystals reversibly change colour in the temperature range from –30 °C to 120 °C and are sensitive to slight temperature changes, even 0.2 °C. By modifying rod-shaped molecules with optically active (chiral) groups or by mixing optically active molecules among the rod-shaped molecules of liquid crystals, nematic optically active liquid crystals with quite satisfactory thermochromic effect are produced (Coates, 2003).

Systems with direct thermochromism require a high temperature for colour formation and change, and are therefore less interesting for application on textile materials. Among the mentioned systems with direct thermochromisms, CLCs are mostly used. Much more interesting, and more used in practice, are the systems with indirect thermochromism. Typical of such systems is that they are not inherently thermochromic but they respond to changes in the environment triggered by changes of temperature, e.g., ionochromic substances yield colour in the presence of certain ions. For application on textile materials, thermochromic organic pigments are of particular interest.

Thermochromic organic pigments

In most cases, thermochromic organic pigments are composed of three components. The first component is the dye, which is sensitive to the change of pH in the environment (colour former). Such compounds are, for example, spiropyrans and fulgides. Another component is the colour developer, which has the function of a proton donor. Usually, this function is discharged by weak acids, e.g., derivatives of phenols. The third component is the co-solvent, which serves as a hydrophobic, non-volatile medium in which the dye and the colour developer are distributed. Hydrocarbons, fat acids, amides and alcohols can appear in the role of colour developers. For application on textile substrates, these three components are embedded into microcapsules (Fig. 7.4). At low temperatures, the components appear in the solid state. In such state, the interactions between the dye and the colour developer may occur, which leads to the formation of colour. At a higher temperature, the system starts to melt and the interactions between the dye and the colour developer are not possible and the colour disappears. Although lots of dyes, colour developers and co-solvents have been registered so far, the precise mechanism of colour formation has not yet been explained completely. By incorporating a specific compound, a colour change temperature regulator, to conventional thermochromic organic pigments composition, it is possible to delicately regulate the temperatures of colour change (Fujita, 2002).

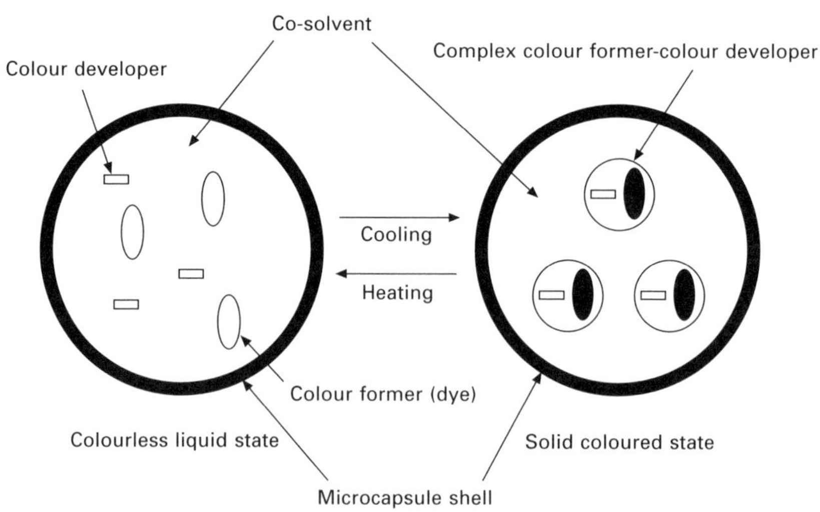

7.4 A microencapsulated complex system of organic thermochromic pigment with a representation of changes under heat and cooling.

7.2.3 Electrochromic compounds

Electrochromism is induced by the gain or loss of electrons. It is a reversible change of colour, which occurs due to the electrochemical redox reaction, oxidation and reduction. A redox reaction is triggered by weak electric currents at a voltage below one to a few volts. Under the influence of electric current, electrochromic materials change their colour from a colourless to a coloured state, from one colour to another or to a few different colours. The example of a multicolour electrochromic compound is polyaniline, which appears in yellow, dark blue or black colour, depending on electrical potential.

Electrochromic substances are:

- inorganic oxides of transition metals: tungsten (WO_3), iridium, rhodium, ruthenium, magnesium, cobalt
- Prussian blue (Fe (III) hexacyanoferrate (II), which is an inorganic pigment for dyes, lacquers, printing inks
- metallic phthalocyanines
- viologen – 4,4′-dipyridinium compounds
- Buckminsterfullerene (C60 – in the presence of alkaline metals as antiions, thin fullerene films change their colour from yellow-brown to silver-black)
- electroconductive conjugated polymers (polypyrrole, polyaniline, polythyophene, polyfurans, polyarbasols etc.) (Somani, 2002).

Measurement of electric current and voltage in electrochemistry was one of the first application fields of electrochromic dyes. Electrochromic dyes change their colour under the influence of electric current and are therefore suitable for application in electrochromic devices that are functioning as batteries. Such devices are composed of an electrochromic cathode, which is separated from the opposite electrochromic anode with adequate solid or liquid electrolyte. The anode is covered with an electrochromic substance that has the same colour in the oxidized state as the other selected electrochromic substance on the cathode in the reduced state. After starting the cell with an electric current pulse of a few volts, the redox reaction takes place, which leads to the colour change of the electrochromic dye on electrodes. The redox reaction is automatically maintained with little or even without outside electric current. Usually, electrodes are made of conductive glass and covered with a compound the colour of which in the oxidized state differs from the colour in the reduced state.

7.2.4 Solvatochromic compounds

Solvatochromism is a reversible change of the absorption or emission spectrum of a material that is induced by the action of solvents. The colour change is the consequence of the absorption maximum shift, which occurs due to differences between the solvation energy of the initial and excited state in various solvents. The excited state, which is more polar than the initial state, is more stable in more polar solvents. Such systems require lower energy for excitement, which leads to bathochromic shift of the absorption spectrum. This phenomenon is called positive solvatochromism. The less polar excited state than the initial state produces a counter-effect and a hypsochromic shift of the absorption maximum. This phenomenon is called negative solvatochromism. The majority of solvatochromic materials are metal complexes.

7.2.5 Mechanochromic compounds

Mechanochromism is a reversible change of colour of compounds because of a deformation action, such as elongation and compression. Strongly coloured polydiacetylenes $/{=}(CR{-}C{\equiv}C{-}CR)_n{=}/$ are the polymers with the system of conjugated π bonds lengthways a polymer molecule. Under the influence of a change in temperature, pH or mechanical stress, they absorb visible light. In the cool, non-extended state, polydiacetylenes (PDA) are blue (the absorption maximum at 640 nm), while in the excited state at 45 °C, solvated with acetone or due to mechanical abrasion, they convert to red colour (the absorption maximum at 540 nm). It is possible to modify the properties and application of PDAs by changing the functional and end groups in a polymer chain. By linking polyurethane chains at the beginning and at the end of a polydiacetylene molecule, its solubility in organic solvents can be enhanced. Side groups and the formation of polydiacetylenes (bulk, crystal, film, vesicle etc.) have an effect on absorption spectra (Carpick, 2004).

The first process of synthesis of mechanochromic polymers based on diacetylene was patented in 1988 (Rubner, 1988). A copolymer film was synthetized from a diisocyanate, a flexible elastomeric prepolymer and a chain extender containing diacetylene units, which has elastic properties and exhibits mechanochromism. Depending on the proportions of a diisocyanate, prepolymer and chain extender it is possible to achieve reversible colour change from blue to red purple at extension to 200%, or from red to yellow at extension to 110%.

7.3 Advantages and limitations of application

The advantages of smart dyes are closely connected with the special properties they have in comparison to conventional dyes, such as spectral characteristics of certain dyes and their intensities, colour change rate at the change of environmental factors, rate of reversion to the original colour state, stability of the excited state and degree of fastness. The parameters that describe the properties of photochromic dyes are colourability, the wavelength of the dye absorption maximum, number of cycles, cyclability, fade time or half time of reversion, half time of exposition and fatigue.

Colourability is the ability of a colourless or slightly coloured chromic material to develop colouration. The standardized method for determining the colourability of photochromic dyes is based on the colour evaluation of a sample when it is exposed to illumination and when it is left in the dark by using the Gray Scale for Colour Change (Textiles ..., 1993). λ_{max} describes the wavelength of the dye absorption maximum.

The number of cycles means the number of reversible transitions from the colourless state to the coloured state, which is highly dependent on the dye degradation degree. If the degradation degree in one cycle is x, the content of the non-degraded colour Y can be calculated by using eqn 7.5:

$$Y = (1-x)^n \qquad 7.5$$

Cyclability (Z_{50}) is the number of cycles required for the decrease of the initial absorbance by 50% at a specific wavelength.

Fade time or half time of reversion ($t_{r,1/2}$) estimates the colour fade rate during the reversion to the original colour state. This is the time that is required for the decrease of the coloured form absorbance at certain wavelength in one cycle to the half value. Half time of exposition ($t_{e,1/2}$) represents the time required for the development of colouration of a dye at excitement to the half value of maximum absorbance at a certain wavelength in one cycle. Fatigue describes the decrease of the efficiency of chromic compounds through usage due to the degradation of dyes.

In general, spirooxazines are highly resistant to photodegradation but sensitive to high temperatures. Chromenes exhibit good stability to high temperatures but have only moderate fatigue resistance. Fulgides exhibit moderate fatigue resistance and are resistant to high temperatures. The tendency of photochromic dyes to degradation due to oxidation considerably limits their potential for application on textile materials, where they are exposed to repeated washing.

In a wide range of thermochromic dyes, only few are capable of developing colour changes in the temperature range between –15 °C and +40 °C, which is very important for usage on textiles. In the temperature range between 5 and 15 °C, CLCs exhibit substantial colour changes (Nelson, 2002). Thermochromic organic pigments have poor stability under the influence of daylight and UV rays and their usage for outdoor purposes is therefore limited. Because of sensitivity to heat they can stand only a limited number of washing and drying cycles.

Photochromic and thermochromic dyes can cause allergies and can be dangerous if they are not used in compliance with instructions. The main properties of electrochromic compounds are contrast ratio, switching speed/

time, electrochromic memory, colouration efficiency and electrochromic stability (Argun, 2004). Contrast ratio is the difference in transmittance in the visible spectrum. It is often given as a percent transmittance change at a specifed range of wavelengths, where the compound has the highest optical contrast.

Switching speed is expressed with time required for the colour change (colouring/bleaching) of the electrochromic compounds. It may be defined as the time to become 75% of the ultimate change in per cent transmittance. Switching time depends on ionic conductivity of the electrolyte, ion diffusion, applied voltage and the morphology of the polymeric material. Electrochromic memory is the ability of the electrochromic compound to retain its colour without current. It is very short for solution-based electrochromic compounds such as viologens and very long (days or weeks) for solid-state electrochromic compounds.

Colouration/electrochromic efficiency η gives the power requirements of an electrochromic compound. It is determined as the change in optical density ΔOD per unit area of the electrode Q_d for a given wavelength (eqn 7.6).

$$\eta = (\Delta OD)/Q_d \tag{7.6}$$

Electrochromic stability is the ability of the compound to retain its electrochromic properties (especially electrochromic contrast) over a large number of switching cycles. It is reduced because of irreversible oxidation or reduction at extreme voltages, voltage drop due to the internal resistance of the electrode or the electrolyte, side reactions in the presence of water or oxygen and heat release.

7.4 Examples of application

7.4.1 Main application fields

The application of smart dyes is based on the phenomenon of reversible colour change and other related chemical and physical changes triggered by external factors. Smart dyes offer the possibility of enhancing the attractiveness and functionality of existing products. The ability of photochromic dyes to reversibly change their colour provides potential for new designs, decorations and fashionable effects. Typical examples of such applications are clothing, shoes, jewellery, cosmetics (nail varnish), toys and furnishings. Photochromic dyes are widely used for the protection of money, cheques, documents and brand names. Specific reversible colour changes enable application of photochromic dyes for camouflage purposes. The sensitivity of certain photochromic dyes to UV ray intensity enables the development of actinometers, dosimeters and self-developing photography. Widely used products, which are sensitive to UV ray intensity, are sunglasses. Photochromic dyes in the lenses of sunglasses darken under the influence of intense sunlight and lose colour with low UV ray intensity. Photochromic dyes are successfully used for windows and transparent façades to control sunlight and diminish dazzling. They also enable architects to design colour change façades. (Addington, 2005) Heat sensitive photochromic dyes are convenient for heat measurement, as temperature indicators and as pyroelectric materials.

Reversible changes in the refractive index, dielectric constant, oxidation/reduction potentials and changes in geometrical structure are the basis for the application of photochromic dyes in high-tech technology for optical memories and switches, photochromic microimages, information encoding, stenography and filters. Organic thermochromic pigments are used as indicators of adequate storage and consumption temperature for food and drinks, such as thermochromic dyes on the packing of children's food, milk, beer, non-alcoholic drinks, wine, on coffee and tea cups, etc. In the field of identification, thermochromic dyes may provide additional protection for personal documents, credit cards, prescriptions, etc., because it is difficult to photocopy the thermochromic dyes. Thermochromic dyes based on CLCs are used for decorations, in cosmetics, thermodiagnostics such as thermography, for aquarium thermometers, for skin thermometers, in optics and electrooptics, etc.

The main application fields of electrochromic dyes are car mirrors and smart windows, which regulate the incoming light, and visual displays that compete with LCD monitors. Polydiacetylenes are physiologically acceptable solvatochromic polymers that are used on food products and packaging, etc.

7.4.2 Examples of applications on textile materials

In the textiles sector, smart dyes are less used than in other sectors. The application of organic thermochromic pigments has been increasing, although the selection of dyes that are capable of developing colour changes in the temperature range from –15 °C to +40 °C remains very limited. CLCs are very expensive, have low colour density and poor colour selectivity. In order to obtain high colour density, these dyes should be used in relatively high amounts. Photochromic dyes are less used than thermochromic dyes due to poor stability. There are only few examples of using solvatochromic and mechanochromic dyes on textiles. The application of electrochromic dyes on textiles is in progress. Besides diversified fashion and decorative application, many special functions such as thermoregulation, camouflage, product labelling, medical and security, applications of smart dyes in textiles are on the increase.

Uses of smart dyes for fashion and decorating purposes

The first fabrics with photochromic dyes appeared on the market in the 1980s. The Japanese producer Kanebo Ltd. used microencapsulated spiropyrans, which were printed on textile materials. Under the influence of UV rays with wavelength 350–400 nm, the dyes reversibly changed colour from light blue to dark blue (Hongu, 1997). At the end of the1980s, unstable spiropyrans were replaced with more stable spirooxazines (Yoshihiko, 1989). At this time, Toray Industries Inc. developed the process of coating fabrics with photochromic dyes. The fabric, which came to the market under the trade name Sway UV®, was able to turn blue or violet under the influence of UV rays with wavelength 350–380 nm. When the effect of UV rays ceased the colour disappeared in 30 seconds. Sway UV® was used for T-shirts, polo shirts, jumpers etc. (New ..., 1989).

On the basis of thermochromic organic pigments Toray Industries Inc. developed a multicolour fabric Sway® in 1988. This fabric enabled 64 colour hues in temperature intervals of 5 °C in the temperature range –40 °C to + 80 °C. They used the technology of microencapsulation of four thermochromic pigments, which were capable of changing colour from white into pink, blue into black, yellow into blue and pink into grey. Depending on end-use, colour changes were designed to occur at 11–19 °C for ski-wear, at 13–22 °C for women's clothing and at 24–32 °C for window shades (Masuko, 1987).

The Japanese company Matsui-Shikiso Chemical Company developed the Hypercolour® process for printing cotton fabrics with thermochromic organic pigments with negative thermochromism (Shimizu, 1988). The exclusive right to use this process was held by the Generra Sportswear Company, which manufactured T-shirts with several colour change choices in the late 1980s and early 1990s. Today, organic thermochromic pigments are mostly used for embroidery on apparel, such as weaving threads, and for thermal printing on a variety of fabrics.

In the 1980s, the process of leather and skin coating with thermochromic liquid crystals was patented (Ruggeri, 1983). The process includes preparing a water dispersion of microencapsulated thermochromic CLCs with emulgated synthetic binder (vinyl, acrylic, methacrylic or amide resin), which is screen printed on a dark coloured material and protected with a transparent film. The colouration of the printed sample takes place at the temperature change in the intervals 16–22 °C, 22–28 °C and 26–31 °C depending the weight percentage of cholesteric substances. A recipe with 73.2 wt.% of cholesteryl nonanoate, 11.7 wt.% of oleyl cholesteryl cargonate and 15.6 wt.% of cholesteryl chloride is given as an example of colour changes in the temperature range 16–22 °C. The visual effect of the fabric depends on the angle of observation.

Thermochromic dyes, which are applied on yarns containing metal fibres, are activated by heat that is released during the heating of metal fibres under voltage. By combining woven electronic circuits from electroconductive yarns, thermochromic inks and drive electronics, it is possible to design various dynamic textile patterns, which are electronically controlled. Electric

Plaid™ is the first such programmable colour-change textile display technology, which enables colour changing of fabrics similarly to computer displays. By fabric surface structuring into 64 (8 by 8) electrical areas or animation cells, which undergo a programmed colouration by means of control electronics, it is possible to design various visual effects on the fabric surface, i.e., various animations (Orth, 2003).

Very interesting fashionable effects can be obtained with mechanochromic dyes. Polydiacetylenes, which are bound to elastic polyurethanes, enable colour change at stretch or compression. The process of manufacturing electrospun specifically shaped clothes, shoes and other related garments, which develop colour on the deformation area was patented. Colouration of material on the deformation area can be used for evaluating the comfort of clothing and shoes (Bowlin, 2002).

Thermoregulation

The reversible colour change of thermochromic dyes also indirectly changes the heat absorbance of a textile. Lighter shades and white colour of thermochromic pigments increase heat reflectance, whereas darker shades increase heat absorbance. These effects can be successfully used for the coatings of firemen's uniforms which become white at high external temperatures and consequently reflect heat (Hibbert, 2002) and for covering buildings (Reinaldo de Oliveira Neves, 2001).

Thermochromic dyes can hasten substantial dimensional changes of fibres. At higher external temperatures, fibres which contain thermochromic dyes shrink. The pores in a fabric enlarge and enable passage of a higher amount of air and, consequently, cooling down of the body. In a cold ambient temperature, fibres expand and close pores, so that a fabric can retain as much body heat as possible (Hibbert, 2001).

Smart dyes for camouflage purposes

Camouflage is the disguising of persons or objects by imitating patterns and colours in the environment. Today, it is used for military purposes and in sports hunting to conceal people, abodes, military and other equipment. The camouflage patterns and colours match with the background (environment). Conventional dyes, which are not able to develop reversible colour change, do not provide sufficient camouflage in the conditions of different light intesity (in the morning, in the evening, in cloudy weather, etc.) despite highly precise imitation of the environment and many various colours. The intensity of colours, colour type and pattern remain the same regardless of the sunlight intensity. The beginnings of the development and application of photochromic dyes on textiles for camouflage date back to the 1960s when

American Cynamid Co. first developed photochromic spiropyrans (Hongu, 1997; Fisher, 1967).

In 1998 Conner patented the process of photochromic dye application on textiles, which were previously dyed with conventional dyes. This process enables improved camouflage effect at various degrees of light intensity. Additive mixing of the colour of photochromic and conventional dye produces various colours of the camouflage pattern in the shade and at direct sunlight. Photochromic dyes, which are colourless in a closed place and in the open air protected from direct sunlight or in the shade, and which develop colouration under the influence of the increasing sunlight illumination, have advantages over other photocromic dyes. According to Conner, suitable photochromic dyes for camouflage purposes are, e.g., acryl-substituted heterocyclic photochromic dyes marketed under the trade name Reversacol® (Conner, 1998).

Scientists at DuPont are developing ways to manipulate light in such a way that soldiers could actually be invisible. EIC Laboratories is working on electrochromic camouflage, a chameleon fabric that would change colours instantly to blend in with its surroundings (Newman, 2003).

Smart dyes as detectors of forgery

Smart dyes are frequently used to prevent forgery or as protective elements for documents or money. Likewise water print on paper, hidden markings based on photochromic and thermochromic dyes on textiles provide protection from forgery. Such markings are usually protected brand names, which are screen printed on demarcated areas on the top or underside of a textile product. The demarcated area has a different appearance from its surroundings. The marking is made up of microparticles with an appropriate binder. Microparticles are composed of microencapsulated thermochromic dyes and phosphorescent dyes, which appear in different combinations with ceramic, glass and transparent plastic materials. Glass, ceramic and plastic materials in the form of tiny particles also contain smart dyes and represent more expensive protection.

By selecting a suitable binder, it is possible to impart permanent or temporary protection to the products. Water-soluble binders enable removal of protection at the first washing. Thermoplastic binders provide permanent fixing of protection at ironing. Markings and demarcated area appear in various conditions depending on the composition of microcapsules. Thermochromic dyes that change their colour within the body temperature range induce colour change of the clothing during wear. When photochromic dyes are used, the protected marking on clothing will appear in the open air (Tebbe, 2002).

7.5 Application processes

Photochromic and thermochromic dyes are usually available as microcapsules in pulverized form. The shell of microcapsules acts as protection and improves stability of dyes to detergents in particular, and extends their lifetime. A special problem related to most organic photochromic dyes is that they show great colour change when they are dispersed in solutions or in a macromolecular melted state, whereas colour changes are minimal or do not occur at all in the crystalline form. Also for some photochromic dyes such as spirobenzopyrans, which exhibit all their photochromic properties even though they are not present as a solution and can be added directly into a polymer resin, microencapsulation is a more convenient method. Microencapsulated organic photochromic dyes, spirooxazines and others maintain their photochromic properties much better when they are dissolved or dispersed into hindered amine-type compounds than in other forms, e.g., in polymer resins (Kamada, 1993). Newly developed spirooxazine-based sulphonic dyes can even be used in a water solution directly as a conventional dye (Shah, 2005).

The change of colour of thermochromic dyes, which are used on textile materials, is closely connected with the change of aggregate state. Organic thermochromic pigments and CLCs are always microencapsulated.

Microencapsulation

Microencapsulation is the process by which an active substance, which represents the core of a microcapsule, is protected with a special wrapper or shell. A microcapsule is a tiny particle with a size of one to 1000 μm, which has the core composed of a thermochromic or photochromic system and the shell made of polymer material. Conventional microencapsulation processes can be mechanical (spray drying, centrifugation, co-extrusion, etc.) or chemical (co-acervation or interfacial polymerization). Chemical processing is more suitable for thermochromic and photochromic dyes. To obtain satisfactory shelf-life and durability on textiles interfacial polymerization is nearly always used.

For microencapsulation of organic thermochromic pigments by complex co-acervation, two polyelectrolytes are used (e.g. gel and gum Arabic). In the initial phase, at pH below 4.7, gel is positively charged and gum Arabic negatively. The active substance (core material) is dispersed in a gel solution to which the solution of gum Arabic is added. By regulation of pH to the value 4, the formation of a liquid complex co-acervate, which is composed of gel with active substance and gum Arabic and water, is induced. This liquid complex co-acervate encloses an active substance to produce the core of a microcapsule. Gelatinization of the shell occurs during the system cooling down phase. Usually, additional cross-linking of the shell with glutaralaldehyde takes place as well. After drying, microcapsules in pulverized form are produced (Sen, 2001).

The formation of the shell by the interfacial condensation process starts with polycondensation on the active substance surface, which represents the core of a microcapsule. By mixing active substance and one of the reactants (e.g. polyfunctional acid chloride or isocyanate), a water-insoluble blend is produced, which is subsequently dispersed in water by means of an emulsifier. The other reactant (e.g. polyfunctional amine or alcohol) is added to the water phase. During interfacial polymerization, which takes place on the core surface, the shell of the microcapsule is formed. This process is used for the formation of aminoplast-based microcapsule shells. A solid substance, which represents the core of the microcapsule, is dispersed into water, which contains urea, melamine or water-soluble condensate of formaldehyde. With the addition of anionic polymer and at proper temperature and pH, the aminoplast-based shell is formed.

Many different substances can be incorporated into microcapsules by using chemical processes. However, it is important that certain basic requirements are fulfilled. The active substance should not be soluble in the carrying medium and should not react with the shell or exert some other influence on it, the active substance should be properly dispersed in the carrying medium and should be resistant to the changes of pH, temperature or other conditions required by the microencapsulation process.

Application methods

Besides different printing (screen, transfer and electrostatic) and coating techniques, some other methods of application of photochromic and thermochromic microencapsulated compounds, such as spraying, impregnation (Kamata, 1993) and dyeing, are used in practice. In order to obtain good stability and the colour effect of microencapsulated dyes applied on textiles, it is necessary to consider also the fineness of fibres. The relationship between the diameter of microcapsules, the diameter of fibres and the density of fibres is proposed by Shibahashi (1987). Microcapsules can be used as conventional pigments and are applied on textile substrates by using polymer binders, or are added to polymer resins.

7.5.1 Microcapsules fixed with polymer binders

The choice of binder is highly important for the quality and stability of dyes, particularly at washing and ironing. Mostly used are water-soluble polymer binders, (starch, modified starch, carboxymethyl-cellulose, polyvinil alcohol, xanthates), synthetic latexes (such as styrene-butadiene copolymer, poly(vinyl acetate), polyacrylates with anionic or nonionic emulsifiers) and aminoaldehyde resins (such as urea- and melamine-formaldehyde resins, dimethylolethylene-urea, dimethyloldihydroxyethylene-urea, dimethylolpropylene-urea and silicones) (Boh, 2003). For application of microcapsules on nonwovens, fibres, yarns and woven materials, a suspension which, besides microcapsules and binder, contains also antifoaming and viscosity controlling agents is prepared.

Water dispersion of microencapsulated thermochromic CLCs and an emulsified synthetic binder (vinyl, acrylic, and methacrylic or amide resin) can be applied by screen-printing, coating or spraying on a previously dyed dark material and which is then protected with a transparent film (Ruggeri, 1983). Better stability of the coating can be obtained by adding a thermoplastic polymer into the coating medium. The example of a coating medium for application on a dark dyed polyester/cotton fabric by using a screen printing technique presented by Sage contains 30 parts by weight of the microencapsulated thermochromic CLCs dispersion, five parts by weight of an acrylic polymer, 30 parts by weight of fusible polyamide powder, five parts by weight of ammonia solution and 30 parts by weight of water. The coated fabric was dried for ten minutes at 50 °C and then hot pressed at 120 °C at pressure 1.2 N/cm^2. After 20 washing cycles in a 1% solution of commercially available washing powder at 40 °C, the fabric still retained bright colours (Sage, 1994).

The addition of polyurethane latex improves the softness of the fabric handle, whereas the addition of melamine/formaldehyde resins produces stiffer handle. The addition of a UV absorber into a coating medium improves the stability of thermochromic dyes in the open air. For printing photochromic and thermochromic dyes on textile materials, the influence of the substrate on the visual effect of photochromic or thermochromic dyes should be taken into account. Light coloured substrates are more suitable for photochromic dyes and dark coloured substrates for certain thermochromic compounds, such as CLCs.

7.5.2 Microcapsules in polymer resin

Surface abrasion is one of the reasons for low durability of the microencapsulated organic thermochromic pigment applied by printing or coating. Another reason, which applies particularly to nonwovens, is the difficulty of applying the coating uniformly. By incorporating the encapsulated organic thermochromic pigment into the polymer melt of polyesters, polyamides or polyolefines (Kamata, 1995; Ishimura, 2004) the uniformity as well as the fabric durability is enhanced. The patent applies to the manufacture of melt spun nonwovens with 0.5–5% of an incorporated microencapsulated organic thermochromic pigment, which changes in the temperature range 40–60 °C (Carlyle, 2003).

For the formation of thermoplastic fibres, organic photochromic pigments in the form of a dye concentrate are added to the polymer (masterbatch). In this way the photochromic properties of the dyes are retained. The method of making thermoplastic fibres from a master batch containing photochromic pigments is described in the patents (Hwu, 1993, 1995). At 210 °C, the microencapsulated photochromic pigment is blended with polypropylene of the melt flow index 35 (or low melting nylon 8, nylon 12, nylon 6, nylon 6.6 and others) to prepare a master batch with 1% of a photochromic dye. A master batch and polypropylene are blended in the one-to-twelve weight ratio for extrusion into fibres.

A quite new process of preparing photochromic polypropylene resin for fibre formation describes the process of dissolving a photochromic compound (chromene, spiroxazine and spiropyran based compounds) into an organic solvent mixture containing 20–70% by weight of toluene, 20–65% by weight of methylethylketone and 5–35% by weight of normal-hexane, and adding polypropylene resin into the solvent mixture at a temperature of 60 °C to 90 °C for six to nine hours. By using this process, a photochromic resin is produced, which represents a sufficient effect even when added in a relatively small amount of 0.0005–0.005% by weight to the polyproplylene resin, because the dye is uniformly distributed. Photochromic resin is appropriate for fibre formation by the conventional meltspun process (Lim, 2004).

Microencapsulated organic thermochromic pigments can be added to the solution of acrylonitrile copolymer in aqueous sodium thiocyanate. The resulting mixture is uniformly dispersed into the spinning dope so that it contains only 1% by weight of a thermochromic pigment (Ono, 2002).

7.6 Future trends

The colour of textiles is highly important and is practically always the decisive factor for the customers' decision to buy. In the 1990s, photochromism and thermochromism were widely used, particularly in fashionable textiles. At present, on-going research investigates the usage of chromism on textiles in order to create functional passive smart materials, which can only sense the environmental conditions, and functional active smart materials, which can sense and react to the environmental conditions by changing their colour (camouflage, thermoregulation).

Microcapsules and the dyes inside them generally do not endure more than about twenty laundering cycles. High temperatures at tumble drying and ironing accelerate deteorioration of the microcapsules' properties. For a wider application of photochromic and thermochromic dyes it would be necessary to improve their light stability, their resistance to detergents, particularly oxidation ones, and their yield of colour (to achieve deeper hues). Beside this, the high price of smart dyes in comparison to conventional dyes due to microencapsulation and poor selection of appropriate binders for textile substrates, represent challenges for future research. There is potential for the development of new smart dyes, such as water-soluble photochromic dyes. The necessity for pressure-sensitive smart dyes (Kanakkanatt, 1996) for application on textiles, which reversibly change their colour under the influence of tensile or compressive stress, is growing.

7.6.1 Flexible UV sensors

Flexible UV sensors based on photochromic dyes, which are integrated in clothing, warn the wearer of exposure to various intensities of UV rays. It is a simple and user-friendly way of active smart protection. Coupled with the information about the sun protection factor (SPF), it would enable safer movement of the wearer in the open air. The results of the research carried out so far (Viková, 2005a) show that certain photochromic dyes, in which light or UV rays induce substantial changes in their structure and, consequently, the change of their reflectivity, can be used as flexible textile sensors. Under the influence of illumination with UV rays, the reflectance curve shape changes in the visible part of the spectrum and colouration takes place. At reversion to the original state in the absence of UV rays, the shapes of the reflectance curves exhibit the changed time dependence and hysteresis occurs. With certain light stable dyes from the spiroindolino-naphthaoxazines and naphthapyrans group, linear dependency between the hysteresis surface and the intensity of illumination occurs and their reaction is similar to that of the conventional illumination measuring devices. At illumination, the halving time changes with the intensity of illumination – at 1000 luces, it is more than 35 minutes and at 10,000 luces, it is less than ten minutes (Fig. 7.5).

Ultraviolet absorbers are the substances, that are capable of absorbing hazardous ultraviolet irradiation. In this way, the UV ray transmittance of the fabric is decreased. Simultaneous application of a UV absorber in concentrations, which provide efficient protection on textiles from hazardous ultraviolet irradiation, does not affect linear responsiveness of photochromic dyes as photosensors. From the user's viewpoint, it is important that a UV absorber imparts to a textile product efficient protection and that at the same time a photochromic dye warns of hazardous irradiation in the environment. Further investigations should focus on the dyes with quicker responsiveness and higher photosensitivity, which would provide a more user-friendly method of UV protection for people with sensitive skin, particularly children.

7.6.2 Smart chemochromic dyes

ECI Biotech of Worcester developed the first biosensors on the basis of smart chemochromic dyes, which can be applied on textile materials. New

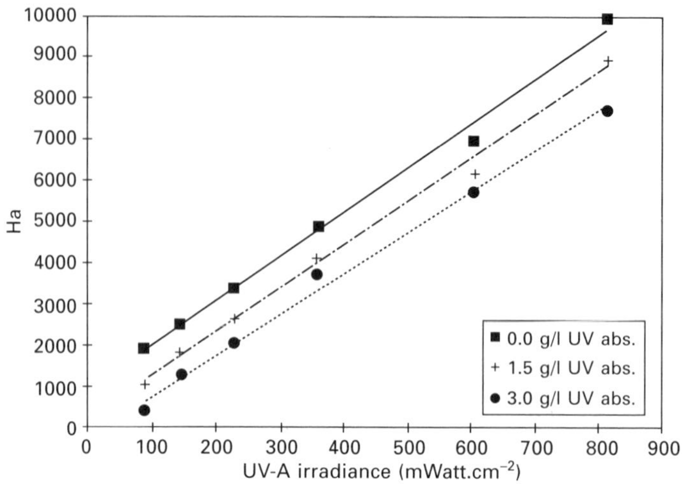

7.5 A variation of a colour hysteresis area Ha with an intensity of illumination. Courtesy: Martina Viková.

technology is based on colour identification of proteins, which are specific for certain pathogenic microbes. In the patent application (Sanders, 2003) the process of detecting prokaryotic microorganisms (bacteria, blue-green algae, actinomycetes, mycoplasma) which frequently develop on animals is described. A biosensor identifies proteins, such as microbial specific protease, in the outer membrane of pathogenic bacteria or unique secreted proteins. A biosensor is a specific chromogenic substrate, which undergoes cleavage in the presence of a specific protease. The result is the change of colour, which warns the user of danger. The product is marketed under the name ExpresDetect™. A biosensor (detector) can be applied on the surface of practically any material, including textile materials. Possible application fields are dental flosses, diapers, swabs, feminine pads, wipes, wound dressings, catheters, specimen containers, etc.

Protective underwear with chemochromic dyes for identification of dangerous gases is in the phase of development. A colour change informs the user about the area of incoming toxic gas, about the direction of its expansion and about its intensity. In comparison with the local dosimeters that are used today, this is a simpler, more cost-effective and faster method of detecting danger, which is particularly important in exposure to very toxic gases (Viková, 2005b).

7.6.3 Electrochromic fibres

Dynamic colour-responsive 'chameleonic' fibres are electrochromic fibres based on intrinsically conductive polymers (ICPs) and molecules that contain chromophores. Electrically conductive polymers with the structure composed of many conjugated double bonds, which oxidize from the colourless state to the coloured electrically charged state in the presence of antiions, exhibit colour changes within a narrow range of the visible spectrum. With graft copolymerization of a conductive polymer with molecules, which contain chromophore groups, ICPs become more sensitive and exhibit colour changes in a wider range of the visible spectrum. These molecules contain chromophore groups that change light absorbance in the visible, UV or infra-red range under the influence of electric field. Such molecules are, for example, porfirins and ring-shaped porfirin structures. With copolymerization of these molecules, electrochromic systems, which dynamically change colour, were produced. They can be used for the manufacture of chameleonic fibres or for direct application on textiles. Under the influence of static or dynamic electric or magnetic fields, these fibres can quickly change colour, colour shade, colour depth or light transmittance. They have potential for coatings and additives, on carpets, curtains, wallpapers, camouflage clothing, T-shirts, smart uniforms, etc. Chameleonic fibres have not been introduced to the market yet (Hardaker, 2003).

7.6.4 Wearable textile CLCs displays

The technology of fully coated CLCs displays on single textile substrates is extending to the field of intelligent textiles or wearable electronics. These new flexible, multi-colour displays with a thickness of 30–35 μm are fully integrated with textile materials. They are composed of a few layers, which are applied on a textile substrate one upon another by a coating process. The first layer is a levelling layer made of polyurethane or acryl. The next layer is a patterned electrode made of electroconductive polymer, which is applied onto the levelling layer by screen-printing. Then, microencapsulated CLCs are applied and another layer of electroconductive polymers printed. On the top, the display is protected with a durable clear coating. Poly(3,4-ethylenedioxythyophene)-poly(styrene sulphonate) (PEDOT-PSS), which excels in perfect adhesiveness, low electrical resistance and high optical transmittance, is used as electroconductive polymer. The colour of liquid crystals is closely related to reflectance and bistability of CLCs under a controlled electric field. By applying several layers of liquid crystals with different stable pitch properties under an electric field, multi-colour displays are obtained (Shiyanovskaya *et al.*, 2005).

7.6.5 Water-soluble photochromic dyes

The development of new water-soluble photochromic dyes represents an important move forward in the development of less expensive photochromic dyes for textile and leather materials. We speak of a series of spirooxazine-based photochromic dyes containing a sulphonate group, which imparts water solubility to dyes. These dyes are designed for dyeing protein substrates, such as fashionable leather shoes and accessories, silk apparel and furnishings. Under the influence of UV irradiation (maximum wavelength 370 nm), a dyed silk substrate (at a dye concentration of 2% of weight of fabric) exhibited a change in colour from its original natural pale yellowish to green. The colour changes are much more distinct immediately after dyeing when the fabric is still wet than after drying. The wash fastness and photostability of dyed silk fabrics are moderate (Shah, 2005).

7.7 Sources of further information and advice

Important smart dyes are listed in Table 7.1 and commercial products producers in Table 7.2.

Table 7.1 Commercial smart dyes

1. Photochromic dyes Color Change Corporation (IL, USA)/ http://www.colorchange.com/ SolarActive International (CA, USA)/ SolarActive™/ http://www.solaractiveintl.com/ PPG Optical Products (Pennsylvania, USA)/ Photosol®/ http://corporate.ppg.com/PPG/opticalprod/en/photosol/default.htm James Robinson Ltd. (Huddersfield, UK)/ http://www.james-robinson.ltd.uk/index.htm Matsui International Inc. (California, USA)/Photopia®/ http://www.matsui-color.com/ Matsui Shikiso Chemical Co. Ltd. (Kyoto, Japan)/ Keystone Aniline Corporation/Reversacol®/ http://www.dyes.com/products/transprinting.html
2. Thermochromic dyes Color Change Corporation (IL, USA)/ http://www.colorchange.com/Matsui International Inc. (California, USA)/Chromiccolor®/ http://www.matsui-color.com/ Matsui Shikiso Chemical Co., Ltd. (Kyoto, Japan) Merck (UK)/ http://www.merck.co.kr/english/product/product-frame.asp?Level=6-1

Table 7.2 Commercial smart textiles

Producer	Textiles
SolarActive International/ http://www.solaractiveintl.com/ SolarActive™/	Threads for embroidery and weaving; clothes (T-shirts, wedding dresses, children's clothes), buttons, jewels, toys
Detco Enterprise (NC, USA)	Clothes
Super Textile Corp. (Taiwan)/ http://www.supertextile.com/	Umbrellas, shoes, caps
International Fashion Machines (WA, USA)/ http://www.if machines.com/	Exclusive textiles, future design, artworks
ECI Biotech Expressive Constructs, Inc. (Worcester, USA)/ http://www.ecibiotech.com/detection.php	Wound dressing

7.8 References

Addington D M, Schodek D L (2005), *Smart materials and new technologies*, Amsterdam, Elsevier.

Aitken D *et al.* (1996), 'Textile applications of thermochromic systems', *Rev Prog Coloration*, 26, 1–8.

Argun A A *et al.* (2004), 'Multicolored electrochromism in polymers: structures and devices', *Chem Mater*, 16, 4401–4412.

Bamfield P (2001), *Chromic phenomena*, Cambridge, The Royal Society of Chemistry.

Boh B *et al.* (2003), 'Microcapsules in textile industry', in Arshady R and Boh B, *Microcapsule patents and products*, London, Citus Books, 236–262.

Bouas-Laurent H, Dürr H (2001), 'Organic photochromism (IUPAC Technical report)', *Pure Appl Chem*, 73 (4), 639–665.

Bowlin G *et al.* (2002), *Electroprocessing polymers to form footwear and clothing*. World Intellectual Property Organization WO 02/032642 A3.2002-04-25.

Burkinshaw S M *et al.* (1998), 'Reversibly thermochromic systems based on pH-sensitive spirolactone-derived functional dyes', *J Mater Chem*, 8, 2677–2683.

Carlyle T, Rivera M (2003), *Meltspun thermochromic fabrics*. World Intellectual Property Organization WO 03/035948 A1. 2003-05-01.

Carpick R W *et al.* (2004), 'Polydiacetylene films: a review of recent investigations into chromogenic transitions and nanomechanical properties', *J Phys: Codens Matter*, 16, R679–R697.

Coates D *et al.* (2003), *Thermochromic liquid crystalline medium*. United States Patent US 6,660,345 B2. 2003-12-09.

Conner K H (1998), *Methods for increasing a camouflaging effect and articles so produced*. United States Patent 5,846,614. 1998-12-08.

Fisher E *et al.* (1967), *Stabilization additives for photochromic compounds*. United States Patent 3,322,542. 1967-05-30.

Fujita K, Senga K (2002), *Thermochromic microencapsulated pigments*. United States Patent 6,494,950 B1. 2002-12-17.

Hampp N (2005a), *Method for guaranteeing the authenticity of documents*. United States Patent Application Publication US 2005/0047593 A1.2005-03-03.

Hampp N (2005b), *Optical data store and method for storage of data in an optical data store*. United States Patent Application Publication US 2005/0111270 A1. 2005-05-26.

Hardaker S H, Gregory R V (2003), 'Progress toward dynamic color-responsive "Chameleon" fiber systems', *MRS Bulletin*, 28, 8, 564–567.

Hibbert R (2002), *Textile innovation*, London, Line.

Hongu T, Phillips G O (1997), *New fibres*, Cambridge, Woodhead, 56–59.

Hwu Y-R *et al.* (1993), *Method of making synthetic fibers containing photochromic pigment*. United States Patent 5,213,733. 1993-05-25.

Hwu Y-R *et al.* (1995), *Synthetic fibers containing photochromic pigment and their preparation*. United States Patent 5,422,181. 1995-06-06.

Ishimura N (2004), *Temperature-sensitive color-changeable composite fiber*. United States Patent 6,794,935 B2. 2004-06-15.

Kamada M, Suefuku S (1993), *Photochromic materials*. United States Patent 5,208,132. 1993-05-04.

Kamata, M *et al.* (1993), *Thermochromic dyeing method and cellulose product dyed thereby*. United States Patent 5,221,288. 1993-06-22.

Kamata, M *et al.* (1995), *Reversibly variable color patterning composition for synthetic resin articles*. United States Patent 5,431,697. 1995-07-11.

Kanakkanatt S V (1996), *Method of using multichromic polymers in packaging*. United States Patent 5,501,945. 1996-03-26.

Lim J *et al.* (2004) *Process for preparing polypropylene resin containing photochromic compounds and polypropylene yarn produced using polypropylene resin*. World Intellectual Property Organization WO 2004/065464 A1. 2004-08-05.

Masuko T (1987), 'New materials speed up skiers; heat-activated dye adds color', *Japan Economic Journal*, 25, 1291, 10.

Nelson G (2002), 'Application of microencapsulation in textiles', *Int J Pharm*, 242, 55–62.

Newman C (2003), 'Dreamweavers', *National Geographic*, 203, 50–73.

'New textile change color depending on sunlight' (1989), *Japan Chemical Week*, 30, 1501, 18.

Ono, Y *et al.* (2002), *Thermochromic acrylic synthetic fiber, its processed article, and process for producing thermochromic acrylic synthetic fiber*. United States Patent 6,444,313. 2002-09-03.

Orth M A, Berzowska J M (2003), *Electronically controllable, visually dynamic textile, fabric, or flexible substrate*. United States Patent Application Publication US 2003/0224155 A1. 2003-12-04.

Reinaldo de Oliveira Neves J (2001), *Use of thermochromic black pigments on white textile or coating materials, to save energy in buildings or other closed spaces*. World Intellectual Property Organization WO 01/92633 A1. 2001-12-06.

Rubner M F (1988), *Diacetylene segmented copolymers*. United States Patent 4,721,769. 1988-01-26.

Ruggeri C (1983), *Textile material coated with liquid crystals*. UK Patent Application GB 2 116 578 A. 1983-09-28.

Sage I C (1994), *Surface coating medium*. United States Patent 5,376,699. 1994-12-27.

Sanders M C (2003), *Device for detecting bacterial contamination and method of use*. United States Patent Application Publication 2003/0096315 A1. 2003-05-22.

Sen A K (2001), *Coated textiles*, Lancaster, Technomic, 187–189.

Shah M R B *et al.* (2005), 'Photochromic protein substrates', *Mol Cyst Liq Cryst*, 431, 235/[535]–239/[539].

Shibahashi Y *et al.* (1987), *Thermochromic textile material*. United States Patent 4,681,791.1987-07-27.

Shibahashi Y *et al.* (2004), *Method for alternately expressing color-memorizing photochromic function in toy element, and an alternately color-memorizing photochromic toy*. United States Patent Application Publication 2004/0135097 A1. 2004-07-15.

Shimizu G, Hayashi Y (1988), *Thermochromic composition*. United States Patent 4,717,710. 1988-01-05.

Shiyanovskaya I *et al.* (2005), 'Single substrate encapsulated cholesteric LCDs: coatable, drapable and foldable', *SID 05Digest*, 1-4. http://www.kentdisplays.com/corporate/print/2005SID.pdf

Somani P R, Radhakrishnan S (2002), 'Electrochromic materials and devices: present and future', *Mat Chem Phys*, 77, 117–133.

Tebbe G (2002), *Textile material for garments*. United States Patent Application Publication US 2002/0137417 A1. 2002-09-26.

Textiles – Tests for colour fastness – Part B05: Detection and assessment of photochromism. ISO 105 – B05: 1993.

Towns A (1999), 'The heat is on for new colours', *JSDC*, 115, 196–199.

Viková M (2005a), 'Colour change kinetic behaviour of photochromic smart textile sensors', in *4th Central European Conference 2005 Fibre-grade polymers, chemical fibres and special textiles: book of abstracts*. Eds Militký J, Maršálková M. Liberec, Technical University of Liberec, 129–130.

Viková M *et al.* (2005b), 'Textile based sensors – identification of dangerous gases penetration', in *4th Central European Conference 2005 Fibre-grade polymers, chemical fibres and special textiles: book of abstracts*. Eds Militký J, Maršálková M. Liberec, Technical University of Liberec, 139–140.

White M A, LeBlanc M (1999), 'Thermochromism in commercial products', *J Chem Ed*, 76 (9), 1201–1205.

Yoshihiko K *et al.* (1989), *Photochromic fiber*. JP1111007. 1989-04-27.

Part II

Smart medical textiles for particular types of patient

8
Intelligent garments for prehospital emergency care

N LINTU, M MATTILA and O HÄNNINEN,
University of Kuopio, Finland

8.1 Introduction

Prehospital emergency care is an essential part of the chain of survival in cases of trauma or acutely exacerbated diseases. An emergency is a more or less urgent and dangerous situation, because of weakening of some or many vital functions. Prehospital means the period before arrival at hospital. Prehospital emergency care includes all diagnostic and therapeutic procedures carried out by the ambulance (emergency care) team. This team consists of a paramedic and emergency care technician. In some organisations also an emergency physician or nurse can be involved. Appropriate medical control is crucial to guarantee high-quality prehospital care (Holroyd *et al.*, 1986). The organisation of emergency services differs greatly in different countries, and even in different areas of a country (Suserud *et al.*, 1998). For this reason the facts included in this chapter cannot apply to each national organisation. In order to understand the specific features of applications of smart textiles in prehospital care some of its basic characteristics will be described.

The working circumstances in prehospital emergency care are difficult and the tasks are demanding. The ambulance team gets its actual 'mission' by alarm centre personnel, the initial information on the particular 'case' is based on the alarm call and compiled mostly by someone who is inexperienced in health care. Each case is individual and diagnosis can be initially obscure on arrival at the patient. What has happened, what is the situation, how has it developed and what should be done, are logical questions in this situation. Based on patients described symptoms and signs, a preliminary diagnosis and estimation of degree of urgency are completed, but only on some certainty level. Clinical assessment includes patient's observations, measurements and palpations. However, these manual operations, based on human sensation, cannot detect deviations from the norm of all vital functions. Human senses can be clarified by patient monitors, which greatly supplement the clinical picture and open new areas for applications of smart textiles and intelligent garments.

8.2 Different cases and situations

Emergency care services provide care and transportation for a range of different categories of cases. There is a scale from extremely urgent, through urgent to non-urgent missions. There is also a great variation in the disease or trauma that has caused the emergency and of which vital functions deviate from normal and by how much. It will be necessary to estimate these deviations from the normal range. If possible, it includes the stabilisation of vital functions and hopefully returning them to a normal level before transportation.

8.3 Circumstances

The location and circumstances of incidents varies greatly. In most cases they occur at home, but often also outdoors in different circumstances. The weather can be very cold, rainy and windy. Also during transportation the patient is often exposed to outdoor conditions. A smart protection against variable conditions is thus a challenge for emergency care services.

8.4 Vital functions

It is important that every organ in the human body has continuously optimal oscillating homeodynamics under continuous neuronal and hormonal control. These are functions that are essential and vital for wellbeing. With the aid of intelligent garments it is possible to monitor different vital functions, such as ECG, circulation, respiration, EMG and skin temperatures.

8.4.1 Consciousness

Central and peripheral nervous systems monitor and control the body's functions and adapt them to surrounding ambience and its variations. They protect the body against external/internal influences and dangers. A fully conscious person can greatly facilitate the evaluation of a situation and survey its possible reasons by expressing sensations of the body and explaining their development. His/her important protective reflexes are active. Decrease of consciousness level means always decrease of body security linearly with the loss of perception. Then the danger of occlusion of airways increases as well as the probability of aspiration of gastric contents to bronchi.

Degrees of consciousness can be scaled based on eye opening, verbal and motor response (Glasgow coma scale). The opening of eyes can be spontaneous, a response to voice or to pain, or it is absent. The verbal response can be orientated, confused, inappropriate, and incomprehensible or absent. There is practically no instrumental method to monitor the level of consciousness.

8.4.2 Circulation

It is essential that every organ receives continuously enough oxygen and nutrients from blood circulation. Equally important is the removal of waste products including carbon dioxide. This situation requires normal blood volume, cardiac output and optimal circulatory distribution. The heart pumps blood to tissues through a vascular system consisting of arteries, capillaries and veins. Every contraction of the left ventricle creates a systolic pressure wave in great arteries, and the elasticity of arterial walls maintains the diastolic pressure in circulation. Blood pressure varies greatly between individuals and depends on physical activity (Thomas *et al.*, 2005). Blood pressure is necessary to create blood flow to tissues by overcoming the peripheral vascular resistance. Tissue circulation is controlled by dilation and constriction of local small arterioles. The heart acts according to the rhythm dictated by the sinus node. The impulse proceeds through atria to ventricles. Heart rate adapts to circulatory needs in accordance with the stroke volume which is the volume of blood pumped by one beat.

8.4.3 Respiration

Respiration requires rhythmic movements of the thoracic cage. This is necessary for the exchange of alveolar air and interchange of oxygen and carbon dioxide between alveolar air and blood in pulmonary capillaries. As a result arterial blood haemoglobin will be nearly completely saturated with oxygen. Haemoglobin in the red blood cells carries oxygen to tissues delivering part of the bound oxygen in the capillary to adjacent tissues. Alveolar ventilation also removes carbon dioxide from the body that is produced in tissues.

8.4.4 Body temperature

Thermal balance means that the temperature of the body is optimal for organ function. Core temperature, i.e., the temperature in the central inner parts of the body, is maintained within a narrow range, as human beings are homeothermic. In contrast to the core temperature, the temperature in the peripheral parts of the body, such as in the extremities, varies greatly in accordance with the ambient temperature.

8.5 Monitoring of vital functions

With our own senses we can estimate only roughly if vital functions are performing adequately or if they are deviating from the normal level. In some trauma cases the casualty is stained by blood and mud. Moreover, stress can cause a paleness of the face that can complicate visual estimation of the casualty's state. We can greatly augment our understanding of the actual situation of vital functions by recording parameters electrically, which represent cardiac function, circulation, oxygenation, ventilation and thermal balance (Konstantas *et al.*, 2004, Lymberis, 2004). Patient monitoring is based on probes and wires that can measure electric voltage or current, pressure or light flow. The necessary number and location of electrodes (probes) depends on which phenomenon (parameter) is recorded and how exact data are needed.

8.5.1 Electrocardiogram (ECG)

ECG measures voltage differences created by electric discharges in the heart during each cycle. From different leads of the electrocardiogram one can estimate the impulse propagation, heart rhythm, vascular resistance and possible lesions in the heart muscle as well as their location and extension. Myocardial infarction and cardiac arrhythmias can be detected with an ECG. The recorded ECG represents electric functions of the heart and has no direct correlation with the blood pumping action of the heart. The most impressive pathological evidence is given by a difference in present ECG compared with an earlier recorded one. The exact location of ECG electrodes is a prerequisite for the utilisation of the method in morphologic diagnostics. The probes should have a firm skin attachment and should not be allowed to move at all.

8.5.2 Pulsation

Pulsation is a quite informative circulatory parameter in different situations. Pulsation is recorded at the wrist (radial pulsation), at the inguinal channel (femoral pulsation) or at the neck (carotid pulsation). Pulse rate can be counted by pressing lightly with a finger on an artery but this manual method is laborious. As well as the rate in beats per minute, the strength (strong, weak or absent) and rhythm (regular or not) can be detected.

8.5.3 Pulse oximetry

Pulse oximetry is a highly respected measurement among patient monitoring methods (Nuhr *et al.*, 2004). Oxygenation is such an essential and vulnerable function, that a non-invasive method providing reliable information on oxygenation status is more than welcome. At present the measurement is based on the differences in light absorbance between oxyhaemoglobin and reduced haemoglobin. They are measured with two different emitted wavelength lights (Sinex, 1999). The probe is located usually on a finger, light emitter and detector on opposite sides. A specific algorithm calculates oxygen saturation and pulse rate (Barker, 2002, Gehring *et al.*, 2002, Tobin *et al.*, 2002). Moreover, a visible pulse wave can be reproduced on the screen. The amplitude of the pulse wave mirrors circulation changes at the measuring site (finger) and gives information on the peripheral circulation.

In the interpretation of saturation values one must master the oxygen dissociation curve characteristics. As the normal saturation is 95–98%, 92% means an imminent hypoxaemia and at the 90% level hypoxaemia is already real. Changes in oxygenation are fast in many emergency cases, and active treatment of hypoxia is both essential and effective. Pulse wave amplitude is a relative parameter, which strongly reacts to several different stimuli.

8.5.4 Measurements of body temperature

The measurement of core temperature from rectum, tympanic membrane or oesophagus is technically easy. Skin temperature measurements are a totally different entity. Both individual data and their differences serve as valuable material in the interpretation and conclusions. Temperatures and their textile-integrated measuring sensors are intrinsic components of intelligent garments for prehospital emergency care.

8.6 Selection of monitoring methods

In prehospital conditions all actions should be undertaken easily and quickly because of shortage of time and manpower (Birk and Henriksen, 2002). The selection of methods and parameters in patient monitoring starts from the real needs and benefit/effort ratio of the parameter. In each case it must be considered, which of the vital functions are absolutely necessary to evaluate and which parameters are the most informative for the diagnosis and status estimation. This type of intelligently and individually tailored patient monitoring would greatly increase the benefit/effort ratio. At the same time it reduces the flow of information which is also a very important aspect in emergency care.

8.7 Interpretation of monitored parameters

The interpretation of recorded data requires clinical experience, knowledge and good familiarity with the monitoring method and physiological background of the function that it measures. Very seldom the recording expresses directly what the diagnosis is and the actual patient situation. There is a need to interpret symptoms, signs and monitored parameters together and thus obtain a diagnosis by utilising all relevant means. Correct diagnosis and treatment is the main purpose of prehospital care.

8.8 Telemedicine

Therapeutic decisions require deep expertise in the interpretation of findings. There is clearly a need for teleconsultation to have an expert's advice on line (Bhatikar *et al.*, 2002). Telemedicine application for prehospital emergency care includes transmission of all recorded data to an expert, who can reconstruct the situation, give the correct diagnosis and send treatment and action advice in real time (Anantharaman and Swee Han, 2001). The essential contents of a patient's chart are anamnesis, status, measurement and recording data, all in structured digital form. Thus an interpretation is possible and reliable for an experienced emergency physician to make therapeutic decisions that are transmitted in digital form as a reply to consultation.

The best solution for the organisation of telemedicine services in prehospital emergency care would be one national expert centre, which would always be ready to add high-quality expertise to emergency care both for ambulance and health centre personnel. In the evaluation of a situation correctly monitored and recorded parameters and their trends are valuable because they can be transmitted to experts' computer screens. The effects of therapeutic procedures can also be followed in real time (Gallego *et al.*, 2005).

Presently, the teleconsultation in emergency care in Finland is limited to suspected myocardial infarctions. Twelve lead ECG is transmitted from the field to the nearest central hospital for evaluation and decision of starting thrombolysis is received back from the hospital before patient's transportation. This practice of immediate action has had a positive effect on the infarction outcome. In ECG transmission usually telefax is used.

8.9 Negative effects of transportation on vital parameters

The aim of prehospital emergency care is to stabilise a patient's state to a safe level, before the start of transportation, if it is possible. In an apartment building, carrying the patient on a stretcher from the upper floors is a physically demanding task both for paramedics and the patient. Carrying the patient in the head-down or up position can seriously influence his/her blood circulation. Elevators, on the other hand, are often so small that the patient must be carried in a sitting position, which can be fatal for the patient. During carrying and transportation the paramedic needs to supervise the situation by continuous patient monitoring, and intelligent clothing would be a valuable resource to detect the dangerous development of a situation in real time.

If the patient is well stabilised at the scene there is no need to drive him/her to hospital with maximal speed. Angular acceleration, acceleration and deceleration of the ambulance vehicle all have harmful effects on circulation (Sagawa and Inooka, 2002). These physical factors can also provoke nausea and vomiting, which can lead to dangerous aspiration of gastric contents into bronchi.

8.10 Patient chart

Presently anamnesis, symptoms and signs, observations and measurements are written on patient charts in analogue form. This form contains also notes on times of dispatch, of arrival at the scene and start of transportation and arrival at hospital. It also includes remarks on therapeutic procedures and medication. It is difficult, however, to include information of continuous monitoring in this written form. Its contents are not in transmittable form. A digital patient chart would be a radical improvement for the chain of information (Meislin *et al.*, 1999). All data would be in digital form as a database in the network, simultaneously available in real time for all involved in this particular patient's care. In this networking, a selected abstract of patient's case history could also be augmented before arrival at the scene. These facts could decisively improve diagnostics in prehospital care. The monitoring system based on intelligent clothing would offer valuable assistance to prehospital care.

8.11 Data security

When patient data and case history are handled, data security and privacy have always seriously to be taken into consideration. There are very strict regulations concerning patient data secrecy, which should be known and obeyed. These secrecy rules should not, however, prevent the patient getting optimal treatment, especially in emergencies. It is also important that only authorised health care personnel have direct access to patient data. If the paramedic asks for advice from a national expert centre, patient identity can be omitted so the interchange of data is fully legal and acceptable.

Because decisions on treatment are made based on values and trends of monitored parameters, they must be highly reliable and real. The treatment decisions also include great responsibility because they concern human health and possibly even life. All artefacts are harmful and potentially dangerous. The chain of information includes many points where the registered data can be corrupted. One of the critical points in this chain is the interface between the human body and the probe, just in the area of smart textile applications. Motion easily causes disconnections in tight contact as well as variations in the mobile net intensity. On the other hand, movement may be one characteristic of the emergency care.

8.12 Day surgery

Post-operative care has fundamentally changed in recent years. Earlier, patients were under close supervision after surgical operations in hospital for days, whereas nowadays some patients are returned home only a couple of hours after completion of surgery. Also new anaesthesia methods and anaesthetics have made earlier discharge from hospital possible. The adaptation of vital functions to so short post-operative observation is demanding. The most critical periods are the transportation home and the first twenty-four hours there. Patients' safety would require established reliable monitoring services after day surgery.

These monitoring services would benefit from a smart garment, which would include sensors, connectors, collector and emitter as a patient interface. The smart collector would continuously record and save trends as well as analyse monitored parameters to detect all impending deviations from normal. These functions require a large amount of artificial intelligence because many factors should be simultaneously noticed. The emitter unit would send the data to a call centre for further interpretation in case a parameter or its trend seems to be suspicious. At this level artificial intelligence inevitably requires support from top medical expertise. The most important is the appropriate response of emergency medical services to every alarming situation (Bhatikar *et al.*, 2002). This post-operative monitoring service is a special short-term application of home monitoring services for elderly ill patients (Dittmar *et al.*, 2004, Prentza *et al.*, 2004). In this way an intelligent garment can enhance the safety and wellbeing of the users and support health care.

8.13 Protective covering

One example of the multidisciplinary approach in the development of better patient protection in health care has been the Ergovaate-special clothing for health and social sector-process at the University of Kuopio during 2001–2003. Its aims have been to incorporate technology into clothing for use in emergency care and first aid by developing a protective covering for injured casualties with integrated patient monitoring and data networking. A new concept for emergency care was developed (Mattila *et al.*, 2003). The concept consisted of three different parts: (i) protection of the patient with rescue covering, (ii) monitoring the vital functions of the patient and (iii) connecting the patient data to a digital patient chart and wireless transmission. The developed and tested prototype of the rescue covering is currently in everyday use in, e.g., rescue services and helicopters in Finland (www.telespro.fi). A demonstration prototype of the patient monitoring and data transmission system was also developed. The protective covering is easy to use in typically demanding emergency circumstances. It does not hamper emergency care procedures. It is possible to touch, examine and treat separate parts the body while exposing only the relevant part to the effects of weather.

The selected special materials of the covering allow maintenance after each use. It is easy to remove contaminated blood and other body fluids and to clean the covering without damaging its protective and operating characteristics. This requires a high-class service system. When a casualty is transported to hospital in the protective covering, a replacement covering should be provided for the ambulance staff. This is the only way to guarantee uninterrupted preparedness for prehospital protection against hostile conditions, such as cold and rain. It is also essential that effective cold protection continues in the hospital during the first hours of stabilisation.

8.14 An integrated monitoring of vital functions

Integrated patient monitoring, data collection and data transmission systems are separate additional modules, which are most important and beneficial in multiple casualty traffic accidents, but they are useful also in single case emergencies. The final goal is a smart integration of probes and cables within the protective textile. A digital patient card would offer obvious advantages in the evaluation of the state of vital functions and their development over hand-written notes. In multiple casualty situations digital patient charts serve as a guideline for setting casualties in priority order to emergency care procedures and transportation. Digital information is not site limited, and is simultaneously available in the same form to all those who understand and need it for decision making. The principal implement in the utilisation of digitalised information could be a Palm PC.

The follow-up of location (accident scene, emergency care tent, local hospital, trauma centre) of casualties in the chain of rescue should be totally automatic, utilising wireless phone networks or special tags and detectors.

8.15 Mobile isolation

Some severe infectious diseases require efficient isolation to protect health care personnel and to prevent infection dissemination and a serious epidemic. The isolation need covers the time from the first suspicion of possible infection, through verification to full recovery. Because care of these infections demands special expertise, they are usually nationally concentrated on special units. As a consequence, suspected cases are often transported long distances and in a critical condition. This requires special preparedness of emergency care both to simultaneously care and isolate, and protect emergency care staff. A seamless isolation of infected patients is the most effective way to prevent the distribution of the problem. Efficient preventive and disinfecting measures are necessary during the whole chain of transportation from home to final isolation room in a central hospital. This includes public stairways, transportation vehicles and long hospital corridors.

The contamination risk concerns both the emergency care personnel and interior of the vehicle and all pathways the patient is carried through. It is difficult to clean the whole area and impossible to disinfect it. It is much easier to isolate the patient within an individual containment (Hänninen *et al.*, 2003). Such containment should be clean and ready to use and provide good isolation. It should integrate the opportunities for monitoring and care and be 'portable' to fit in the vehicles and elevators. The protective clothing should be impermeable to microbes and washable at high temperature without losing its benefits. This offers a challenge to materials.

8.16 Optimal smart solution for prehospital emergency care

Because time is the critical factor in sudden emergency situations all the components of the monitoring chain should be instantaneously applicable. As a matter of fact, all the time spent on attaching separate sensors, connecting separate cables, looking at separate screens and trying to get connections for real time devices means delay in diagnosis and appropriate treatment. This point alone provides an opportunity for an intelligent garment to provide all essential components in one entity (Anliker *et al.*, 2004) (see Fig. 8.1).

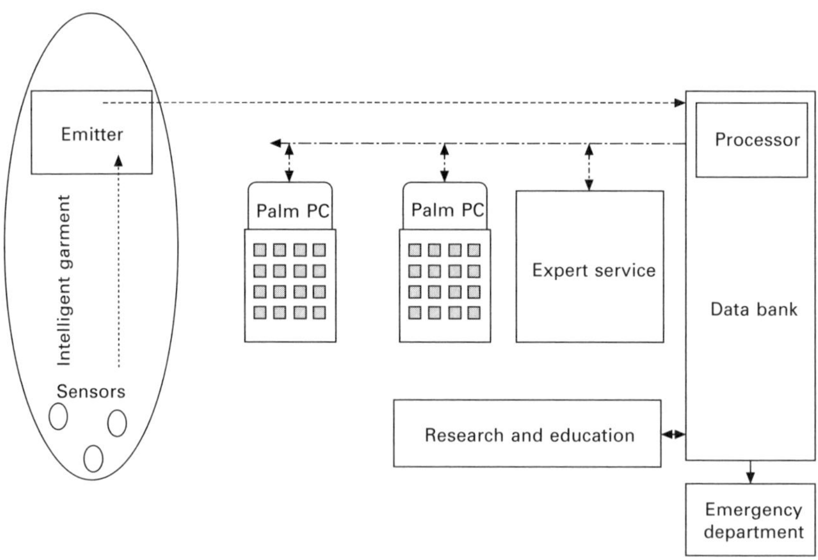

8.1 Schematic presentation of information pathways. The links make patient data available to all participants in medical rescue with the aid of sensors in the intelligent garment. Expert service is connected on line to the accident scene and databank. The databank serves current problem solving and research as well as educational needs.

8.16.1 Sensors

Many of the monitoring sensors can be integrated into textiles, e.g., a shirt or a thorax-surrounding belt so that a firm touch with the body at appropriate points can be achieved. Subsequently, the time of probe application would be greatly decreased. The differences in thorax size would provide inbuilt difficulties. All important parameters cannot be recorded from the thorax area, but need some other specific points of recording, e.g., for blood pressure, skin temperatures and end tidal carbon dioxide.

8.16.2 Cables

Different cables and wires that connect probes to collector units disturb measurements and they can become loose and be a source for faults in measured data. Textile integrated electrodes and wireless connections can solve the present problem of lead agglomeration.

8.16.3 Patient chart

Treatment decisions are based on different components of information such as actual anamnesis, case history, status, observations, monitored parameters, procedures and medication. This information should be in easily readable structured form, preferably in graphic phenotype. This entity is called a digital patient chart (electronic patient chart) and it represents a modern high-tech information tool as a completion to an intelligent garment. The same real-time information can be seen on the screen of the Palm PC of the paramedic at the scene, in the emergency department of the responsive hospital and in the experts' telemedicine office. If all digital charts are collected in one national archive, it could serve as a comprehensive source for research, development and education. So far this reliable documentation of different cases in prehospital care has been lacking.

8.16.4 Teleconsultation

The cases in emergency situations are often complicated and the need for expert advice for diagnostics and optimal treatment is urgently needed (Soysal *et al.*, 2005). This requires a standby advice service system, instantly ready to give appropriate medical advice on a wide range of problems. In a small country a national expert centre would be a justified solution to guarantee a high quality of teleconsultation round-the-clock seven days a week.

8.17 Conclusions

The presently available sensor and information transfer technologies make the follow up of the vital functions possible. Nevertheless, only a minimal part of the technically possible applications is in routine use in prehospital emergency care at present. Prehospital emergency care opens distinctive challenges for the application of modern technology and design in extremely demanding conditions. The applied monitoring technique can be decisive for survival through correct diagnosis to appropriate therapy enabling also teleconsultation on line. A partial solution could be an intelligent garment, which would provide integrated probes, cables and wireless connection to Palm PC (mobile PC screen) in one entity (Barnard and Shea, 2004). The adoption of the potentially valuable technologies takes time because of the difficult and multidimensional working conditions.

There is a need for efficient services from alarm to response, whenever intelligent garments are used in home care for elderly sick patients and postoperative monitoring after day surgery. Smart applications for emergency care require multidisciplinary cooperation of top experts in emergency care, in smart textile solutions and monitoring/information technology because end products and organisations should be usable in difficult field conditions.

8.18 References

Anliker U, Ward J A, Lukowicz P, Troster G, Dolveck F, Baer M, Keita F, Schenker E B, Catarsi F, Coluccini L, Belardinelli A, Shklarski D, Alon M, Hirt E, Schmid R and Vuskovic M (2004), 'AMON: a wearable multiparameter medical monitoring and alert system', *IEEE Trans Inf Technol Biomed*, 8 (4), 415–27.

Anantharaman V and Swee Han L (2001), 'Hospital and emergency ambulance link: using IT to enhance emergency pre-hospital care' *Int J Med Inform*, 61 (2–3), 147–61.

Barker S J (2002), Motion-resistant pulse oximetry: a comparison of new and old models', *Anesth Analg*, 95 (4), 967–72.

Barnard R and Shea J T (2004), 'How wearable technologies will impact the future of health care', *Stud Health Technol Inform*, 108, 49–55.

Bhatikar S R, Mahajan R L and DeGroff C (2002), 'A novel paradigm for telemedicine using the personal bio-monitor', *Biomed Sci Instrum*, 38, 59–70.

Birk H O and Henriksen L O (2002), 'Prehospital interventions: on-scene-time and ambulance-technicians' experience', *Prehospital Disaster Med.* 17 (3), 167–9.

Dittmar A, Axisa F, Delhomme G and Gehin C (2004), 'New concepts and technologies in home care and ambulatory monitoring', *Stud Health Technol Inform*, 108, 9–35.

Gallego J R, Hernandez-Solana A, Canales M, Lafuente J, Valdovinos A and Fernandez-Navajas J (2005), 'Performance analysis of multiplexed medical data transmission for mobile emergency care over the UMTS channel', *IEEE Trans Inf Technol Biomed*, 9, (1), 13–22.

Gehring H, Hornberger C, Matz H, Konecny E and Schmucker P (2002), 'The effects of motion artifact and low perfusion on the performance of a new generation of pulse oximeters in volunteers undergoing hypoxemia', *Respir Care*, 47, (1), 48–60.

Holroyd B R, Knopp R and Kallsen G (1986), 'Medical control. Quality assurance in prehospital care'. *JAMA*, 256 (8), 1027–31.

Hänninen O, Lintu N, Holopainen J, Seppälä S, Mattila M A K (2003) 'Preparedness needed to isolate suspected severe infection patients during transportation' in NBC 2003 symposium on *Nuclear, biological and chemical threats – a crisis management challence,* K. Laihia (ed.), U Jyväskylä Research Reports 98. 154–7.

Konstantas D, van Halteren A, Bults R, Wac K, Widya I, Dokovsky N, Koprinkov G, Jones V and Herzog R (2004), 'Mobile patient monitoring: the MobiHealth system', *Stud Health Technol Inform*, 103, 307–14.

Lymberis A (2004), 'Research and development of smart wearable health applications: the challenge ahead', *Stud Health Technol Inform,* 108 (1) 55–61.

Mattila M A K, Lintu N, Holopainen J, Seppälä S and Hänninen O (2003), 'Smart protection of trauma patients against weather influences in prehospital care', *Acta Anaesth Scand,* 47, Suppl 116, 57.

Meislin H W, Spaite D W, Conroy C, Detwiler M and Valenzuela T D (1999), 'Development of an electronic emergency medical services patient care record', *Prehosp Emerg Care*, 3 (1), 54–9.

Nuhr M, Hoerauf K, Joldzo A, Frickey N, Barker R, Gorove L, Puskas T and Kober A (2004), 'Forehead SpO2 monitoring compared to finger SpO2 recording in emergency transport', *Anaesthesia*, 59 (4), 390–3.

Prentza A, Angelidis P, Leondaridis L and Koutsouris D (2004), 'Cost-effective health services for interactive continuous monitoring of vital signs parameters – the e-Vital concept', *Stud Health Technol Inform*, 103, 355–61.

Sagawa K and Inooka H (2002), 'Ride quality evaluation of an actively-controlled stretcher for an ambulance', *Proc Inst Mech Eng,* 216 (4), 247–56.

Sinex J E (1999), 'Pulse oximetry: principles and limitations', *Am J Emerg Med*, 17 (1), 59–67.

Soysal S, Karcioglu O, Topacoglu H, Yenal S, Koparan H and Yaman O (2005), 'Evaluation of prehospital emergency care in the field and during the ambulance drive to the hospital', *Adv Ther*, 22 (1), 44–8.

Suserud B O, Wallman-C:son K A and Haljamae H (1998), 'Assessment of the quality improvement of prehospital emergency care in Sweden', *Eur J Emerg Med*, 5 (4), 407–14.

Thomas S H, Winsor G, Pang P, Wedel S K and Parry B (2005), 'Near-continuous, noninvasive blood pressure monitoring in the out-of-hospital setting', *Prehosp Emerg Care*, 9 (1), 68–72.

Tobin R M, Pologe J A and Batchelder P B (2002), 'A characterization of motion affecting pulse oximetry in 350 patients', *Anesth Analg*, 94, (1 Suppl), S54–61.

9 Smart medical textiles in rehabilitation

J McCANN, University of Newport, UK

9.1 Introduction

This chapter looks at applications for smart wearable textiles in rehabilitation from a design perspective. It proposes that good design is key in the development of textile related products that aid rehabilitation. To promote compliance in self-monitoring and remote monitoring of aspects of fitness and training during rehabilitation, products must be comfortable, look stylish and attractive and function reliably in relation to the medical and cultural needs of the wearer. The application of technical textiles with wearable technology, that is ubiquitous within the clothing 'system', provides a new generation of monitoring and responsive devices that aid rehabilitation and enhance the lifestyle of an inclusive market.

The current markets for clothing and electronics are separate. Medical devices are developed for 'ill people' with little aesthetic appeal. Technological advances are not readily accepted by some of their intended markets due to badly designed interfaces. To date the incorporation of technology into clothing has been crude at best, and has consisted of marrying existing consumer products into branded clothing lines primarily for sports such as snowboarding, running and fitness. Little has been done to address the design requirements of an inclusive market in terms of sizing, age and culture. Emerging electronic and textile related technologies are confusing to traditional clothing and textile development teams, while electronics and medical experts are not normally conversant with textile and clothing technology. There is a need for a shared 'language' and vision that is easily communicated between these sectors that is informed by end-users and their carers.

It is recognised that a rise in obesity, diabetes and heart disease is resulting with an ever-increasing financial burden on government and private organisations. For the age group 18–36 the continuing growth in obesity is creating 36% rise in medical expenses (Finkelstein, 2006). In order to reduce the level of illness and death associated with obesity and heart disease, governments are recognising the link between sport and fitness and the health of the nation through initiatives such as the Welsh Assembly's 'Food and Fitness Grant Scheme', and the 'Exercise Referral Scheme'. In Finland employees are funded to attend health research centres for tests, evaluation, and consultation regarding individual training programmes. The European Union (EU) is promoting the adoption of information technologies that promote 'Ambient Assisted Living' and independence from hospitalisation. This chapter stresses the need for smart wearable textile products that help to make activities more accessible and positive for those who find themselves sometimes rather abruptly referred for either individual or group rehabilitation.

The worldwide growth for biophysical monitoring wearable systems will grow from $192milion in 2005 to $265million in 2007, within three distinct market areas, health/fitness, medical and government/military (Krebs *et al.*, 2005). 'Baby boomers', who are remaining physically active well into their retirement, are sometimes defined as the 'worried well'. This group has a desire to ensure their own continued wellbeing by monitoring vital signs such as heart rate, temperature and blood pressure. 'The Baby Boomer Generation' (Promostyl, 2005) have lived with design all their lives with icons such as pop stars, film stars and models still prominent. These, and younger users, who do not want ugly, uncomfortable medical devices perceived to be for the ill, provide longer-term demands for well designed rehabilitation aids.

Good design, driven by end-user research, can help exploit niche markets where form and function work in harmony in the research and development of comfortable and attractive products that promote rehabilitation, (see Fig. 9.1).

9.2 Smart textiles used in rehabilitation

The design of smart textile products for rehabilitation must be informed by an understanding of a range of wearable textiles, their properties and constructions, appropriate textile assemblies and an awareness of the increasing blur between textile and garment manufacture. Textiles for use in rehabilitation will be determined by the type of smart fibre and yarn characteristics, textile structures and finishes that may be engineered and placed in relation to zones on the body, preferably to suit the demands of individual figure types, predominant postures and inclusive sizing. Closer fit and appropriate protection can be enhanced by stretch fibres, moulding, bonded seams or components and reinforced areas of support essential in effective rehabilitation. Stretch, in terms of both elastomeric yarn content and by means of mechanical stretch attributes and fabric construction, must be one of the most valuable characteristics for enhanced comfort, fit and movement in garments related to health and wellness. Technical fibre and yarn developments are key

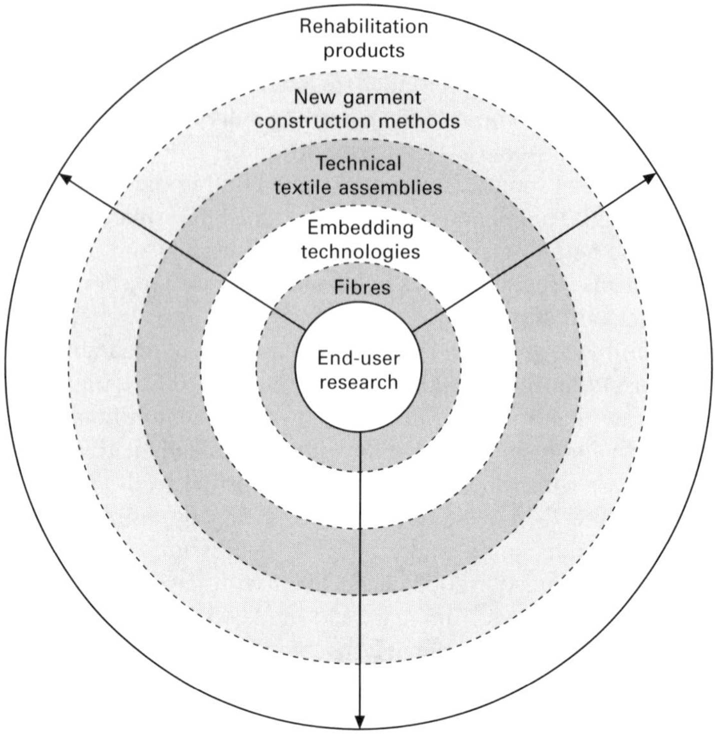

9.1 End user driven design research and development process for rehabilitation products.

characteristics of all fabric innovation but will not be covered in detail within this chapter. Major yarn producers cooperate directly with the machinery developers for the innovation in the production of knitted, woven and non-woven materials.

9.2.1 Knitting technology

There are two basic forms of knitting technology, weft or warp knit constructions both with attributes that are applicable to smart textiles and wearable technology for medical applications. Weft knitted fabrics can be produced in either flat bed or tubular form and may be highly elastic and highly drapeable while two-dimensional warp knitting progresses lengthwise, through the intermeshing of loops in the direction of wale. Unlike weft knit, warp knit is not easy to unravel but these fabrics are not as elastic as weft knit.

The clever use of circular weft knitting has been available in thermal underwear to keep older people warm for some years. Courtaulds, for a major high street chain, introduced a two-sided interlock construction brought together with a third yarn in every seventh stitch. This created columns down the length of the fabric, to trap still air and provide insulation, and could be knitted tubular to body diameters. Yarns could be selected according to Tog ratings with cotton at Tog value of 1, Polyviloft 2 and Silk/Viloft 3. Further Courtaulds developments involved the encapsulation of aromatherapy, for relaxation and encouraging sleep and muscle-easing and finally in antihistamine allergy remedies. Other relevant forms of microencapsulation in textile processing embrace skin cooling and moisturising agents, the delivery of vitamins and the incorporation of biosensors.

Recent innovation in thermal regulation has been in the encapsulation of phase change materials (PCMs). These microcapsules are embedded in textile fibres and, when worn close to the body, change their physical state when the temperature rises or drops beyond a preset level. In theory they enable the body to remain in a comfortable temperature range for longer, with no sweating or excessive chill, as the PCM either absorbs excess heat or releases it as required. PCM technology can be used in panels or zones, where the body loses or over heats, or in whole garments. The appropriate type of 'wax', or PCM, has to be selected according to the requirement of the end-use.

One of the most innovative 'pile' construction producers continues to be Malden Mills in the US. In 2002, in collaboration with the North Face, they developed the M5 battery powered fleece jacket providing 'warmth on demand' with a control unit allowing the user to adjust the heat level. Patagonia's recent development, 'Biomap™' (2005), informed by human anatomy and physiology, seamlessly combines areas or of thick variable knits, that provide insulation and padding, with areas of open construction for breathability, wicking and thermal regulation in relation to the needs of different 'zones' of the body. Engineered shaped channels and areas of reduced bulk, in combination with stretch, enhance movement and protection. The functionality of this variable knit technology can be enhanced with the application of different fibre types and finishes.

The introduction of computer aided design (CAD) in weft knitting is particularly of relevance in whole garment knitting. Shima Seiki has developed whole garment machines, where a pattern or garment specifications can be fed into the knitting machine and a seam-free garment can be knitted to end-user requirement in terms of measurement, yarn selection and stitch positioning. This new technology opens up the possibility of mass manufacturing techniques with opportunities for the designing of bespoke clothing for those who have mobility restrictions or who simply find conventional clothing inappropriate. Sophisticated 'seam free' structures comprise symmetric or asymmetric 'zones' around the body with variable attributes with regard to stretch and stability, moisture management, weight and/or density, all enhanced by fibre and yarn selection. The incorporation of conductive properties and textile sensors for monitoring vital body signs can also be strategically embedded into the textile structure (e.g. Wealthy, Textronics, Adidas/Polar).

Stoll promotes flat knitting machines that can produce 'three-dimensional, spherically curved products with all the reinforcements, openings and pockets that you require' in a single manufacturing process. The flexible protection of individual variations in patterns and jacquard applications, in two- and three-dimensional complex shapes can be produced 'quickly and completely with material savings and no waste'. Tubes and pockets, with finished selvedges, can accommodate pads and reinforcement splints while dense two needle bed constructions 'prevent penetration by foreign bodies'. The inlay of threads or yarns, can be altered from row to row and spacer structures can be incorporated during the knitting process. A breadth of fibres, monofilaments and multifilament threads, including 'wires and cables for heating elements, screening and the conduction of electricity', can be processed in single- or double-faced products. (Stoll, 2006)

9.2.2 Spacer textiles

Warp knitted spacer fabrics are structures that consist of two separately produced layers that are joined back to back. The two layers can be produced from different materials and can have completely different structures. The yarns that join the two face fabrics can either fix the layers or space them apart. It is this three-dimensional space that is the special feature of these structures. It can be easier to process high performance and high strength fibre yarns on knitting equipment in comparison with weaving equipment due to lower abrasion and tension and to shorter yarn paths during manufacture. Spacers can also be knitted on weft machines, the advantage being that it can be knitted in three-dimensional structures on a circular machine or on electronically controlled flat machines. There are limitations of the thickness of the fabric that can be produced and the range of structures. Spacer fabrics provide an added dimension and are being widely used as for their airflow and breathability and for their compression strength for the replacement of foam, cushioning and neoprene products. With the possibility of knitting different fibres on different faces, in different thicknesses and surface designs, many properties can be achieved for a range of end uses. They may be heat moulded with relevant applications including footwear soles, compression bandages, body armour to include orthoses. Yarn selection can be from natural to synthetic fibres, and micro-fibres, to include polyester, polyamide, Kevlar and Nomex.

9.2.3 Weaving technology

Woven fabrics can be designed to have many different aesthetic and performance characteristics as desired. Determining factors have to be considered at every stage of the design process from the fibre, the spinning of the yarn, woven structure, warp and weft density and any finishing technique. A woven fabric may be decided upon for several reasons, the most likely being its potentially superior strength and stability over other knitted or non-woven textile constructions.

As a general rule woven structures do not to have the inherent multiaxial stretch of a knit, which is a critical property when a textile is required to support and conform to the body shape. However, this can be challenged not only through the use of elastomeric yarns in both the warp and the weft, but also through selective use of leno structures, which also offer the possibility of a very open and lightweight fabric that retains a high level of stability. The stretch properties can be further enhanced by using an over twisted crepe weft yarn in instances where the use an elastane yarn would be inappropriate. 'Added value' characteristics can either be applied at the fibre or spinning stage, or as coatings or finishing treatments after the fabric has been woven, with ever greater research been done at the nano level. Such characteristics include: anti-static; stain resistance; anti-microbial; UV protection; and wicking, to name but a few.

A large number of branded fabrics with chemical anti-bacterial finishes have been on the market for some time, primarily aimed at the sportswear, uniform, and healthcare sectors. However, the jury is still out amongst healthcare professionals as to whether relying on anti-bacterial textiles is sensible, as they may encourage bacteria to develop resistance or mutate into stronger strains. It is also feared that hospitals may become too sterile for those recovering from illness, making them vulnerable to the bugs that abound in the 'normal' environment once discharged from hospital. Nevertheless, textiles containing yarns with inherent characteristics that promote healing are becoming ever more common in contemporary healthcare. Natural materials such as chitosan (derived from crab and shrimp shells), alginate fibres (seaweed) and silver, all share healing characteristics and are starting to be widely used in a variety of woven wound care dressings including bandages, gauzes and lint, as well as being used in clothing for those suffering from skin complaints such as eczema.

Pure silver has remarkable healing properties, but also boasts an enviable number of other extremely useful characteristics making it ever more popular. It has been proven to eliminate over 800 micro-organisms including MRSA (Methicillin Resistant Staphylococcus Aureus). It is anti-static, anti-electromagnetic radiation, anti-odour, highly conductive and also has excellent thermodynamic properties. Silver can be applied as a coating, or more efficiently used as a yarn (whereby it is bonded to a polyester core) and selectively woven into a fabric of a different fibre quality if required. 'See It Safe' by Toray is one such branded woven silver content textile aimed at the healthcare industry for use in bedding, curtains, uniforms, patient-wear, etc. Textiles that facilitate transdermal medicine delivery are another interesting area of research. Whilst still in the research stage, Re-Midi, founded by Diana Irani, is a fashion company that will release herbal remedies from clothing as soon as it comes into contact with skin, by responding to the natural pH of bodies (British Council, 2005).

9.2.4 Nonwovens

Nonwovens are textile materials often made from high quality fibres with versatile properties which can transform a two-dimensional substrate into a three-dimensional product. They function, often hidden away, as inserts, paddings, or as backings to give support to outer shell fabrics or three-layer assemblies or used as linings or insoles. In the context of rehabilitation, shock-absorbing foam is used for orthopaedic and medical products. It is claimed that visco-elastic polyester foam is breathable and, dependent on temperature and humidity, will absorb impact pressure, while slowly regaining its original shape on release. (Foampartner, 2006) The production of three-dimensional deep moulded products, such as Novolon™, can be digitised in a continuous moulding process in various patterns and mould depths adjusted to the desired properties. Novolon works with nonwoven, knits and woven products with the mould pattern and height determined to the performance specifications desired with regard to parameters such as airflow, absorbtion, compression resistance and weight. Virtually any colour, shape or density can be created. The d3o laboratory develops innovative protective material, with 'intelligent molecules that flow with you as you move but on shock lock together to absorb the impact energy' with applications into body, head, feet, gloves and hard shell products (d3o, 2006).

9.2.5 Ink-jet printing

It is reported that, in addition to artificial skin that can be grown a few millimetres thick, it may soon be a reality to produce 'made-to-measure skin and bones, which could be used to treat burn victims or patients who have suffered severe disfigurements' by using ink-jets that can print human cells. Professor Brian Darby and his team at the university of Manchester, can scan in dimensions into a computer to aid the placing of cells in any specified position to grow tissue or bone. Using ink-jet printers to print 'thin layers of a material repeatedly on top of each other' they can create three-dimensional 'tissue scaffolds' (Hunter, 2005).

9.3 Applications

9.3.1 Areas of rehabilitation specialisation

The emerging integration of advanced sensors and technologies into wearable textile structures provides a platform for a range of applications and end uses within functional apparel to promote health and wellness. To simplify the subject for those concerned with the design of textiles, clothing and textile related products, Fig. 9.2 identifies some important areas for consideration. The potential for the application of smart textiles cannot be contained exclusively within one category but examples are given that provide a link between certain textile constructions, and their particular attributes, with certain medical conditions.

9.3.2 Compression hosiery

A number of diseases can lead to a disruption in the flow of fluids leading to swelling in the legs, ankles and feet known as oedema. Varicose veins, veins that have been stretched out and do not move the blood back to the heart efficiently, result in a back up of blood in the legs. Congestive heart failure also leads to trouble with swollen legs when the weakened heart muscle is unable to operate efficiently as a pump that leads to blood stagnating in the veins, especially in the extremities such as legs and feet. A blockage of the lymphatic system resulting from cancer or lymph gland inflammation can also lead to leg and wrist swelling. As well as increasing the amount of

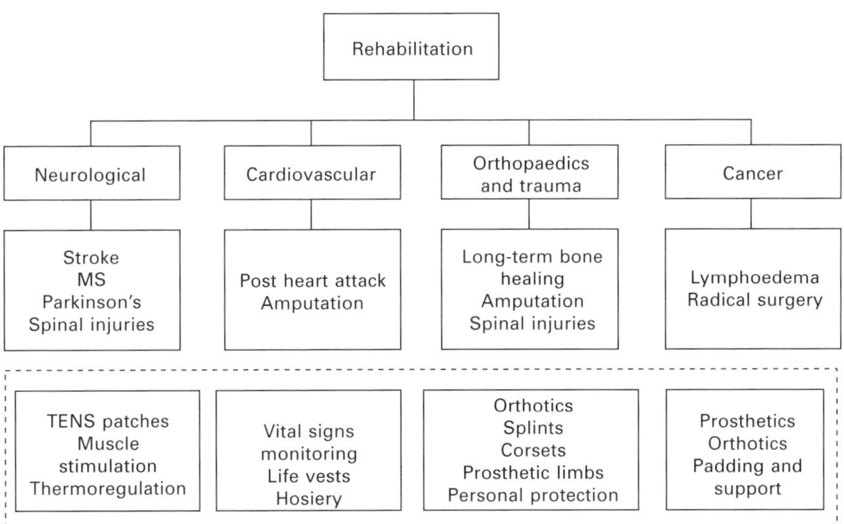

9.2 Areas of rehabilitation specialisation and smart textile related products.

exercise, to promote weight loss and strengthen muscles in the legs, to help the circulation of blood and other fluids back through the veins to the heart, one of the most effective means of treating the problem of oedema is to wear high-quality compression hosiery. This type of support hose provides the highest degree of compression support at the ankles, with the compression gradually decreasing up the leg. This improves venous return in the leg and helps lessen the pooling of fluid in lower extremities. In addition weight loss will reduce strain and pressure on veins in the legs and abdomen and improve circulation.

Compression garments are normally provided in standard sizes rather than made to measure. The William Lee centre, in Manchester, has created a system called Scan to Knit based on Shima Seiki technology. Bespoke medical compression garments are being developed for people who have developed severe ulcers through age, infection or injury. The project aims to improve the effectiveness of compression bands, that apply pressure which forces lymphatic fluid towards a functioning lymph node, by using a specialised computer-assisted manufacturing process. The leg is scanned, in a few seconds a three-dimensional (3D) model is constructed from the scans and then this model is fed into a knitting machine to produce a seamless garment. Much of this process will occur online, making easy communication possible between the hospital (where scans will be conducted) and the garment manufacturer. The whole garment technique is ideal as there are no seams to aggravate the ailment. When implemented commercially, this technology will save costs nursing time within the UK Venous Ulcer units and bring great long-term benefits of comfort and compliance for individual end users.

Custom-made compression stockings and support braces are knitted to anatomical shapes 'for general medical and orthopaedic use as well as stump socks, textile implants and spacer fabrics for use with orthoses'. Stoll technology produces 'articles for the prevention and treatment of disorders of the lymphatic and blood vessel systems and their consequences, as well as the treatment of hypertrophic wounds'.

9.3.3 Vital signs monitoring

Self and remote monitoring products will benefit a range of different areas of rehabilitation. The 'MyHeart' collaborative research project has developed a sensing garment for health surveillance based on a conductive woven structure, incorporating textile sensors, developed by Sefar Inc (MyHeart Project, 2006). The prototype has been trialled since 2004 at the Hospital San Raffaele in Milan. The textile sensors monitor the body's vital signs, to include electrocardiograpic (ECG), body temperature, blood pressure, respiration, activity and electromyogram (EMG). The record is 'digitised and evaluated by on-body electronics' and the results sent wirelessly to a mobile phone and from there to a server to be analysed by healthcare professionals. The commercialised version, promoted through Smartex, defined as 'intelligent biomedical clothes', aims primarily at identifying risk factors for the prevention of major cardio vascular diseases. It claims to interact with the user, as well as with professional services, in helping 'to avoid heart attack and other acute events by personalized guidelines and giving feedback' providing the necessary motivation for a new lifestyle. The potential for this technology to become available in attractive inclusively designed garments, would encourage compliance in exercise for rehabilitation (Smartex, 2006).

Subsequent stages in the MyHeart development of biomedical clothes focuses 'on the user motivation and the individual benefit' (MyHeart Project, 2006). The main objectives have been defined along five different application areas some with particular relevance to textiles with the potential to aid rehabilitation. 'CardioActive' will look at improved physical activity with products that stimulate users to be lead a more active lifestyle. The system will determine speed, distance and height levels, postures and gestures and dedicated physical training with relevance to sport and fitness. 'Specific training plans and recommendations for training will be personalised on the individual condition and ambition level of the user'. 'CardioBalance' will look at improved nutrition and dieting while 'CardioSafe' focuses on 'applications for early diagnosis and prediction of acute events'. Other groups involved in bio-monitoring include BodyMedia, Vivometrics, Sensatex Inc. and Textronics.

9.3.4 Pain relief

Pain relief accessories include TENS machines (transcutaneous electric nerve stimulation) and electro-muscle stimulation machines. Cefar claims that their 'Cefar Easy Belt' is effective for quick and easy targeted electrostimulation, to the lower back or abdominal muscles, or for gentle massage. This shaped black neoprene support is held in the desired position with a Velcro closure and with the stimulator positioned in a pocket on the belt. Currently electrodes are attached to rather than embedded in the neoprene. Another textile related form of pain relief is in the introduction of dressings with built-in pain medication that 'alleviate ongoing pain for people with chronic wounds' such as leg ulcers and pressure sores. A precisely engineered dressing can slowly and constantly deliver an appropriate dosage of pain-reducing drug directly into the wound. The Danish medical device manufacturer, Coloplast, launched 'Biatain-Ibu' at London's Royal College of Physicians in March, 2006 (Biatain-Ibu Coloplast, 2006).

9.3.5 Braces and splints

Orthopaedic braces include supports for knees, ankles, wrists and backs for a variety of conditions. An extensive splinting device, 'The Body Splint' has been developed by Second Skin, designers and manufacturers of medical custom made Lycra garments and splints. This 'garment' is both for children and adults who may have 'the neurological diagnosis of post traumatic head injury, CVA, post immersion injury or cerebral palsy'. It is designed 'to promote better arm and hand function by addressing issues of postural stability at the pelvis, trunk and shoulders. It controls trunk posture and addresses tonal issues of the upper limbs ... for clients whose trunk and pelvic instability, in addition to their arm tone, limits their upper limb function.' It is a highly interactive, educative device that covers the body with the design dependent upon the individual wearer's functional needs and objectives. Worn for between six and eight hours per day, the splint enables the wearer to perform daily activities in a modified position 'allowing their muscles to have the opportunity to perform at greater biomechanical advantage.' (Second Skin, 2006) The splint must be close fitting, cut to enable freedom of movement, and has extensive zips for donning and doffing.

9.4 Future trends

9.4.1 Smarter textiles – smarter design

In order to promote compliance in rehabilitation, traditional barriers that have existed between design and technology must be removed. As well as knowledge of technical textiles and sophisticated garment manufacturing techniques, such as moulding, bonding and welding, designers need an awareness of the technology of wearable computing. A generic glossary of terms is needed for those new to this hybrid area of design in the encapsulation of micro-electronics into textiles that explains sensors, data processing, actuators, communications and issues to do with power. The design research and development team of the future demands a shared language to bring attractive product to market that is accessible and affordable without being boring, stigmatising or over protecting. Wearable textile products, with smart and/or embedded technologies must be comfortable, easy to use and should look good. Designing for the physiological and biomechanical needs of the body must be indivisible with aesthetic considerations that are sympathetic to the particular culture and lifestyle of the wearer (Fig. 9.3). If successful, this new hybrid design area has recognised growth potential providing strategic business opportunities for industry partners to develop future markets.

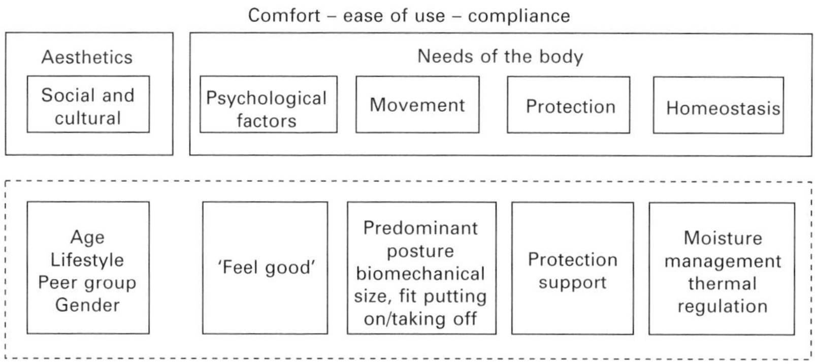

9.3 Identification of end-user design requirements relevant to illness.

9.4.2 Taking inspiration from performance sports apparel

There is an obvious opportunity for the transfer of technically and aesthetically innovative design principles from an early adopter of smart textiles and wearable electronics, the performance sports industry. Sports brands, also concerned with health and wellness, have been leading innovation in the application of technical textiles with attributes that include moisture management, antimicrobial properties, thermal regulation, protection from the weather and the environment and extreme personal protection. The cut and comfort of sports clothing with articulation for extreme movement and predominant posture has been enhanced through the use of stretch fibres and fabric constructions and seam free knitting. Innovation in laser cutting, garment moulding bonded and welded seams and textiles sprayed onto the body form are all more prevalent in the performance sportswear sector than in everyday clothing or fashion. Wearable electronics are emerging in products from leading sports brands and this provides an exciting and positive design led image to promote in the area of textiles for rehabilitation. These design principles could be extended to a more inclusive market in terms of size, age range, culture and lifestyle requirements.

At the Penn State Center for Sports Medicine, Dr William Kraemer, a distinguished sports medical expert, and DuPont of Wilmington, USA, conducted a five-year study from 1991–1995, into the relationship between compression garments and muscle performance. Garments for men and women in Lycra Power were intended to reduce muscle vibration, a major cause of muscle fatigue, to improve the feedback between body and brain, increasing accuracy and efficiency of movement. A series of findings from the research program claimed a measurable impact on performance with a direct link between wearing compressive sports apparel and an athlete's performance by reducing muscle fatigue and improving proprioception. The research showed that all types of fatigue (strength, endurance, and power) can be significantly reduced by wearing compressive garments and increased the accuracy of the athlete's movements or body positioning. The results were found to be even more remarkable with untrained subjects.

In performance monitoring, an Adidas and Polar partnership has launched 'Project Fusion' that combines Polar's heart rate, speed and distance monitoring equipment into Adidas apparel and footwear. To eliminate a hard chest strap, special fibres bonded into Adidas running tops work in conjunction with the relatively small Polar WearLink connector to monitor heart rate. Polar's stride sensor is placed in a cavity in the AdiStar Fusion shoe. (Anon, 2005a) The data is sent to a wrist-mounted computer that records and displays information in real time with the possibility to download and analyse data after the activity is over. In another collaboration with Polar, the NuMetrex™ heart rate monitoring sports bra uses seamless knitting techniques to incorporate a strapless heart rate monitor. Sensors embedded in the Nylon/LYCRA® knit construction replace electrodes and relay the heart beat signal by means of the Polar WearLink™ transmitter. This is snapped into the inside of the bra support band and communicates to Polar and other compatible analog watches and to fitness machines with integrated monitoring that provide training information. Numetrex claims that this bra gives a second-skin feel with superior comfort and support, moisture management and freedom of movement. Making clothing more comfortable, and the functionality easy to use with precise personalised feedback, has obvious benefits in effective exercise programs for individuals in rehabilitation.

Seamless knitted garment technology, applied to functional sportswear, demands a multidisciplinary mix of expertise 'as all the materials and processes have to be considered holistically as they interrelate and depend on each other for a satisfactory garment to be produced.' The fibre specialist, Unifi Inc., led collaboration between a specialist group of industry partners in the development of performance tennis garments from 2003–2005. The design research was driven by Nike's garment concepts that balanced performance with aesthetics in addressing the needs of top athletes. Wykes Ltd provided the precise yarn characteristics 'inextricably linked to knitted structures, quality settings, finishing techniques and sizing' appropriate for Shima Seiki 'WholeGarment' technology. Quantum Knitwear produced the garments and Stevensons Dyers carried out the garment finishing and testing. Despite the women's garment being worn at Wimbledon in August 2005, subsequent commercialisation of this development has been dropped by Nike 'on the basis of cost and lack of "wow" factor' (Knitwear Development, 2006). The future product development mix becomes even more complicated with the emergence of wearable technology with additional layers of legal protocol related to ownership of intellectual property. The testing and compliance associated with standards for health and wellness products introduces a whole new culture to be addressed by traditional textile and garment producers.

A leading innovator in body protection for sport, Lino Dainese, maintains that 'Design effects all human beings, from birth to death. Design is around us, on us and in us.' (Briatore, 2004, p. 33). The main focus of this company is 'the safeguarding of the body and of life' for extreme sport in making personal protection more comfortable and wearable. They aim for more natural movement with less impression of restraint 'to protect the parts of the body most subject to harm in case of a fall'. The Dainese Procom 'electronic under suit' is a system which measures biometric data with the monitoring of parameters, such as blood pressure, perspiration, adrenaline, etc., that determines the physical state and comfort of a rider (p. 110). Lino envisions a future where his aim is to bring project development at Dainese 'to an everyday level, because everyone needs protection. Elderly people fall down, they slip, almost always in their homes ... and they break bones.' Lino states that 'we feel closer to medicine than to fashion' (p. 25/26).

9.4.3 Linking technical textiles to eHealth

The area of sports rehabilitation, especially for high-risk groups such as elite athletes with a disability, has direct relevance. Companies involved with the development of textile related applications for rehabilitation have become involved in the promotion of health and wellness particularly in the sponsorship of international sporting events. Otto Bock Health Care, founded in 1919, a brand leader in the development of innovative wheelchairs, took on the role as 'Official Service Provider for the Turin 2006 Winter Olympic Games'. The company's international team for Turin was composed of 60 technicians who offered their services free of charge for athletes from all countries. Johnson and Johnson, with major business in medical devices, also pledged commitment as 'Official Health Care Products Sponsor' of the Turin games and as 'Official Partner to the Beijing 2008 Olympic and Paralympic Games'.

Performance sports clothing technology can be adopted in aiding the rehabilitation of certain disabilities. The characteristics and physiological requirements of the body change in relation to specific disabilities resulting in more extreme clothing demands. For example, injuries to the spinal cord prevent temperature regulation, through perspiration, from below the injury and, in some cases with quadriplegics, this also occurs above the injury as the information is not transferred to the brain and therefore it does not respond. For active wheelchair users the importance of moisture management, thermal regulation and protection from both the weather and the environment becomes paramount particularly when participating in sport. The comfort of clothing for disabled sport demands cut and articulation related to predominant posture and the required manoeuvrability. The demand for functional and aesthetically desirable inclusive design is recognised and increasing with social enterprises, such as Equal Adventure, providing the opportunity for disabled people to participate in sports.

Applications of seamless knitwear have real impact for inclusive design. The use of seamlessness allows for the subversion of normal ideas of back, front and left-right symmetry and for the distorting of the garment shape and the rules governing the placing of seams is completely avoided for the disabled or unconventional body shape. Claire O'Brien, a graduate, from Central Saint Martin's BA Knitted Textile Design, has challenged the convention of the traditional jumper by creating a jumper for an amputee, with the potential for this experimental work to be translated into mass production. The future scenario can be envisaged of people sitting in the comfort of their own space with a 3D scanner set up by the computer system. Once a chosen area of the body has been scanned the information can then be translated through the web to a receiving manufacturing unit for the resulting product to be mailed to the 'customer' within a given period of time.

eHealth is acknowledged as the major challenge facing Europe's healthcare systems. It could potentially become the third largest industry in the healthcare sector. At the 'eHealth 2005' conference Europe's Health and Innovation ministers concluded that they need to raise awareness of the pressing need for a more integrated and interoperable European health information space with a staged and structured approach over the next five-year period (Europe's Information Society Thematic Portal, 2006).

This chapter argues that improved design, in the functionality and aesthetics of textile related devices, will encourage individuals obliged to engage in rehabilitation, for a range of conditions, to comply with their prescribed activities. The potential exists for smart textile related devices to be more comfortable, in terms of moisture management and protection, to be tailor made and with enhanced functionality enabling the wearer to self-monitor or be monitored by their carers through the remote monitoring of vital signs such as heart rate and/or skin temperature. The link between eTextiles and eHealth has been made and this points to the potential for the mass customisation of textiles and clothing employing the innovative production methods promoted for the whole textile and garment chain by the European Union's Leapfrog Project (2006).

9.5 Sources of further information and advice

9.5.1 Power sourcing for smart 'wearables'

Konarka has a development programme to create portable wearable power-generating capabilities based on a technology that converts light to electrical energy combined with electronic textile systems to provide renewable, wearable energy sources for personal electronic devices. Benefits will include 'increased levels of convenience, freedom of use and performance while minimally affecting the garments' overall weight, size or appearance'. Daniel Patrick McGahn, Executive Vice President, Konarka (Anon, 2005b). Academic research is being undertaken into a 'flexible thin-film thermoelectric converter' wearable energy system to provide a promising solution in microscale thermal management and power generation and temperature sensing. 'In particular it will have impact on the design of future functional clothes that use body heat for power generation or personal climate control for medical condition monitoring of outpatients' (Guo Min, Cardiff University Engineering Department).

9.5.2 Internet links to health and wellness related products

BodyMedia:	http://www.bodymedia.com/main.jsp
Sensatex Inc:	http://www.sensatex.com/
Second Skin:	http://www.secondskin.com
Vivometrics	http://www.vivometrics.com
Textronics Inc:	http://www.textronicsinc.com/ourproducts.html
Numetrex:	http://www.numetrex.com
Dainese:	www.dainese.com
Equal Adventure:	www.equaladventure.co.uk
d3o protection:	http://www.d3o.com/ index.php?cont=21_technology&section=1
Coloplast:	http://www.coloplast.com

9.6 References

Anon (2005a) Seamless Integration Sportech (Future Materials) Issue 5 10–11.

Anon (2005b) Wearable power-generating technologies. *Technical Textiles International*, October/November 2005 p 6 [URI http://www.technical-textiles.net/htm/f20051015.088864.htm accessed 10th April 2006].

Biatain-Ibu Coloplast, 2006, The world's first wound dressing with built-in pain medication, Press Release [URI http://www.biatain-ibu.com/ECompany/BiatainIbu/homepage.nsf/(VIEWDOCSBYID)/726F2BCDE20EFE73C1257137003AE817 accessed 10th April 2006].

'Biomap^{TM}', (2005) Material Gains SGB Sporting Goods Business UK June 30th [URI http://www.connectingsport.com/news/fullstory.php/aid/89/Material_Gains.html accessed 24th April 2006]

Briatore, V (2004) Dainese II design salva la vita edizione billingue', Abitare Segesta.

British Council (2005) Feelgood Fashion, Culture Lab July [URI http://www.britishcouncil.org/russia-science-culture-lab-july.htm accessed 10th April 2006].

d3o Technology [URI http://www.d3o.com/index.php?cont=21_technology&section=1 accessed 10th April 2006].

Europe's Information Society Thematic Portal (2006) [URI http://europa.eu.int/information_society/text_en.htm accessed 10th April 2006].

European Union's Leapfrog Project (2006) [URI http://www.leapfrog-eu.org/ accessed 24th April 2006].

Finkelstein (2006) *The bare bones of obesity*. WSA March /April 32–3.

Foampartner (2006) Line of Foam materials. [URI www.foampartner.com accessed 24th April 2006].

Hunter S (2005) Scientists use ink-jet printers to create made-to-measure skin, *Technical Textiles International*, March/April, p. 8.

Knitwear Development, *Knitting International*, December 2005–January 2006.

Krebs D, Shomka, S (2005) 'Mobile and Wireless Practice, A White Paper on wearable systems – global market demand analysis, Second Edition', Venture Development Corporation, October 2005 [http://www.vdc.corp.com]

MyHeart Project, 2006, [URI http://www.hitech-projects.com/euprojects/myheart/ accessed 10th April 2006].

Promostyl, 2005 *BBG, Baby Boomer Generation*, Paris.

Second Skin (2006) Body splint [URI http://www.secondskin.com.au/content.aspx?tabid=4&itemID=4 accessed 10th April 2006].

Smartex (2006) Smartex, Woven Smart system, Electrotextile, Smart materials, fibers and fabrics, body tracking, piezoresistive fibers, graphite coated fibers, sensing garments, sensing seat [URI http://www.smartex.it/ accessed 10th April 2006].

Stoll (2006) The right way to knit, Technical Textiles with Stoll Flat Knitting machines [URI http://www.stoll.com/ accessed 10th April 2006].

10
Smart medical textiles for monitoring pregnancy

P BOUGIA, E KARVOUNIS and D I FOTIADIS, University of Ioannina, Greece

10.1 Introduction

Pregnant women living in remote areas work during pregnancy and face certain health problems (e.g. high blood pressure, kinetic problems requiring immobilisation, kidney or heart diseases, multiple pregnancy). Usually they feel uncomfortable with frequent visits for prenatal monitoring. The inaccessibility of the fetus, the sensitivity of fetal and maternal health status and susceptibility to psychological conditions pose significant difficulties in monitoring the progress of the pregnancy effectively. Furthermore, bulky or invasive equipment and long examinations in clinical settings affect both the mother and the fetus causing additional stress which influences their health. The use of a wearable platform able to monitor non-invasively fetal and maternal vital signs could improve significantly their living conditions. LIFEBELT is a transabdominal wearable device for long-term health monitoring that facilitates the parental monitoring procedures for both the mother and the fetus.

Hospitals and obstetric clinics, on the other hand, might avoid the frequent visit of additional patients (most of them hypochondriacs), so the remote health monitoring provided by LIFEBELT will contribute to a significant reduction of the hospitals' load. The hospitals' efficiency in that way can be increased as well as the quality of the provided services. LIFEBELT is also a valuable decision support tool for the obstetrician, who is enabled to monitor patients remotely, evaluate automated preliminary diagnosis of their condition based on collected and analysed vital signs, access patients' medical data at any time and most importantly be alerted when potential pregnancy complications require physical examination of the patient. Furthermore, the obstetricians are able to use mobile units and portable devices to organise their work and increase their work efficiency and effectiveness.

Another important goal for LIFEBELT was to foster an efficient collaboration link between medical research activities and Information Society Technology areas in order to produce innovative technological systems that are not only driven by fundamental medical requirements but can be effectively applied to serve daily individual needs (both for citizens and health professionals). Towards this goal LIFEBELT approach carried out mid-term multidisciplinary research on IT health application systems and disease detection mechanisms. Apart from the technological development, research aspects were supported and extended through the application of algorithms for medical diagnosis (and in some cases prognosis). Research on knowledge-based methods and intelligent classification algorithms for the signal processing and automated diagnosis were a major goal for LIFEBELT. Extensively tested algorithms and knowledge-based approaches were used to evaluate the maternal and fetal health status and detect potential risks for fetal hypoxia, pre-eclampsia, distress, intrauterine growth restriction, as well as maternal physical and psychological health problems (including congenital and other heart diseases). The processing and analysis of fetal and maternal heart rate and the analysis of cardiotocographic or simple ECG traces provide valuable clinical information about the health condition and progress of the pregnancy.

Finally LIFEBELT could be a precious tool for health professionals and medical researchers since it provides quantified information including analysis and prediction of trends, easy retrieval of case studies for education purposes and medical statistical data.

10.1.1 State of the art

Various commercially available devices and systems (either stand-alone or interconnected to hospital centres) have already provided vital sign monitoring and recording. These refer mainly to portable devices accompanied with special visualisation and processing systems as well as health services targeted at pregnant women [1–3].

The potential of measuring fetal (and maternal) ECG throughout most of pregnancy and labour is rightly identified as a unique development which could have ground-breaking clinical significance. It has two broad applications, one detecting hitherto undiagnosed abnormalities of cardiac function (congenital heart diseases, as well as those acquired during pregnancy such as twin to twin transfusion) in early fetal life, and the other, a new approach for the assessment of fetal well being during pregnancy and delivery. The first is a small but challenging application whereas the second is a large application and they should be assessed separately.

The ECG is an essential tool in the diagnosis and treatment of cardiac conduction abnormalities. Currently it is very difficult to isolate the fetal ECG, particularly between 28 and 35 weeks of gestation, probably because of the increase in vermix covering the fetal skin which 'insulates' the fetal cardiac electrical activity from the exterior. A capability to achieve a reliable and accurate fetal ECG recording throughout pregnancy has long been considered to be important in fetal medicine. ECGs can also be important in monitoring some high risk pregnancies, e.g., twin to twin transfusion. A third application of a fetal ECG is that it enables the accurate measurement of fetal heart rate, again not routinely possible, which in turn enables clinicians to monitor fetal heart rate variability (HRV) as a guide to fetal well being.

In such a wearable system fetal electrocardiogram (fECG) must be processed. Various techniques have been used for fECG detection and extraction. The most recent ones include algorithms based on adaptive filtering [4], FIR neural networks [5], fuzzy logic [6], IIR adaptive filtering combined with genetic algorithms [7] and a wavelet-transform based method using a bi-orthogonal quadratic spline wavelet [8]. A statistical method has been used for simultaneous measurement of fetal and maternal heart rates in real time for ambulatory monitoring [9]. Independent component analysis (ICA) for blind source separation (BSS) techniques have been successfully applied [10]. BSS is based on the assumption that the original (source) signals are linearly mixed and that these mixed signals are available. BSS finds in a blind manner a linear combination of the mixed signals and recovers the original source signals, possibly rescaled and randomly arranged in the output. ICA algorithms were tested and performed well.

10.1.2 Benefits resulting from LIFEBELT

LIFEBELT provides an innovative, intelligent, personalised health monitoring system to safeguard the health of both the mother and the fetus, resulting in tangible and measurable improvements in terms of 'quality of life'. It is an integrated solution for long-term health monitoring of the mother, enabling her to actively participate in the management of her own health during pregnancy and to respond to potential risk factors. Through the use of LIFEBELT, monitoring will become more frequent and will be achieved without unnecessary and embarrassing physical intrusions. More frequent monitoring will also result in a greater sense of 'safety' in the mother and contribute to a 'sounder' psychological state. LIFEBELT permits monitoring to be done on a regular basis, even when the mother is located in remote areas where access to properly equipped health facilities is difficult, time consuming, costly or where transportation is curtailed or rendered impossible due to local weather conditions. LIFEBELT liberates future mothers, by providing an advanced and safe, wearable monitoring device providing direct feedback to the attending physician 'anytime and anyplace'.

In the case of women who work, the empowerment is even greater as they increase their sense of safety in their working environment, minimise unnecessary absenteeism and disruptions to their working schedules resulting from frequent visits to the attending physician, while it further facilitates pregnant women by enhancing their ability to continue to travel for personal or professional reasons. LIFEBELT increases the chances of early detection through facilitating monitoring in a more congenial environment and saves time, effort and associated costs related to visits to healthcare professionals and hospitals. As mentioned above, this feature is essential in the case of pregnant women who live in remote and isolated areas. Finally, it improves the overall level of health services provided to pregnant women by reinforcing new and more effective monitoring procedures and promoting the use of IT in this particular medical field.

In the case of the attending health professional and hospital/medical centre, LIFEBELT provides an additional, innovative early-diagnostic and decision support tool which allows for personalised monitoring of a wide variety of parameters of both the mother (maternal heart rate, blood pressure, temperature, weight, oxygen saturation and abdomen growth) and the fetus (fetal ECG, fetal heart rate) all in the format of a convenient report, which can be received at any time. It increases efficiency and minimises unnecessary, time-consuming, one-on-one visits aimed solely at monitoring and allows for the provision of higher quality medical care to pregnant women. Additionally, LIFEBELT provides medical statistical data useful in generating studies of great value to the entire European health sector, assists in the introduction of additional, advanced IT solutions amongst health professionals and increases IT related skills in the European health industry allowing for further introduction of innovative techniques and products.

10.2 Methodology

LIFEBELT is an intelligent, personalised health monitoring system that will safeguard the health of both the foetus and the pregnant woman, thus contributing to early illness detection and disease prevention. The end product consists of the wearable device and the centralised system (Fig. 10.1). The wearable device consists of two components, the sensing module and the handheld device. The sensing module is a multi-sensor signal recorder jacket that uses two electric boards. These boards acquire in digital form the abdominal fECG and mECG, the maternal oxygen saturation (SpO_2), the temperature and the blood pressure. The chosen sensors are accurate, lightweight, and easy to use. As far as the ECG electrodes are concerned, these are disposable, pre-gelled, and simple to apply. CHEOPE (Chip for HEalth mOnitoring of PrEgnancy) is the ASIC chip used in the main board, which is able to acquire signals from different sensors and digitise them in order to transmit all the acquired measurements to the handheld device. A 16-bit microcontroller unit is used for data processing.

All the electronic parts and the sensors are collocated on a jacket to obtain a comfortable vest that is easy to wear. The garment was realised by cotton

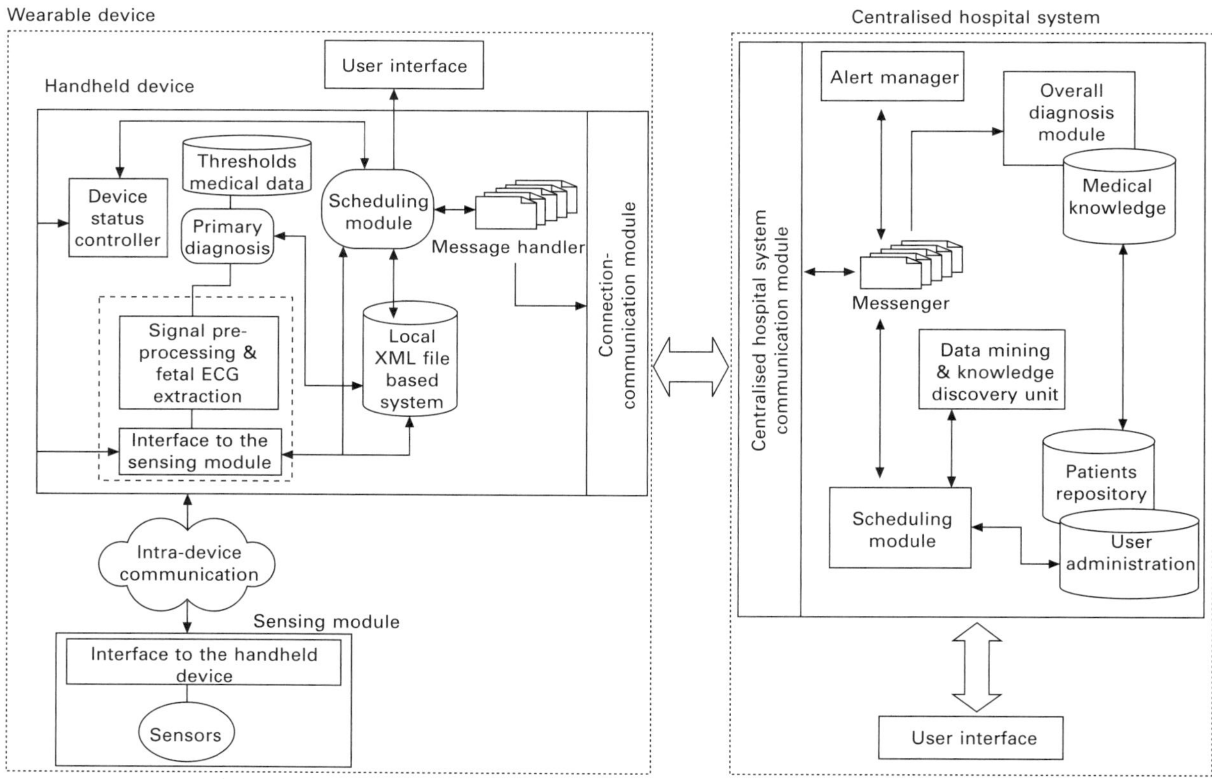

10.1 The LIFEBELT architecture.

to avoid any allergic reaction for the pregnant woman. As illustrated in Fig. 10.2, the garment looks like a vest with only one sleeve where the cuff for pressure measurement is attached; on this sleeve also the temperature gauge is connected. The vest has two pockets where the main board and the auxiliary board are accommodated (Fig. 10.3). Some cuts in the vest help the pregnant woman to identify the right position when applying the ECG electrodes (Fig. 10.4).

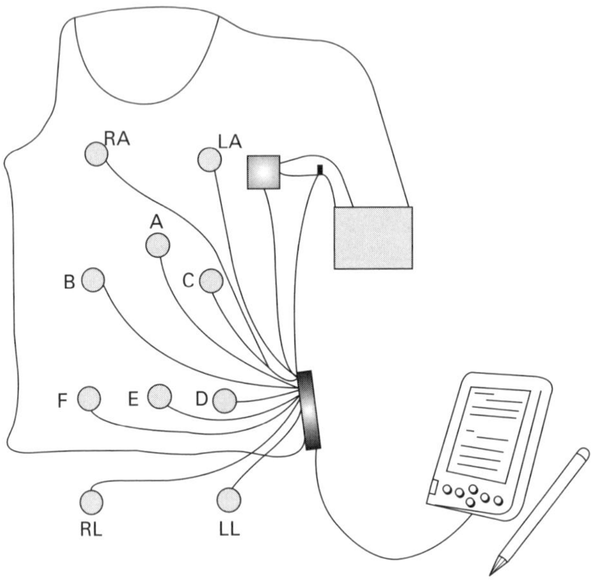

10.2 Sketch of the garment.

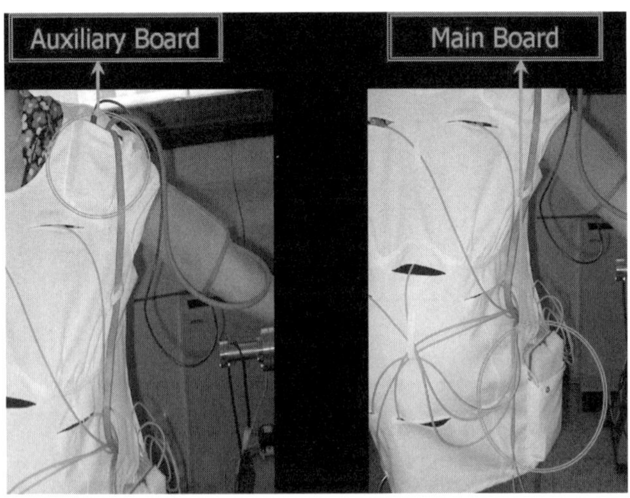

10.3 Electronic boards positioning.

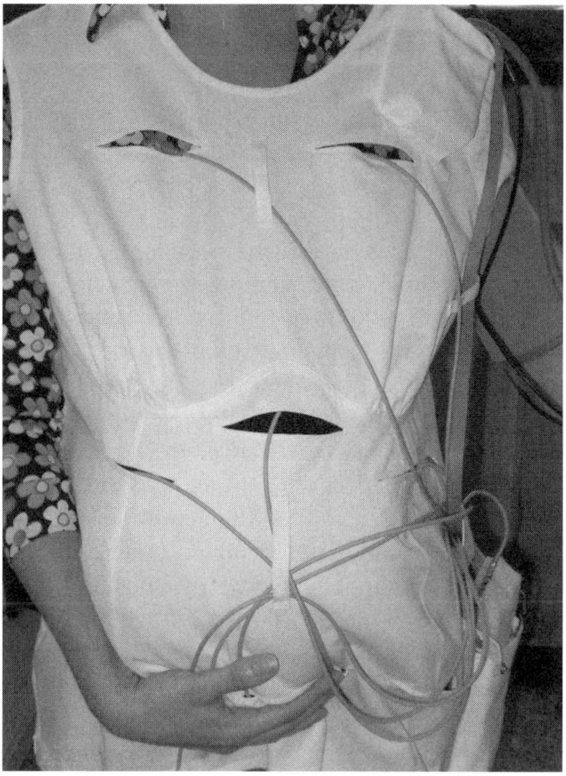

10.4 Frontal view of the vest.

The handheld device is a Tablet PC where signal pre-processing and fECG extraction is implemented. It performs preliminary diagnosis based on medical knowledge and predefined thresholds. It checks the schedules of monitoring and commences the monitoring procedure holding all the necessary data for the operation of the modules running in the Tablet PC. In addition, it manages communication with the centralised system. The handheld device incorporates a user interface, a signal pre-processing and storage unit and the communication module. The pre-processing unit records all acquired signals, checks the signal status (to verify that recordings of vital signs are not interrupted or corrupted) and make any necessary signal transformation (signal enhancement, preliminary filtering and A/D conversion). The processed signals are temporarily stored in the handheld device.

The user interface is pre-programmed by the health professional and customised for each specific user. It enables the pregnant woman to start the monitoring procedure (according to a pre-defined schedule) and input textual information regarding physiological and psychological symptoms or observations (special textual reports). The device also alerts the user, in case the signal levels are not up to the desired level, to re-adapt the monitoring belt or in case there is no reason to start measurements (e.g. the number of measurements per week predefined by the doctor is exceeded). The communication module is responsible for sending all collected medical information (multi-signal measuring reports and special textual reports) to the centralised hospital system through a GSM/UMTS (or other) cellular infrastructure.

The centralised system includes the system repositories and the modules to perform other functions. The modules comprising the centralised system fuse the individual measurements in order to provide a combined diagnosis on pregnancy status, manage the communication between the centralised system and the wearable devices and the algorithms for knowledge discovery and data mining in order to generate statistical anonymous data and trend identification. In addition, alerts and messages are generated in case of potential problems and abnormalities. The most crucial functions of the platform are signal processing and diagnosis (Fig. 10.5). More specifically the following functions are provided: (i) maternal and fetal ECG extraction, (ii) noise removal, (iii) arrhythmia detection, (iv) myocardial ischemia diagnosis, (v) data fusion and overall diagnosis.

10.2.1 Maternal and fetal ECG extraction

Our system's main concern is to extract both the maternal and the fECG using recordings of eight leads (three thoracic bi-polar and five uni-polar on the abdomen). The thoracic signals contain primarily the mECG, with little

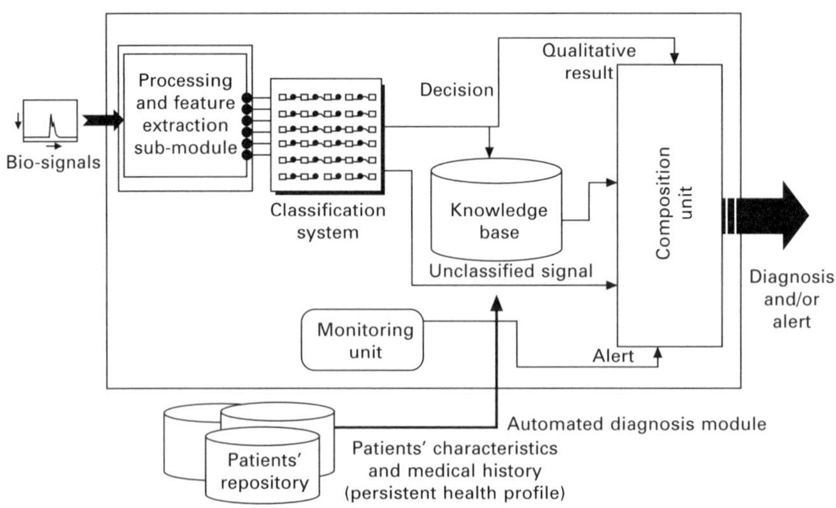

10.5 The automated diagnosis module.

if any contribution from the fECG. On the contrary, the abdominal leads record a composite signal, consisting of the contributions from both the mECG and the fECG. The extraction of maternal and fetal ECGs is based on the processing of all recordings (from eight channels) taken during an ECG measurement. Both thoracic and abdominal recordings are used for the separation of the composite signal and the analysis to its main components.

In the processing stage, the separated ECG signals (fECG and mECG) are filtered in order to remove noise. In the analysis stage all the main ECG characteristics are detected (P wave, QRS complex, T wave, ST segment, isoelectric line) and their features (time duration and amplitude) are estimated. The separated ECGs' (fECG and mECG) processing and analysis provide the extraction of key features such as decelerations, accelerations and short-term variability. This is especially important for the detection of foetal abnormalities and dysfunctions. The analysis of the HRV and characteristics extraction results are fed to an appropriately trained knowledge-based expert system that interprets and classifies the input signals, leading to a preliminary diagnosis for both foetal and maternal health disorders (e.g. pre-eclampsia, foetal distress, arrhythmia, maternal ischemic episodes, etc). Since this is one of the most crucial parts of the LIFEBELT project, several techniques were applied to the acquired signals and their performance was compared in order to choose the one which gives the best results.

Blind source separation techniques

Blind source separation (BSS) methods are used to extract unobserved signals (called sources), assumed statistically independent, from a few unknown mixtures of these signals. The main advantage of these techniques is that they do not require any prior knowledge about the signals (contrary to main filtering methods), only their statistical independence. Exploiting statistical independence leads BSS approaches to use high order statistics, usually higher than two, corresponding to the decorrelation used in the classical approach.

Three BSS techniques were evaluated: principal component analysis (PCA) [11], fixed-point independent component analysis (Fast-ICA) [12] and Jade-ICA [13]. PCA removes correlation from the observed signals while ICA eliminates higher order dependencies. In general, the ICA of a random vector consists in searching for a linear transformation that minimises the statistical dependence between its components. The concept of ICA may actually be seen as a higher order refinement of the PCA which can only impose independence up to second order (uncorrelation). Furthermore a novel algorithm, the complex continuous wavelet transform (CCWT), was developed for fECG extraction based on the complex continuous wavelet transform and a heuristic algorithm. The CCWT performs continuous wavelet analysis of real signals using complex wavelets [14]. CCWT is implemented following a four-stage schema. First, pre-processing is realised through signal averaging of all the recordings. Then, the mother's heart beats are recognised and in the third stage the candidate fetal QRSs are detected. In the last stage a heuristic algorithm is applied to identify the overlapped fetal QRS points and discard the misdetected (false positive) QRSs.

10.2.2 Noise removal

As far as myocardial ischemia and arrhythmias of the mother are concerned, the QRS complex, the isoelectric line, the ST segment and the T wave must be correctly detected. However, the presence of noise, such as power line interference (A/C), the electromyographic contamination (EMG) and the baseline wandering (BW), in an ECG recording is unavoidable, thus, making the detection process a difficult task. To overcome this problem we have developed a technique [15] to remove BW and to accurately detect the isoelectric line and the J point in cases where the ECG is contaminated with A/C and/or EMG noise.

10.2.3 Arrhythmia detection

LIFEBELT uses an efficient method for arrhythmia beat classification and arrhythmic episode detection and classification [16]. The method is based on the R–R interval signal extracted from ECG recordings. A set of rules is used for beat classification in four beat categories and a deterministic automaton is used for the arrhythmic episode detection and classification into six categories.

In the case of arrhythmia recognition the heart rate variability signal must be constructed at first, thus, the exact location of the main QRS point (peak of the R or S wave) is needed. This point is detected based on the maximum and minimum points of the QRS complex. The interval between two successive QRS complexes is called the R–R interval, even if the peak of the S wave is used. The heart rate variability signal results from the ECG signal and represents the time evolution of the R–R intervals. Our approach for arrhythmia diagnosis employs the information from the R–R interval. The procedure starts with the arrhythmic beat classification which is performed using a set of knowledge-based rules, applied on a three R–R interval duration sliding window. The beat classification results are fed into a knowledge-based deterministic automaton. The arrhythmic episode detection and classification is implemented for six rhythm types: ventricular bigeminy, trigeminy, couplet, tachycardia, flutter/fibrillation and 2nd heart block.

10.2.4 Myocardial ischemia diagnosis

A four-stage procedure was developed for ischemic episodes detection [15]. The four stages correspond to noise handling and ECG feature extraction, beat classification, window classification and identification of ischemic episodes duration. In the first stage, pre-processing of the ECG recording is performed to achieve noise removal and extraction of the signal features to be used for beat characterisation. In the second stage each beat is classified as normal, abnormal (ischemic) or artefact. This information is used in the third stage (the window characterisation stage) where each 30-s ECG window is classified as ischemic or not. In the fourth stage the identification of start and end points of each ischemic episode is performed based on the concatenation of consecutive ischemic windows. It is noted that the whole procedure described above is applied in each lead separately. At the last stage, a merging procedure is followed to identify the overall ischemic episodes from the episodes detected in each available lead.

10.2.5 Data fusion

Electronic fetal heart rate monitoring

This is commonly used to assess fetal well-being during labour. Although detection of fetal compromise is one benefit of fetal monitoring [17, 18], there are also risks, including false positive cases that may result in unnecessary surgical intervention. Fetal heart rate patterns are classified as reassuring, nonreassuring or ominous. After the FECG extraction, through BSS procedure, the mother and fetus waveforms are detected. The maternal and fetal R waves are detected (using a very simple methodology) and they are used in order to extract the maternal (MHR) and fetal heart rate (FHR). The procedure is as follows: the RR interval signal is computed as the difference between consecutive R waves and then the HR is calculated as 60/RR for each RR interval of the RR interval signal.

Baseline fetal heart rate

Baseline FHR is the mean FHR rounded to increments of five beats per minute during a ten-minute segment, excluding periodic changes and periods of marked FHR variability (segments of the baseline that differ by more than 25 beats per minute). Fetal tachycardia is defined as a baseline heart rate greater than 160 bpm and is considered a nonreassuring pattern. Tachycardia is considered mild when the heart rate is 160 to 180 bpm and severe when it is greater than 180 bpm. Tachycardia greater than 200 bpm is usually due to fetal tachyarrhythmia or congenital anomalies rather than hypoxia alone.

If the baseline FHR is less than 110 beats per minute, it is termed bradycardia. Fetal bradycardia is defined as a baseline heart rate less than 120 bpm. Bradycardia in the range of 100 to 120 bpm with normal variability is not associated with fetal acidosis. Bradycardia less than 100 bpm occurs in fetuses with congenital heart abnormalities or myocardial conduction defects, such as those occurring in conjunction with maternal collagen vascular disease. Moderate bradycardia of 80 to 100 bpm is a nonreassuring pattern. Severe prolonged bradycardia of less than 80 bpm that lasts for three minutes or longer is an ominous finding, indicating severe hypoxia and is often a terminal event. If the cause cannot be identified and corrected, immediate delivery is recommended.

Baseline fetal heart rate variability

Variability has been defined as FHR fluctuations in the baseline FHR over one minute. These fluctuations are variable in amplitude and frequency and are visually identified as the amplitude of the peak to trough in beats per minute. If the amplitude is not detectable, then it is described as absent FHR variability; if the amplitude is detectable, but less than six beats per minute, then it is defined as minimal FHR variability; if amplitude ranges from six to 25 beats per minute, then this is moderate FHR variability; if the amplitude is greater than 25 beats per minute, then this is marked as FHR variability. In addition, the presence of a sinusoidal FHR pattern should also be noted. The sinusoidal pattern differs from variability in that it has a smooth sine wave pattern of regular frequency and amplitude.

Acceleration

Acceleration is defined as an abrupt increase in the FHR, 15 beats per minute above the baseline, lasting for at least 15 seconds and less than ten minutes. Before 32 weeks' gestation, accelerations are defined as greater than ten beats per minute above the baseline for a duration of greater than ten seconds. Prolonged acceleration is defined as an increase in the fetal heart rate for greater than two minutes, but less than ten minutes (acceleration of ≥10 minutes is a baseline change).

Deceleration

Deceleration is defined as an abrupt decrease in the FHR with the onset of the deceleration to the nadir usually of less than 30 seconds. The deceleration should be at least 15 beats below the baseline, lasting for at least 15 seconds, but less than two minutes in duration. Variable decelerations are felt to be a response of the FHR to cord compression and are the most common decelerations seen in labour. Variable decelerations may be further divided into reassuring decelerations and non-reassuring or atypical variable decelerations. Table 10.1 summarises the categorisation of FHR traces which is used for the diagnosis of fetal health condition.

Maternal blood pressure diagnosis

This sub-system is responsible for assessing the recorded blood pressure values compared to stored medical thresholds. Normal blood pressure is below 140/90 mmHg. The first number is the systolic pressure. This is the pressure in the arteries when the heart contracts. The second number is the diastolic pressure. This is the pressure in the arteries when the heart rests between each heart beat. The categorisation of the blood pressure values is as follows:

- When a systolic blood pressure is between 140 and 160 mmHg or a diastolic pressure is between 85 and 110 mmHg then the pregnant woman has a mild-to-moderate high blood pressure.
- When a systolic blood pressure is above 160 mmHg or a diastolic pressure is 110 mmHg then the pregnant woman has a severe high blood pressure.

Furthermore, this sub-module categorises the diagnosed complications in relation to their severity, i.e., it generates a more acute alert for a systolic blood pressure reaching 160 mmHg than the one generated for a mild hypertension (140 mmHg) by taking into account the previous measurements.

Maternal SpO_2 diagnosis

Arterial oxygen saturation monitoring in pregnant women is useful in moment-to-moment assessments of therapeutic interventions (ventilator changes, intravenous volume administration, oxygen therapy). The sub-system responsible for SpO_2 diagnosis is based on the rule related to digital oxymetry saturation values; if the SpO_2 value is less than 96% the pregnant woman has hypoxemia.

Maternal temperature diagnosis

Normal body temperature averages about 98.6 °F. In pregnancy, a body temperature of at least 101 °F can be of concern. However, most studies have not shown a concern until maternal temperature reaches 102 °F or higher for an extended period of time. Hyperthermia most often occurs from a fever due to illness. Some studies have shown an increased risk for birth defects called neural tube defects (NTD) in babies of women who had high temperatures early in pregnancy. Studies have suggested that there may also be an increased

Table 10.1 Categorisation of the combined fetal heart rate traces

Feature	Baseline (bpm)	Variability (bpm)	Decelerations	Accelerations
Reassuring	110–160	= >5	None	Present
Non-reassuring	100–109 161–180	< 5 for = > 40 but less than 90 minutes.	• Early deceleration • Variable deceleration • Single prolonged deceleration up to 3 minutes	The absence of accelerations with an otherwise normal CTG is of uncertain significance
Abnormal	< 100 > 180	< 5 for = > 90 minutes	• Atypical variable decelerations • Late decelerations • Single prolonged > 3 minutes	

risk of miscarriage. Possible associations between high fever and birth defects such as heart defects and abdominal wall defects have been suggested, although the potential risk for these problems is small.

During pregnancy the maternal temperature is monitored and a corresponding diagnosis is produced according to the medical rules presented below. The sub-system also categorises the diagnosed hyperthermia in relation to its severity, e.g., it generates a more acute alert for a body temperature reaching 102.2 °F than the one generated for mild hyperthermia. Thus, the following set of rules is utilised:

- IF maternal temperature is between 99.5 °F and 100.4 °F, then the woman has mild hyperthermia and the alert severity is low.
- IF maternal temperature is between 100.4 °F and 100.94 °F, then the woman has medium hyperthermia and the alert severity is medium.
- IF maternal temperature is above 100.94 °F then the woman has severe hyperthermia and the alert severity is high.

Textual reports

A pregnancy report is information whose validity is relatively short-lived, and frequently updated, such as the daily measurements, contact with a health care professional, psychological and physiological status, etc. However, there are some parameters like emotional/physical condition, movement of the baby, etc., that constitute a valuable asset of the overall diagnosis of the pregnancy status but they cannot be evaluated using the monitored vital signals. For this purpose, LIFEBELT allows pregnant women to record this information periodically and send it to her doctor in the form of textual reports, using well-designed interactive software integrated in the small handheld device. The information included in a textual report is associated with bleeding notifications, discharge, bruises, cramping abdominal pains or back pains, sudden cessation of uterine contractions, feeling of dizziness, nausea, anorexia, difficulty in breathing, cough, visual disturbances, etc. This information is essential for the assessment of maternal and fetal health status and it is retrieved through a questionnaire that the pregnant woman completes every time she takes a scheduled measurement.

Medical history

Medical history contains all data needed for a comprehensive medical record providing information on general medical history, obstetrics history, previous pregnancies, family history and even the woman's lifestyle in order to determine predisposition, blood transfusions and operations, heart diseases and allergies. This data is initially recorded during the first contact with the health professional, it is stored in a typical patient record and it remains valid in the long term. This information feeds the LIFEBELT overall diagnosis module and through a rule-based technique is correlated with other types of medical information in order to achieve the current pregnancy status assessment.

10.2.6 Maternal and fetal overall diagnosis

Apart from the separate alerts provided in the preliminary diagnosis module in the form of notifications (e.g. appearance of arrhythmic episodes, increase in blood pressure or body temperature, etc.) the results of the primary diagnosis are combined with the textual reports input by the pregnant woman as well as with her medical history to provide useful diagnostic data about the fetal and maternal health condition and the pregnancy progress.

The overall diagnosis module employs such a process of combining data and knowledge from different sources with the aim of maximising the useful information content in order to produce information of tactical value to the responsible obstetrician and improve the system's reliability. The application of data fusion in LIFEBELT is perceived as essential due to the fact that pregnancy assessment is one of those areas in which the required output of the analysis may not be measured directly. The fusion which takes place within LIFEBELT occurs in the decision fusion stage. This is the stage where the measured data, with (MECG, FECG, blood pressure) or without (temperature, SPO_2) pre-processing, is combined with other data (previous measurements, textual reports, medical history, demographic data) and *a priori* knowledge (medical rules and thresholds) in order to generate a global assessment and suggestions for future monitoring parameters.

A simple example could be the following:

- if the pregnant woman does not have a medical history of hypertension
- if preeclampsia occurred in previous pregnancies (25% chance of recurrence)
- if there is an elevation above 140 mmHg systolic or 90 mmHg diastolic during the final measurements
- if the pregnant woman has headaches, visual disturbances, and epigastric pain (indicated in textual reports).

Then a suggestion for proteinuria examinations will be generated. If the result is higher than 300 mg of protein the system will diagnose preeclampsia. In order to achieve the development of the automated diagnosis module, extensively tested algorithms and knowledge-based approaches were used to examine the maternal and fetal health status and detect potential risks for fetal hypoxia, pro-eclampsia, distress, intrauterine growth restriction, as well as maternal physical and psychological health problems (including congenital and other heart diseases).

10.3 Results

Experimental results were obtained from the use of the previously described algorithms in a dataset of real and simulated recordings. All results for fetal R-peak detection were evaluated from expert cardiologists, who calculated three quantitative results: true positive (TP) when a fetal R-peak is correctly detected, false negative (FN) when a fetal R-peak was not detected and false positive (FP) when an artefact is detected as fetal R-peak. Indices of test performance can be derived from these results, such as sensitivity (Se) and positive predictive accuracy (PPA), as well as accuracy (PPAcc).

Our first dataset was composed of real recordings from a database created from the University of Nottingham. Abdominal signals were acquired from three channels of raw ECG data obtained from the same mother at 24 and 41 weeks gestation. The sampling frequency was 300 Hz and 12-bit resolution was employed. The acquisition system uses three pairs of electrodes placed around the mother's abdomen. Experiments in real ECG data provided results that were more than satisfactory (Figs 10.6 and 10.7). Table 10.2 shows results obtained using our novel algorithm in the dataset of the eight different recordings. The obtained sensitivity (Se) and positive predictive accuracy (PPA) reached almost 100% in fetal R-wave detection.

In the second dataset one real recording [18] and ten simulations were used for the evaluation of the proposed approaches. Each recording consists of eight channels, five abdominal and three thoracic. The real recording had one minute duration while the simulations had six minutes. The obtained accuracy for the PCA and the CCWT were 98.44% and 94.52%, respectively. The ICA methods (fast-ICA and JADE) presented the best results (100% for both sensitivity and positive predictive accuracy). All relative results are presented in Table 10.3.

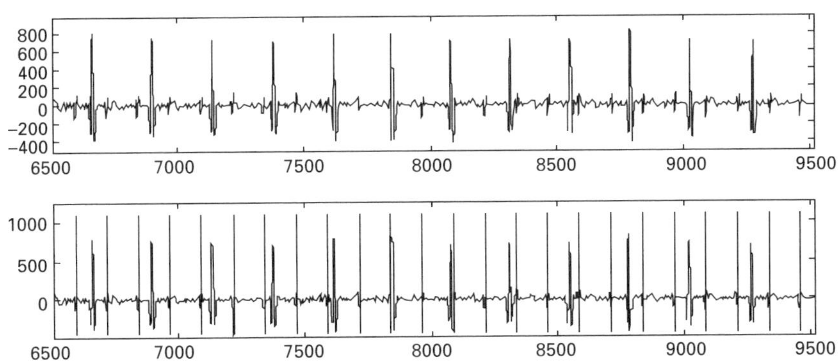

10.6 Observations (sensor signals), one of the three channels of raw ECG data obtained from the same mother at 24 week gestation. (12 bit, 300 Hz).

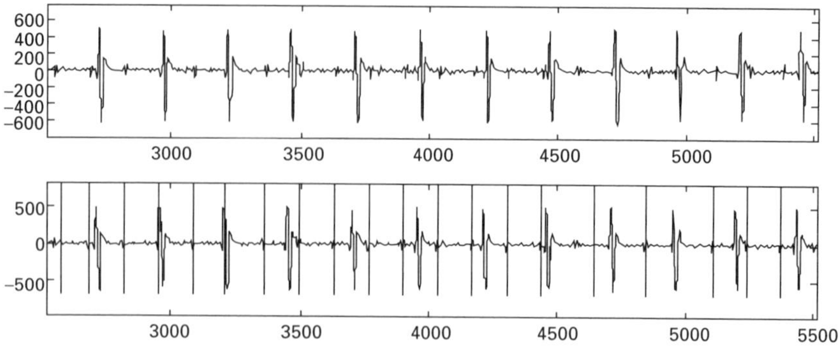

10.7 Observations (sensor signals), one of the three channels of raw ECG data obtained from the same mother at 26 week gestation. (12 bit, 300 Hz).

Table 10.2 Results for fECG extraction using the complex continuous wavelet transform

	TP	FP	FN	Se (%)	PPA (%)
Week 24	143	0	0	100	100
Week 26	139	0	0	100	100
Week 29	137	0	1	99	100
Week 35	128	0	0	100	100
Week 37	134	0	0	100	100
Week 39	143	0	0	100	100
Week 40	141	0	0	100	100
Week 41	121	0	0	100	100
TOTAL	1086	0	1	100	100

Our last dataset consists of real recordings taken by the LIFEBELT sensing module through a series of clinical trials. The ICA method was applied to this dataset since it showed the best performance compared to the other methods. An example of applying the JADE-ICA algorithm to raw data obtained with the LIFEBELT device is illustrated in Fig. 10.8. Clear evidence of fetal ECG presence is observed in the first, second and seventh channels while in the third, fourth and sixth channels the maternal ECG waveform is the dominant feature. Maternal ECG is also observed in the first, second and seventh channels together with the fetal peaks. In the fifth channel the dominant feature is noise. The outcomes of the ICA analysis were examined by medical professionals who validated the presence of fetal ECG.

10.4 Discussion

A wearable system is presented for the monitoring of the health status of the fetus and pregnant mother. The proposed platform acquires several vital signs, such as fetal and maternal heart rate, blood pressure, temperature and

Table 10.3 Results for fECG extraction using four different approaches

Signal	PCA	Fast-ICA	JADE-ICA	CCWT
Recording 1 (1 min) Real recording	TP = 22 FP = 0 FN = 0 **Se = 100%** **PPA = 100%**	TP = 22 FP = 0 FN = 0 **Se = 100%** **PPA = 100%**	TP = 22 FP = 0 FN = 0 **Se = 100%** **PPA = 100%**	TP = 22 FP = 5 FN = 3 **Se = 88%** **PPA = 81.48%**
Recording 2 (6 min) Simulated recording	TP = 875 FP = 0 FN = 0 **Se = 100%** **PPA = 100%**	TP = 875 FP = 0 FN = 0 **Se = 100%** **PPA = 100%**	TP = 875 FP = 0 FN = 0 **Se = 100%** **PPA = 100%**	TP = 875 FP = 24 FN = 10 **Se = 100%** **PPA = 100%**
Recording 3 (6 min)	TP = 716 FP = 26 FN = 2 **Se = 99.72%** **PPA = 96.49%**	TP = 716 FP = 0 FN = 0 **Se = 100%** **PPA = 100%**	TP = 716 FP = 0 FN = 0 **Se = 100%** **PPA = 100%**	TP = 716 FP = 19 FN = 6 **Se = 99.17%** **PPA = 97.81%**
Recordin 4 (6 min)	TP = 756 FP = 0 FN = 0 **Se = 100%** **PPA = 100%**	TP = 756 FP = 0 FN = 0 **Se = 100%** **PPA = 100%**	TP = 756 FP = 0 FN = 0 **Se = 100%** **PPA = 100%**	TP = 756 FP = 18 FN = 6 **Se = 99.21%** **PPA = 97.67%**
Recording 5 (6 min)	TP = 728 FP = 19 FN = 2 **Se = 99.72%** **PPA= 97.45%**	TP = 718 FP = 0 FN = 0 **Se = 0%** **PPA = 0%**	TP = 718 FP = 0 FN = 0 **Se = 100%** **PPA = 100%**	TP = 718 FP = 13 FN = 0 **Se = 100%** **PPA = 98.22%**
Recording 6 (6 min)	TP = 774 FP = 26 FN = 12 **Se = 98.47%** **PPA = 96.75%**	TP = 774 FP = 0 FN = 0 **Se = 100%** **PPA = 100%**	TP = 774 FP = 0 FN = 0 **Se = 100%** **PPA = 100%**	TP = 718 FP = 41 FN = 11 **Se = 98.49%** **PPA = 94.6%**
TOTAL (31 min)	***Se = 99.65%*** ***PPA = 98.44%***	***Se = 100%*** ***PPA = 100%***	***Se = 100%*** ***PPA = 100%***	***Se = 97.29%*** ***PPA = 94.52%***

respiration, and processes them in order to provide diagnosis. The data are transmitted to a centralised hospital system where, among other tasks, the diagnosis is generated. The main function which supports the system is that of fetal ECG extraction. This function uses ECG recordings from the mother's abdomen and for its implementation three techniques based on the theory of blind source separation (PCA, Fast-ICA and JADE-ICA) and a novel algorithm based on the theory of complex continuous wavelet transform, were developed.

It is not an easy task to obtain an accurate and reliable FECG in a non-invasive fashion using several electrodes. Problems develop due to the fact

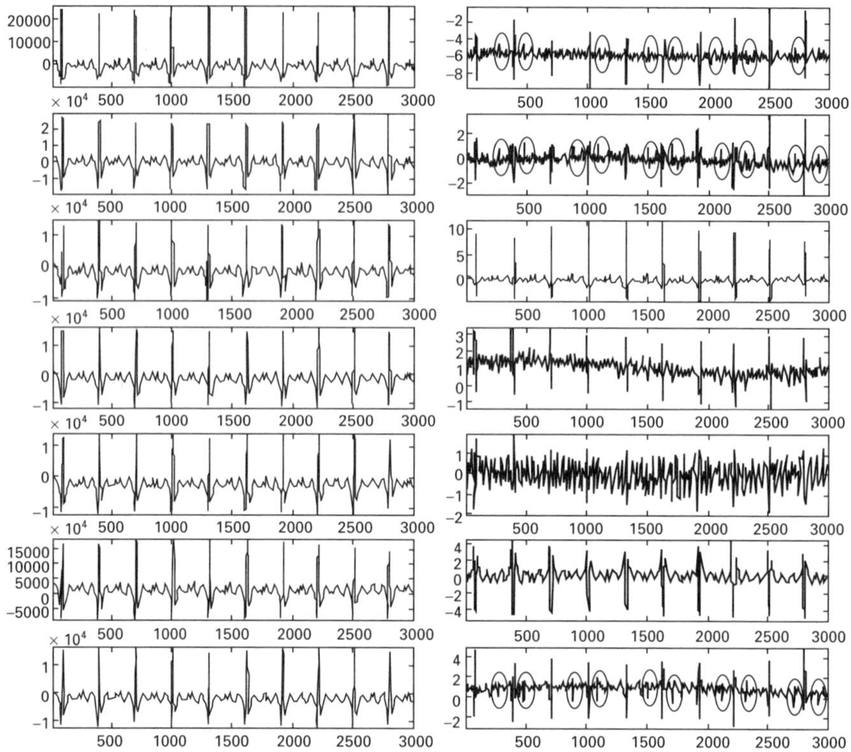

10.8 Left column: observations, eight channels of raw ECG data from LIFEBELT device. Right column: estimated sources or independent components applying ICA algorithm.

that the electrocardiogram (ECG) also contains a maternal electrocardiogram (MECG) which can be from one-half to one-thousandth the magnitude of the MECG. Moreover, the FECG occasionally overlaps the MECG and makes it normally impossible to detect. Along with the MECG, extensive electromyographic (EMG) noise also interferes with the FECG and it can completely mask the FECG.

For this purpose we tested four algorithms using three datasets. One with real data incorporating records from almost all gestation period, from the 20th to 41st week, another one with simulated data and a final one with real recordings from the LIFEBELT device. The proposed algorithms have been proven to be very efficient. The results cannot be compared directly with those of other similar approaches since there is no standard database with MECG recordings. Moreover, most of the detection systems proposed so far evaluate their performance using either simulated signals or a small number of real recordings.

In addition to the ability of extracting accurately the FHR signal, the current monitoring system was also designed to be applied non-invasively.

This feature is highly desirable from both the doctors' and patients' point of view. Moreover, the non-invasive nature of the system combined with its wearability makes the system appropriate for healthcare support at remote settings. The system proposes a major shift from a pregnancy information system based on the hospital setting to one which can always be carried by the pregnant woman and used at any time and place. The main problem in designing such wearable platforms is the elimination of noise from the vital signals. This is performed by the sensing module. Especially in the case of ECG acquisition, we observed that the signal is affected moderately by A/C interference, so better filtering modules could also be used to overcome this drawback. The overall system was evaluated through a series of clinical trials in order fully to examine its potential.

Obstetricians usually utilise Doppler ultrasound as the main tool for assessing the wellbeing of a pregnancy. We propose a wearable platform, which does not replace Doppler but complements accurate monitoring and diagnosis. The system combines several techniques for signal processing, analysis and fusion. It is easy to use and preliminary results indicate good performance.

10.4.1 LIFEBELT innovation

LIFEBELT presents a set of key characteristics that make it innovative both as a concept and practice for remote health monitoring. It is a multi-purpose wearable and not a portable monitoring device. It is 'user aware' and 'user customised' providing personalised service. It is non-invasive and easy to use, requiring minimum user intervention. It combines monitoring of a large range of vital signs (both fetal and maternal). The selection of the monitored biosignals has been made after thorough medical research of indicators and parameters that are crucial during pregnancy and may have a significant preventive, diagnostic or prognostic value for the health of both the fetus and the mother. The LIFEBELT sensors used to measure vital signs were appropriately selected to have absolutely no effect on the health condition of a pregnant woman (e.g. no Doppler ultrasound or other methods that could prove to be harmful for the fetus are utilised). The monitoring device is therefore suitable for long-term monitoring.

The LIFEBELT device is easy to use and cost effective, to allow broad use and distribution by health professionals and hospital centres (no requirements for costly, sensitive and bulky equipment, low-noise or magnetically shielded environment, skilled personnel). LIFEBELT provides a seamless communication link with the hospital monitoring and diagnostic centre, utilising new-generation communication technologies. The communication module is embedded in the hand-held device and is automated (no intervention by the user is required to start sending collected data to the hospital centre). The integration of the biophysical health record (containing both measurement of vital signs and text information reported by the pregnant woman) is integrated to standard electronic patient record (EPR) systems, through a common interface. In this way LIFEBELT enables the utilisation of existing EPR hospital systems.

LIFEBELT supports the use of mobile terminal devices, for all system users; the pregnant woman can insert textual information (about her physiological and psychological condition) and the doctor can access alert messages and patient data. Furthermore, LIFEBELT provides and combines innovative research algorithms for early and effective illness detection, utilising methods for the distinction of fetal and maternal ECGs and researching the separation of twin's fetal ECGs, knowledge-based approaches for detection of arrhythmia and ischemic episodes from the maternal ECG, methods for the detection of various risk factors for the fetus (e.g. pro-eclampsia, fetal distress and hypoxia).

Finally LIFEBELT supports medical research through the study of various indicators' correlation that may lead to diagnostic or prognostic medical decisions (e.g. increased blood pressure, no significant psychological stress of the mother, symptoms of fatigue, increase of weight, for example, may lead to the prediction or diagnosis of pro-eclampsia), the provision of a valuable source of information for the continuous education of health professionals (biophysical health records) and the generation of statistical data concerning various health indicators, symptoms and diagnoses during various stages of gestation.

10.5 Acknowledgements

The present work is part supported by the European Commission, Information Society Technologies (IST) as part of the project 'LIFEBELT (IST-2001-38165) – An intelligent wearable device for health monitoring during pregnancy'.

10.6 References

1. HomeMed, Home Monitoring System (U.S.). Available at: http://www.guthrie.org/Services/homecare/hommed.asp
2. FM-2 Antepartum Foetal Monitor. Available at: http://www.rememuseum.org.uk/electron/equip/elmedi.htm
3. Leeds University Medical School and Jopejo Ltd. Available at: http://www.leeds.ac.uk/media/current/jopejo.htm
4. Mooney, D. M., Grooome, L. J., Bentz, L. S. and Wilson J. D. (1995). Computer algorithm for adaptive extraction of fetal cardiac electrical signal, *Proceedings of the 1995 ACM symposium on Applied computing* (pp. 113–117). Nashville, Tennessee, United States.

5. Camps, G., Martinez, M. and Sofia E. (2001). Fetal ECG Extraction using an FIR neural network. *IEEE Computers in Cardiology* (pp. 249–252). Rotterdam, The Netherlands.
6. Khandaker, A. K. A. (2000). Fetal QRS complex detection from abdominal ECG: A fuzzy approach. *IEEE Nordic Signal Processing Symposium*. NORSIG, Sweden.
7. Kam, A. and Cohen, A. (1999). Detection of fetal ECG with IIR adaptive filtering and genetic algorithms. *IEEE International Conference On Acoustics, Speech and Signal Processing*. Phoenix, Arizona, USA.
8. Khamene, A. and Negahdaripour, S. (2000). A new method for the extraction of fetal ECG from the composite abdominal signal. *IEEE Med Biol Eng Comput*, 47(4), 507–516.
9. Ibahimy, M. I., Firoz, A., Mohd Ali, M. A. and Zahedi, E. (2003). Real-time signal processing for fetal heart rate monitoring. *IEEE Med Biol Eng Comput*, 50(2), 258–262.
10. De Lathauwer, L., De Moor, B. and Vandewallec, J. (2000). Fetal electrocardiogram extraction by blind source subspace separation. *IEEE Med Biol Eng Comput*, 47(5), 567–572.
11. Lathauwer, L. D., Moor B. D. and Vandewalle, J. Fetal Electrocardiogram Extraction by Blind Source Subspace Separation, *IEEE Med Biol Eng Comput*, vol. BME-47, pp. 567–72, May 2000.
12. Gao, P., Chang, E. C. and Wyse, L. Blind Separation of fetal ECG from single mixture using SVD and ICA, in *Proc. of the Information, Communications & Signal Processing and 4th Pacific-Rim Conf. on Multimedia* (CICS-PCM 2003), Singapore, 2003, pp. 15–18.
13. Vigneron, V., Paraschiv-Ionescu, A., Azancor, A., Sibony, O. and Jutten, C. Fetal Electrocardiogram Extraction based on Non-Stationary ICA and Wavelet Denoising, in *Proc. of the seventh International Symposium on Signal Processing and its Applications*, Paris, France, 2003, pp. 69–72.
14. Karvounis, E. C., Papaloukas, C., Fotiadis, D. I. and Michalis, L. K. Fetal Heart Rate Extraction from Composite Maternal ECG Using Complex Continuous Wavelet Transform, in *Proc. of the Computers in Cardiology* 2004 (pp 737–740), Chicago, Illinois, 19–22 Sept 2004.
15. Papaloukas, C., Fotiadis, D. I., Likas, A., Liavas A. P. and Michalis, L. K. A knowledge-based technique for automated detection of ischemic episodes in long duration electrocardiograms, *Medical & Biological Engineering & Computing*, vol. 39, January 2001, pp. 105–112.
16. Tsipouras, M. G., Fotiadis D. I. and Sideris, D. An arrhythmia classification system based on the RR-interval signal, *Artificial Intelligence in Medicine*, vol. 33, March 2005, pp. 237–250.
17. Sweha, A., Hacker, T. W. and Nuovo, J. Interpretation of the Electronic Fetal Heart Rate During Labor, *American Family Physisian*, vol. 59, May 1999, pp. 2487–2506.
18. Moor, D. DaISy: Database for the Identification of Systems, Department of Electrical Engineering, ESAT/SISTA, K.U. Leuven, Belgium. Available at: http://www.esat.kuleuven.ac.be/sista/daisy/

11
Smart textiles for monitoring children in hospital

C HERTLEER and L VAN LANGENHOVE,
Ghent University, Belgium and R PUERS,
Katholieke Universiteit Leuven, Belgium

11.1 Introduction

During the late 1990s, a convergence of developments led to a new era for the textile industry; the introduction of smart textiles. Because the textile industry is invariably looking for new challenges, it meets other innovation-orientated industries on its quest, which results in multidisciplinary research on smart textiles. Together with the emergence of innovatory textile materials, new perspectives are offered for the employment of textiles. Although smart textiles are applicable in a wide range of areas, a great deal of the research focuses on their use in garments. At that time, intelligent textiles were defined as textiles that are able to sense, actuate and adapt themselves to changes in the environment therefore some essential components such as sensors and actuators are required.

Parallel to this evolution, a new concept in healthcare emerged, which aimed at enhancing the quality of life for human beings by providing them with a wearable continuous monitoring system. As a result, the concept of a *wearable smart textile system* made its entry into the textile world. This clothing system typically has monitoring and processing capabilities for bio-physiological signals and provides online data about the health state of the wearer. It is obvious that textiles used for clothing are the ideal interface between the human body and external technologies. Moreover, a successful merging process between new textile materials, wearable microelectronics and advances in telecommunication technologies enables these developments. In order to fulfil the tasks that are assigned to a smart suit, components such as sensors, actuators, data processing and communication devices and an energy supply are essential.

It must be pointed out that the aim of the research is to maximise the possibilities of textiles and to realise as many components as possible in textile material. Moreover, several of these technologies are aimed at facilitating our lives. Implementing them into a garment can therefore considerably increase our level of comfort and safety in a non-obtrusive way. Children especially can benefit from this evolution because today's monitoring methods are not always child-friendly. Generally, children being monitored are prevented from moving freely because wires connect the sensors to the related instruments. By embedding sensors, interconnections, antennas and electronics in the garment, a child-friendly stand-alone suit can be obtained. In addition, the use of embedded textile components guarantees washability (and thus reuse) of the suit.

Based on these ideas, a Flemish project was set up in the late 1990s to develop a smart suit for infants, named the Intellitex suit. A consortium was founded with three partners involved: the Department of Textiles of Ghent University, the Electronics Department MICAS of Katholieke Universiteit Leuven and the Paediatrics Department of Ghent University Hospital. The four-year project was funded by IWT (Belgium). The realisation of the Intellitex suit will be elaborated here. Section 11.3.1 describes the measurements carried out on the respiration sensor, while the two following sections respectively report on the electrodes for monitoring the electrocardiogram and on the inductive data and power link.

11.2 Concepts

Smart textiles belong to a rapidly evolving research area. Throughout the years new prototypes of wearable textile systems have been presented unremittingly. This began in the late 1990s when Georgia Tech (USA) introduced the Wearable Motherboard™.[1] This smart shirt was developed for ambulatory monitoring of soldiers in combat situations. Sensors can be plugged onto the garment for monitoring biosignals. In addition to monitoring vital signs, the shirt can also detect bullet penetration. The garment itself consists of a grid of optical and electroconductive wires, acting as a 'data bus' through which data coming from the sensors is transmitted to a processing unit. The applied weaving process had to be adapted in order not to have discontinuities in this wiring system. The 'textile motherboard' can be tailored to each individual and provides a platform for a suite of sensors. This technology has now been made commercially available by the Sensatex[2] company.

Another smart garment, WEALTHY, has been developed by SMARTEX (Italy).[3,4] It is a wearable monitoring system that fully exploits the possibilities of textiles. Strain fabric sensors, piezoresistive yarns, fabric electrodes and electroconductive interconnections are all knitted into a garment thus allowing the recording of vital signs such as heart and respiration rate, electrocardiogram and temperature. The sensorised garment is completed with a portable electronic unit that processes and transmits the acquired data.

The LifeShirt™ by Vivometrics Inc. (USA) is a stretchable vest whose core sensor system is based on inductance plethysmography. The sensor is a sinusoidally arranged electrical wire mounted on an elastic belt. In addition to this respiration sensor, state-of-the-art conventional sensors are used to record the wearer's electrocardiogram, posture and activity.[5] The complete LifeShirt™ system is composed of three parts: the garment itself, a data recorder and PC-based analysis software.

A final wearable textile system to be mentioned here is a sensorised T-shirt developed within the French project VTAM (Vêtement de Télé-Assistance Médicale Nomade).[6] The T-shirt is equipped with four dry ECG (electrocardiogram) electrodes, a breath rate sensor, a shock/fall detector and two temperature sensors. Sinusoid-like conductors integrated in a textile belt monitor respiration rate, whereas electronic monitoring of the three-component acceleration of the body enables shock/fall identification. A miniature GSM/GPRS module for signal precomputing and transmission, together with a power supply, is stored on a belt that is carried around the T-shirt.

The above wearable textile systems are just a limited selection of ongoing developments. However, few developments are particularly aimed at children. The Mamagoose pyjama was developed by the Belgian company Verhaert. It is a baby suit for monitoring sudden infant death syndrome (SIDS). Three conventional electrodes are integrated to monitor heart rate, together with two capacitive elongation sensors for controlling respiration. This allows a continuous monitoring of the infant's health status and an alarm is sent out in case of potential danger.[7] Also the LifeShirt™ system described above is available in a paediatric size for children from five years of age onwards.

The above-mentioned state-of-the-art smart garments differ in their exploitation of the textile material. Only a few of them use the textile material itself as a sensing device instead of relying on conventional sensors. In a number of applications the textile material is utilised for making the interconnections between the (textile) sensors and the electronics, by knitting, weaving or embroidering them in/onto the garment. Nonetheless, all quoted research efforts express the feasibility and large potential of garments to be used as wearable monitoring systems.

11.3 Smart textiles for children in a hospital environment

The main aim of the research carried out by the Flemish consortium was to explore new textile materials and microelectronics to combine them in a garment for long-term, continuous monitoring of children in hospital. Babies having to be monitored in the prevention of SIDS are only one example in which the garment could be applied. The Intellitex suit is closely related to the Mamagoose pyjamas but clearly distinguishes itself in the more extensive use of textile materials.

Generally, it is an unpleasant experience for a child to stay in hospital. Not only the child but also its parents feel uncomfortable in this unfamiliar situation. Therefore continuous efforts are being made to improve the ambience. Part of this can be achieved by avoiding or decreasing the number of wires that cover the child's body when it is monitored. The electrodes and the wires connecting it to the monitors prevent the child from moving freely and complicate cuddling and hugging the child. Furthermore, monitors using conventional sensor technology often cause skin problems. The monitoring systems currently in use are generally not really 'child-friendly'. But the recent advances in smart textiles can remedy these shortcomings by substituting all these sensors, data processing units, storage and transmission circuitry and interconnections by a single monitoring garment. The patient will not only experience wearing such a garment as normal, but also will be provided with more comfort, mobility and privacy.

From the beginning of the project, we decided to focus mainly on the development of a textile sensor-based system for long-term continuous monitoring of heart and respiration rate. We named it the Intellitex suit. In contrast to other projects we resolved not to integrate conventional sensors but to exploit the capabilities of textile material as such. Therefore, we adopted electroconductive textiles, particularly stainless steel yarns and structures. These yarns are currently being knitted, woven and embroidered by using existing textile technology. The potential of these electroconductive yarns was exploited by integrating them in a garment. The yarn was also used to make the interconnections and the inductive link, hence resulting in an increased integration. In this way the foundations of a washable and child-friendly garment were laid.

11.3.1 Respiration measurements

The respiration rate is measured in various ways, e.g., by sensing pressure, detecting CO_2/O_2 concentration in inhaled and exhaled air, applying body plethysmography (inductance, impedance, capacitance, etc.) and using strain gauges. In the framework of this research, we gave preference to building textile-based strain gauges. In a knitted structure we combined elastic and electroconductive yarns (stainless steel yarns manufactured by the Belgian company Bekintex). Knitted structures were chosen on the one hand because of their inherently elastic properties and on the other hand because undergarments are mainly knitted fabrics. By placing the structure as a coil around the abdomen or thorax, a variation in resistance caused by breathing is obtained. Therefore the highly elastic component is important because it allows the structure to adapt itself to the moving upper body, hence detecting circumference changes.

Several electroconductive, elastic textile structures were successively tested in a controlled environment to evaluate their ability for long-term use and possible property changes after washing.[8] Based on preliminary research, which proved anisotropy in resistance change for knitted structures, they were stretched in the wale direction, as shown in Fig. 11.1. Resistance changes in the course direction are considerably less pronounced because the current flows through one thread uninterruptedly and this conducting path does not change upon stretching. When the structure is stretched in the wale direction, however, the contact points between the successive rows of loops play a prevailing role in the resistance changes. Upon stretching, an increase in contact points results in a decrease of the overall resistance of the structure.

A dynamic resistance measurement set-up was developed to determine these resistance changes. The core instrument was a yarn tensile tester and it was programmed to perform a continuous cyclic elongation which simulates breathing movement. The structure being tested is a circular knitted one, consisting of elasthane as the elastic component and Bekinox stainless steel yarn as the electroconductive component. Figure 11.2 shows the resistance change when the structure is elongated up to 40% and relaxed back to 10%. During the first eight seconds the resistance remains constant, followed by a decrease as the structure is elongated. Subsequently the resistance increases as the structure is relaxed to 10% elongation.

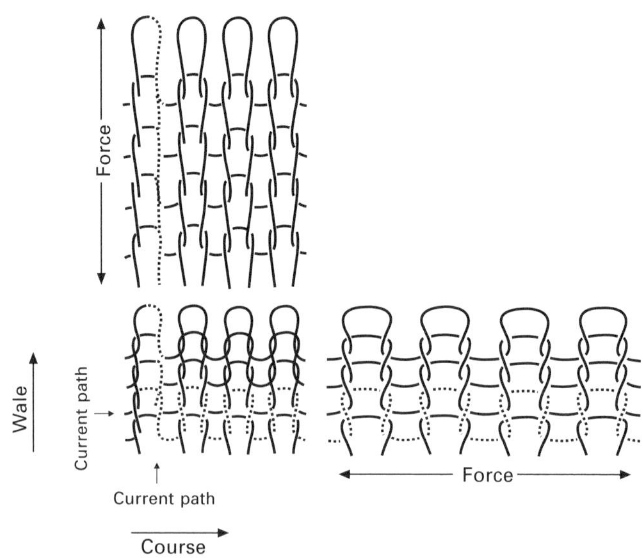

11.1 Conducting path in the course and wale directions upon stretching.

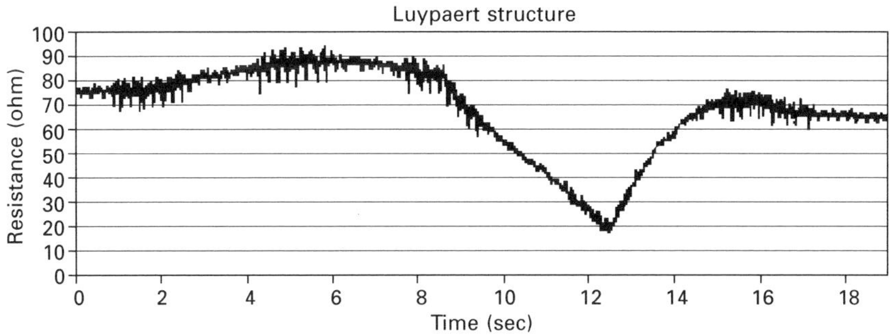

11.2 Change of resistance during one cycle of elongation.

In order to study the evolution of the signal over time, we continued the cyclic elongation for 50 minutes. Figure 11.3 shows the signal at defined times; after 25 seconds and after 5, 25 and 50 minutes. These graphs show a clear drift of the resistance. The signals' amplitude is slowly decreasing after each deformation cycle but the cyclic motion of elongating and relaxing can still be distinguished.

The same series of tests (50 minutes of cyclic elongation) were performed after washing the structure successively 5, 10 and 25 times in a domestic washing machine. An overview of the results is given in Fig. 11.4. This graph represents the evolution of the relative signal amplitude $\Delta R/R_{max}$ as a function of time, where ΔR is $R_{max} - R_{min}$ for each cycle. The graph shows that there is a tendency of the relative signal amplitude of non-washed and washed materials to equalise over time without damaging the reliability of the sensor; however, the influence of washing on the overall resistance of the structure has to be taken into account. It can be concluded that textile structures containing electroconductive material, are useful as strain gauges when they are carefully engineered and characterised.

11.3.2 Electrocardiogram (ECG) measurements

The Textrodes were developed to measure ECG. These Textrodes are a textile structure constituted of stainless steel yarns (by Bekintex), since stainless steel may be used in direct contact with the skin. But stainless steel has some more properties that justify our choice; apart from being a good conductor, stainless steel fibres have a good touch, a low toxicity to living tissue and they can be processed as a textile material.

Because of the intrinsic weakness of the heart's potential that is measurable at the skin (1.5–3 mV), a close contact between electrodes and skin is of major importance. Therefore conventional electrodes are always used in combination with an electrogel. The electrogel establishes a good conductive contact with the skin, thus improving the output signal. However, many

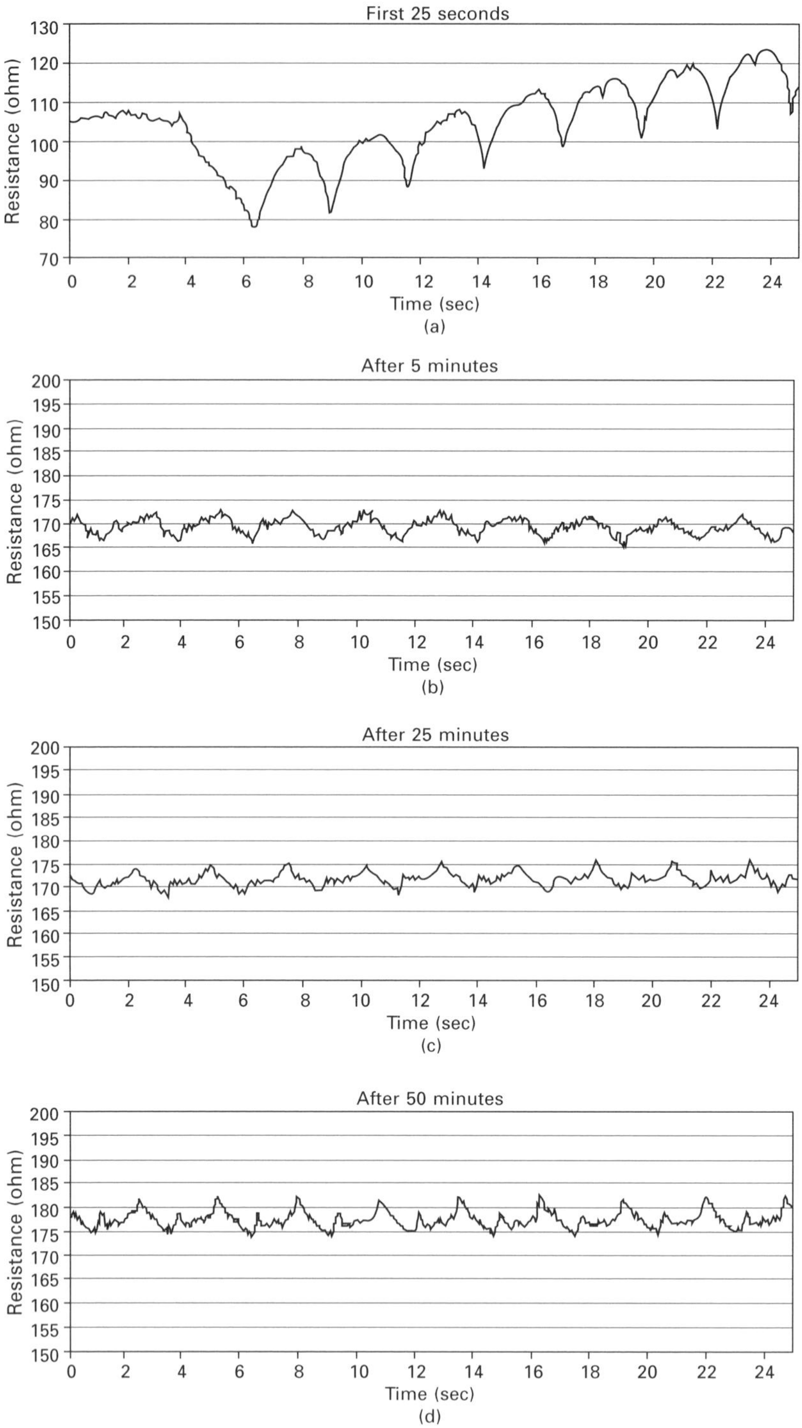

11.3 Electrical resistance change during 50 minutes of cyclic elongation.

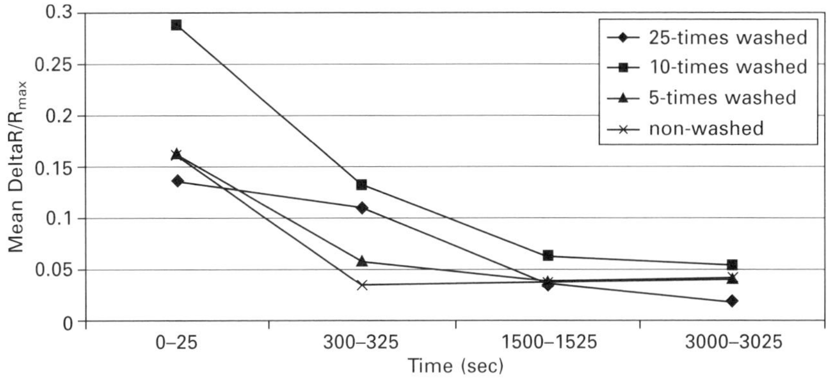

11.4 Relative signal amplitude during 50 minutes of cyclic elongation at selected time for a non-washed, 5-times, 10-times, 25-times washed structure.

patients experience some discomfort because these electrogels may cause skin irritation and softening. These inconveniences impose restrictions on the use of this kind of electrode for long-term monitoring. Using Textrodes could overcome these limitations because the textile material is in direct contact with the skin, hence making electrogel redundant. Therefore elasticity of the garment is a highly required property because it improves close fitting of the suit around the thorax and prevents shifting of the electrodes against the skin.

In recording the ECG and other bioelectric events, the input impedance of the recording system has to be much higher than the impedance of the electrode/bioelectric system. If this is not the case, not only a loss of amplitude of the bioelectric signal will arise, but also a distortion of the waveform.[7] Moreover, low electrode/skin impedance considerably improves the quality of the measured signal as the noise signal is less amplified. This is why the presence of sweat is experienced as beneficial. Since the textile electrodes differ to a large extent from conventional electrodes, the electrode/skin impedance had to be determined. This was done in a frequency domain of 5–100 Hz. As was expected, the textile-electrode/skin impedance had an order of magnitude of 1.5 MΩ cm^2, which is much higher than with conventional gel electrodes, where the impedance typically is 10 kΩ cm^2 in the same frequency range.[8]

Since stainless steel is available in three textile structures, namely a woven, non-woven and knitted one, we decided to investigate the influence of this diversity on the electrode/skin impedance. The development of an electrochemical cell enabled a quality evaluation of the different structures when used as electrodes on the skin. The study is extensively discussed in the book *Analytical Electrochemistry in Textiles*,[9] however, one topic will be highlighted here. The three textile structures were exposed to four concentrations of artificial sweat (10^{-3}, 10^{-2}, 10^{-1} and 0.5 mol/L) for 24 hours and were then analysed to evaluate a possible change in their functioning. The results are summarised in Table 11.1.

It is concluded that the knitted and the woven structures show no significant changes in electrical behaviour as a function of time. The non-woven electrode, however, does reveal some changes, as for the higher electrolyte concentrations the impedance increases considerably. This might be due to corrosion of the structure or adsorption of species at the fibre surface. The phenomenon is more obvious with very high electrolyte concentrations, which means that the influence is limited. Compared to the knitted and woven electrodes, the non-woven one has a more open structure and a much larger surface area owing to individualising of fibres, which makes it more sensitive to chemical and mechanical interaction. This should be taken into consideration when non-woven electrodes are applied as sensing device in biomedical clothing. In relation to the sensation of comfort, non-woven fabrics will perform worse since protruding metal fibres will irritate the skin more easily.

In order to have a good elasticity and, accordingly, an improved contact with the skin, we decided on knitting a sensor integrated belt (Fig. 11.5). Interconnections between the sensors and electroconductive fasteners were knitted in as well. At this stage the electronics were connected to the belt through the fasteners. The belt has a double layer knitted structure; the actual sensing material (stainless steel) is present only at predetermined positions on the inside of the belt, while Viloft/Co is used for the other parts and the outside.

To measure the ECG, a three-electrode configuration was used.[10] Two electrodes were placed on a horizontal line on the thorax, while a third one, acting as a reference, was placed on the lower part of the abdomen (not integrated into the belt). In order to assess their performance, the signal originating from a conventional electrode (gel electrodes by the company 3M) and from the textile electrodes were recorded at the same time. The results of these measurements are shown in Fig. 11.6. Despite the Textrodes generating more noise, the figures show the accuracy of the signal.

The measurements shown in Fig. 11.6 were carried out in a laboratory. Later on clinical tests were performed in an operating room at University Hospital Ghent, Belgium. Anaesthetised children between two and four years old were simultaneously monitored with the textile and the conventional electrodes. The test focused exclusively on the performance of the Textrodes. Because of the ease of handling, a prototype in the form of a belt (as described above) was chosen for the initial clinical tests. The belt can more easily be put on and be removed using a Velcro fastener in the front. It also leaves sufficient space on the body to attach other conventional sensors. However,

Table 11.1 Electrical resistance measured in an electrochemical cell containing knitted, woven or non-woven stainless steel electrodes and different concentrations of artificial sweat. Measurements are done at different exposure times of the electrodes to artificial sweat

Electrolyte concentration (mol/l)	10^{-3}			10^{-2}			10^{-1}			0.5		
Exposure time (hours)	$t = 0$	$t = 12$	$t = 24$	$t = 0$	$t = 12$	$t = 24$	$t = 0$	$t = 12$	$t = 24$	$t = 0$	$t = 12$	$t = 24$
Knitted	31 610	31 530	31 510	3985	3980	3980	316	316	315	26.1	26.8	27.8
Woven	31 510	31 540	31 495	3989	3980	3982	319	316	316	25.9	27.1	27.2
Non woven	31 520	31 510	31 540	3981	3978	3.95	315	330	351	25.9	35.0	60.3

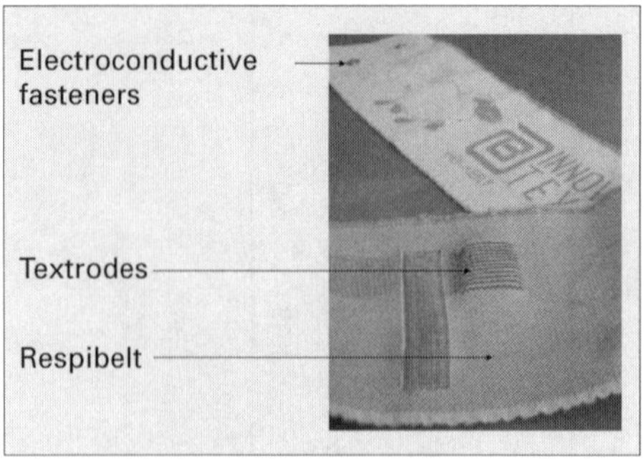

11.5 Belt with integrated sensors and interconnections.

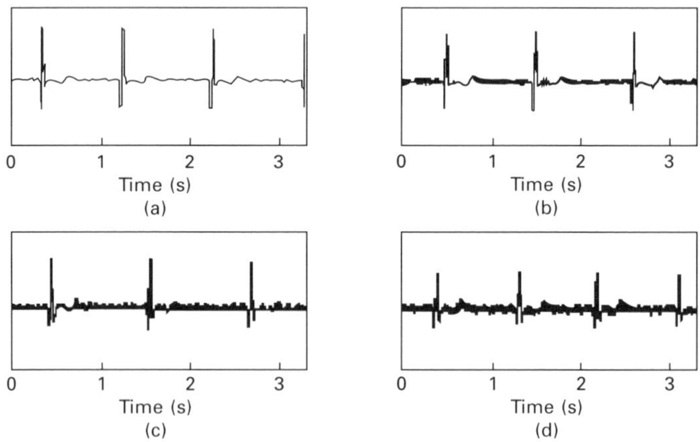

11.6 ECG Measurements using gel electrodes (a) and (b) and using Textrodes (c) and (d).

the aim was to finally manufacture a complete baby suit. The clinical tests revealed the following deficiencies:

- The interconnections between the electrodes and the electroconductive fasteners cause problems after repeatedly opening and closing the belt. Metal fibres stick out of the belt and make contact with the surface of the textile sensor. This causes the signal to be interrupted.
- From the tests, it clearly appeared that a good skin-electrode contact has a very important influence on the quality of the output signal (for ECG measurements).
- The Velcro fastener appeared to be unreliable, coming off too frequently during measuring. A fixed fastening system seems to be indispensable.
- The electrical circuit had to be adjusted because the textile electrodes' signal caused the amplifiers to go into saturation.

11.3.3 Wireless communication and energy transmission

In order to extend the autonomy of the textile-based system, an existing inductive link was modified by using electroconductive textile material.[11] Implementing this inductive link has a double function, enabling wireless bi-directional data transmission on the one hand and power transfer on the other. The data transmission downlink from a base station to the baby is useful, for instance, to change parameters, to determine minimum and maximum respiration rate or to adapt the measuring algorithm to the needs of the patient, while the uplink from the baby to the receiver sends out the measured data. Furthermore, the presence of inductive powering avoids the use of batteries, which reduces the volume of the system and enables continuous measurements. The developed system samples the ECG signal with a frequency of 300 Hz, while simultaneously a power transfer of 50 mW is transmitted from the base station to the suit.

An inductive link requires two coils, a primary coil (the base station) and a secondary coil, operating within a maximal coil separation distance of 6 cm. Since the Intellitex suit is meant for babies, the base station of the inductive link could be hosted in the mattress or the side panels of the cradle, while the secondary textile coil is integrated into the garment. This allows both functions to be realised while the baby is lying in bed. We concluded that the most suitable technique to integrate the coil into the baby suit is embroidery because it allows stitching a very flexible electroconductive yarn with high precision and accuracy onto a textile carrier. The embroidering technique was fully exploited to compromise the conflicting requirements of the coil, which are producing as many turns as possible without them touching each other. A high number of turns makes the coil superior whereas touching turns create a short circuit. The useful area on the baby suit however, also restricts the diameter. The ZSK embroidery machine, equipped with a special W-head, succeeded in manufacturing a 20-turns coil with an external diameter of 10 cm.

11.3.4 Intellitex suit: final prototype

Based on the conclusions drawn from the clinical tests, a subsequent prototype was manufactured. This garment hosts more components than the former belt, as is schematically shown in Fig. 11.7. In this prototype the electronic circuit is the only non-textile component but special attention has been given to its miniaturisation. To prevent damage through washing, these components have to be removed during maintenance of the prototype garment. The Intellitex suit is equipped with textile and textile compatible components (see Fig. 11.8):

- ECG/TEXTRODES (textile): physical interface with the skin to monitor heart, analog front end for ECG amplification and filtering
- respiration/ RESPIBELT (textile): monitoring of respiration rate

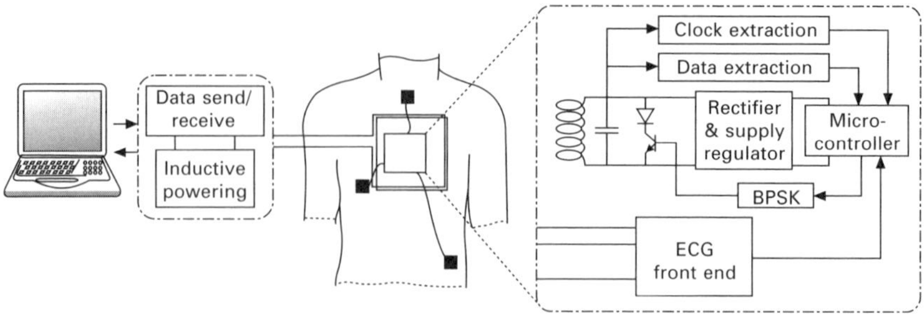

11.7 Concept of the Intellitex suit.

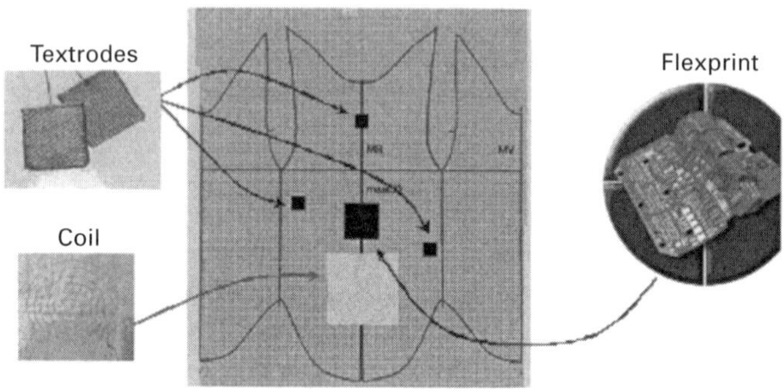

11.8 Build up of the final prototype.

- MICRO-CONTROLLER (on the flexprint): central part of the circuit. A PIC microcontroller has been chosen to perform the following tasks:
  - reading of sensors
  - AD conversion
  - communication
  - takes decisions: e.g. sending out alarm
- MEMORY (on the flexprint): data storage
- ALARM (on the flexprint) : can generate signal-like sound
- INDUCTIVE POWERING/DATA LINK (textile): supplies power required for all the components and ensures the bi-directional data transmission. It is a wireless link that transfers power through inductance.

11.4 Conclusion

The Intellitex suit is an example of a smart biomedical garment exploiting the potential of electroconductive textile materials. It offers a solution to the disadvantages of conventional techniques. As an alternative to conventional electrodes, both knitted and woven stainless steel electrodes (Textrodes) revealed promising results. The main advantages of dry Textrodes are the non-irritating and integrating properties. A disadvantage is the poor skin/

electrode contact which is translated into higher demands on the electronic circuit. Therefore the analogue front-end had to be redesigned and optimised. These electronics were assembled on a flexible printed circuit which can be integrated in the baby suit. A set of clinical tests has on the one hand uncovered some practical deficiencies but has on the other hand proven the usability of textile sensors. An improved prototype was manufactured. The result is a child-friendly garment that allows small patients to be monitored in the best possible conditions (Fig. 11.9).

This work demonstrates that textile materials themselves have a strong potential to be used as sensor elements, interconnections and transmission links in smart biomedical garments. Despite the low quality of the textile sensors, the use of electronics with high requirements provides reliable monitoring. Major benefits are improved patient comfort and the reusability of the sensors. Washable packaging of the electronics and durable interconnections remain major challenges to be tackled, not only for the specific system presented here, but also for all wearable electronics and intelligent textiles developments. There is still a long way to go to obtain reliable commercial smart biomedical garments.

Not only in this study but also in many others, the feasibility of smart textiles has been demonstrated and the prototypes have proved to be really beneficial. The manufacture of truly wearable smart textile systems has made a cautious start but there is still a long way to go. Slowly these new textile-based products are finding their way into our society. Possible problems

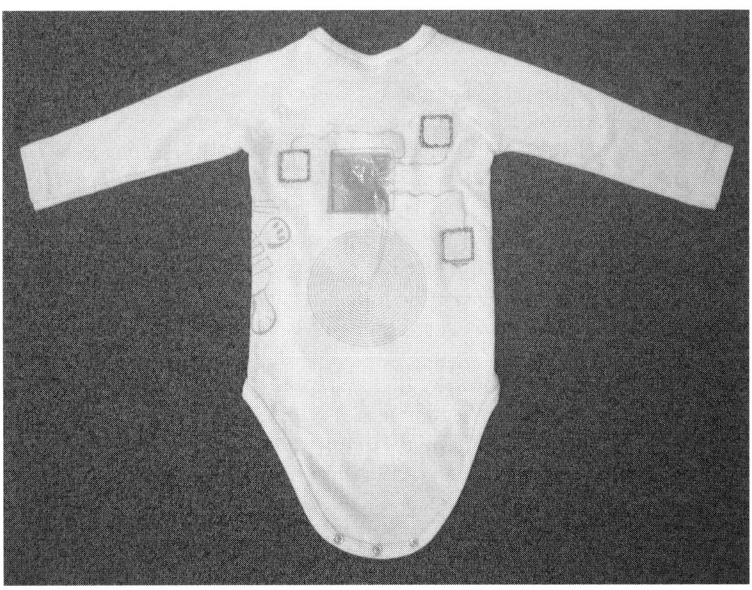

11.9 Final prototype of the Intellitex suit.

however should be recognised and overcome by continuously searching for improved materials and technologies. Treating these systems in the way we treat our daily garments is very demanding and therefore a huge challenge. Consequently, evaluation of long-term behaviour, durability and system performance after repeated laundering should invariably be included in the research tasks. Therefore fundamental research has to support the use of these textile materials sufficiently.

11.5 Acknowledgements

This research project was supported by IWT, in the framework of the STWW programme, contract no. 000160. The authors would like to acknowledge Bekintex and ZSK for their substantial contribution.

11.6 References

1. Gopalsamy, C., Park, S., Rajamanickam, R., Jayaraman, S., 'The wearable motherboard: the first generation of adaptive and responsive textile structures (ARTS) for medical applications,' *J. Virtual Reality*, vol. 4, pp. 152–168, 1999.
2. www.sensatex.com
3. Paradiso R., Loriga G., Taccini N., 'Wearable System for Vital Signs Monitoring', in *Wearable eHealth Systems for Personalised Health Management*, A. Lymberis, D. De Rossi ISBN 1 58603 449 9, p 253–259.
4. www.smartex.it
5. Grossman P., 'The Lifeshirt: A multi-function ambulatory system monitoring health, disease and medical intervention in the real world', in *Wearable eHealth Systems for Personalised Health Management*, A. Lymberis, D. De Rossi ISBN 1 58603 449 9, p 133–141.
6. Weber J.-L., Blanc D., Dittmar A., Comet B., Corroy C., Noury N., Baghai R., Vayasse S., Blinowska A, 'Telemonitoring of vital parameters with newly designed biomedical clothing VTAM', *Proc. of International Workshop – New Generation of Wearable Systems for e-Health: Towards a Revolution of Citizens' Health and Life Style Management*, Lucca, Italy, pp. 169–174, 2003.
7. Verhaert, Mamagoose pyjamas, Information available online at: www.verhaert.com/pdfs/Verhaert%20mamagoose.pdf
8. Lanfer B., *The development and investigation of electroconductive textile strain sensors for use in smart clothing,* E-Team Master Thesis, Academic Year 2004–2005.
9. Westbroek P., Priniotakis G., Kiekens P., *Analytical Electrochemistry in Textiles,* Woodhead Publishing, Cambridge ISBN 1 85573 919 4.
10. Neuman, M.R., 'Biopotential Amplifiers', in: Webster, J.G. (ed.), *Medical Instrumentation – Application and Design*, John Wiley & Sons, 1998, pp. 233–286.
11. Catrysse M., Hermans B., Puers R., 'An inductive powering system with integrated bidirectional datatransmission', *Proc. Eurosens.* (2003) 843–846.

12

Wearable textiles for rehabilitation of disabled patients using pneumatic systems

G BELFORTE, G QUAGLIA, F TESTORE,
G EULA and S APPENDINO,
Politecnico di Torino, Italy

12.1 Introduction

In recent decades, the increase in the number of elderly people and the growing need for rehabilitation therapies have sparked interest in the associated problems. According to several studies, the world's elderly population is growing steadily, and will continue to do so. In developed countries, the percentage of elderly people (over 65 years of age) passed from 11% in 1950 to 17% in 1990, and is expected to reach 25% in 2020 [1]. The same trends are in process in developing countries, though to a somewhat lesser extent. Worldwide, 7.1% of the entire population in 2002 consisted of elderly people, while projections indicate that this figure will increase to 9.5% by 2020 [2]. The number of elderly people living alone has also risen. In the United States, the percentage of people over 75 who live on their own increased from 28.05% in 1970 to 36.35% in 2003 [3].

In addition to the problems due to advancing age, which cause a general slowing of bodily functions, many people also suffer brain lesions leading to cognitive and motor disabilities. These lesions result from pathologies that chiefly affect people over 50 [4]. At the same time, more and more brain injuries of traumatic etiology are occurring, predominately among young people (between 18 and 30) and largely as a result of traffic accidents. Overall, 61% of brain injuries are caused by trauma. In the United States alone, statistics indicate that around 1.5 million cases of cranioencephalic trauma are sustained every year [5]. It follows that the number of people in situations requiring special care, either for rehabilitation or for assistance, is very large. Rehabilitation therapies are needed both for chronic patients, for whom continual exercise prevents their general condition from worsening, and for trauma patients, for whom prolonged exercise may make it possible to regain total or partial muscle function. Rehabilitation therapies and systems can differ widely, and must be personalized for the individual patient. Consequently, there is an enormous demand for assistance and physiotherapy performed by highly trained specialists. Rehabilitation treatments call for a direct relationship between patient and physiotherapist, and are carried out at specialized centers that have their own organizational problems and a limited amount of time available for each patient. All of this entails high social costs.

One possible answer to these problems lies in the use of robotized equipment to provide assistance and perform rehabilitation. Thus, researchers in the sector have begun to design machines meeting the essential requirements of intrinsic safety, high comfort, versatility and adaptability to individual situations. Satisfying these requirements calls for actuators that are safe, compact, lightweight and agile, and can be readily integrated in the system of which they are a part. In general, pneumatic actuators exhibit all of these properties [6, 7]. Pneumatic actuators are favored over electric actuators in biomechanical applications because of their ease of installation, low maintenance requirements, and the fact that they can also be operated without electrical signals of any kind, making them suitable for use in areas involving electromagnetic interference problems.

In the meantime, the textile industry has been developing a host of innovative applications for new sectors, using technical fabrics provided with sensor and actuation functions. These two trends – the use of adaptive pneumatic actuators and the use of smart fabrics – have led to the development of new flexible actuators, true pneumatic artificial muscles whose light weight and wearability make them extremely promising. These fabric-based artificial muscles can be very useful as a power source in rehabilitation equipment, which is usually based on typical robotics concepts, and in controlling aids for the disabled (e.g., hands and upper and lower limbs).

The major issues involved in constructing wearable systems of this kind are weight, power and deformability. Deformability in particular is one of the most important requirements for devices that can be comfortably worn, but are at the same time dependable and durable. Integrating pneumatic muscles and other fabric-based actuation devices in orthopedic braces and other garments makes it possible to develop true active pneumatic clothing capable of supporting disabled people and enabling them to perform rehabilitation exercises in their own homes or workplaces without the direct assistance of physicians and physiotherapists. The main characteristics of pneumatic systems in general and of pneumatic muscles in particular will therefore be discussed below. Their use in a number of biomedical applications will then be described.

12.2 Deformable pneumatic actuators

12.2.1 Types and fabric characteristics

Any active wearable structure must have the adaptability and flexibility typical of clothing; features exhibited by deformable pneumatic actuators. A large proportion of such actuators employ a structure based essentially on reinforced membranes which delimit one or more chambers that can be filled with a pressurized fluid. Depending on type, these membranes may be isotropic, or in other words their mechanical properties are the same in all directions, or anisotropic, i.e., their stiffness will differ in orthogonal directions. In the latter case, the membrane will be able to deform differently in each direction. In its basic form, a membrane consists of a woven structure (for example, a fabric with warp and filling – or weft – yarns) embedded in a layer of rubber or plastic which is impermeable to the fluid and compliant. Anisotropy may be achieved by means of reinforcing fibers strategically oriented in the membrane, or through the use of fibers with differing properties (stiff in one direction and elastic in the other). The same type of behavior can be achieved by means of a knitted fabric or netting surrounding a sort of inflatable elastic balloon.

Introducing pressurized gas into the chamber of a flexible pneumatic actuator can cause an increase in the chamber's volume, resulting in axial, flexural or rotational deformation. The variation in volume can also take place through a change in the membrane's geometry, without requiring significant deformation (as occurs in a bellows, for example). What is achieved, in many cases, is a behavior similar to that of a muscle, and many of these actuators are thus called 'pneumatic muscles'. Though pneumatic muscles can in principle use either compressible or noncompressible fluids, studies and applications have chiefly focused on the first type, and on the use of compressed air in particular. The pressures used are low (typically around 100–200 kPa) so that the membranes' thickness, and hence their stiffness, need not be excessive.

Fluid compressibility provides the compliance desirable for applications involving man-machine interactions. Such 'soft actuators' are particularly suitable for use in wearable systems, as the device is intrinsically safe and pleasant to the touch. In general, flexible pneumatic actuators exhibit the following properties:

- low weight
- absence of internal friction
- inherent compliance
- nonlinear static characteristic
- absence of internal kinematic torques.

The most common types will be described below, where they will be classified according to the type of action that can be obtained. The same principles can be employed in wearable systems, using embedded actuators to produce contraction, extension, bending motions and rotations. Linear actuators are the most widespread type, and feature a constraint at each end whereby they can be connected to the structure to which motion is to be imparted.

Linear tension actuators (pneumatic muscles)

This is the most numerous type, as it has been used in many biomimetic applications, including robotic structures, exoskeletons, atypical devices and so forth. Regardless of construction, these pneumatic artificial muscles, or PAM, operate as illustrated in Fig. 12.1. Thus, for operation at constant load F, we can deduce that a pneumatic muscle shortens by increasing its enclosed volume when the pneumatic pressure is increased. When pressurized at a constant gauge pressure p on the other hand, a pneumatic muscle will shorten if its load is decreased, and increases its enclosed volume until reaching maximum contraction, i.e., minimum length, when load is zero and enclosed volume is maximal. As for conventional pneumatic cylinders, the static characteristic is usually expressed with:

$$F = p \cdot A_e(l) \tag{12.1}$$

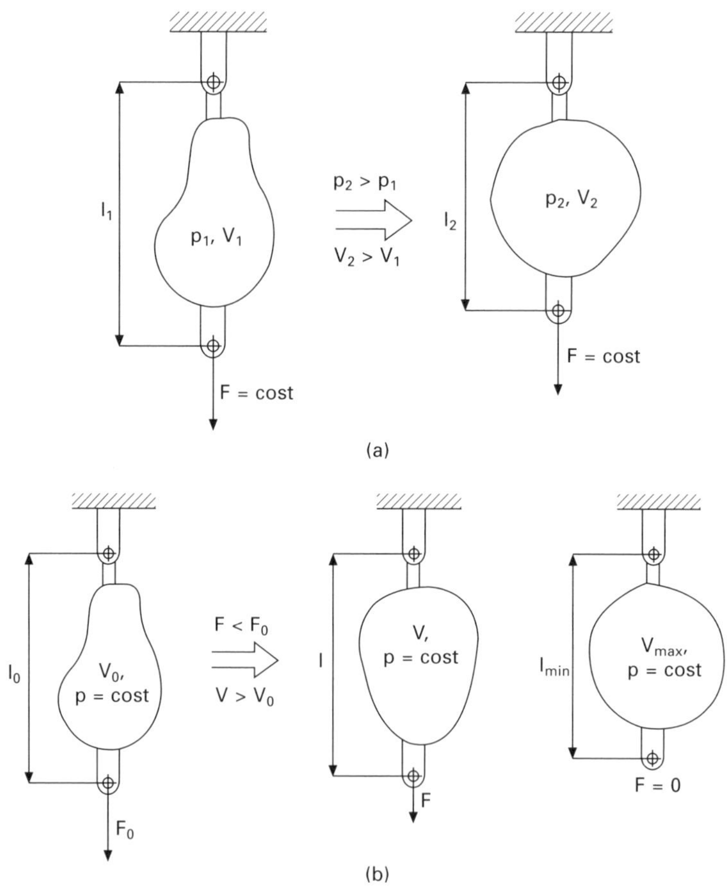

12.1 Pneumatic muscle operation (a) at constant load and (b) at constant internal pressure.

where the only difference is that the effective area A_e is not constant, but depends on the pneumatic muscle's length l.

An identical expression can be used for air springs that generate thrust forces (in this case, $F < 0$ with the conventions used here). Defining percentage contraction C as:

$$C = \left(1 - \frac{l}{l_0}\right) \cdot 100 \qquad 12.2$$

where l_o is the initial length, eqn 12.1 will normally give curves as shown in Fig. 12.2. Here, force F is shown on the ordinate, while percentage contraction C is plotted on the abscissa. The values of C_{max} depend upon the kind of actuator and can be very different among themselves. In order to simplify the analysis, we can say that $A_e(l)$ does not depend on p (or in other words, above a minimum threshold, the membrane's deformation and enclosed volume are not significantly influenced by pressure). In this case, the pressure shown in Fig. 12.2 is simply a scale factor.

As regards stiffness, it is sufficient to derive eqn 12.1:

$$K = \frac{dF}{dl} = p \cdot \frac{dA_e(l)}{dl} + A_e(l)\frac{dp}{dl} = K_A + K_V \qquad 12.3$$

where K_A is correlated to the change in effective area as a function of length, and is thus a stiffness that can be achieved even when the muscle is maintained at p = cost, while K_V (volumetric stiffness) also depends on the change in pressure as length varies. With a constant fluid mass, this type of stiffness is due only to the change in enclosed volume and the type of transformation

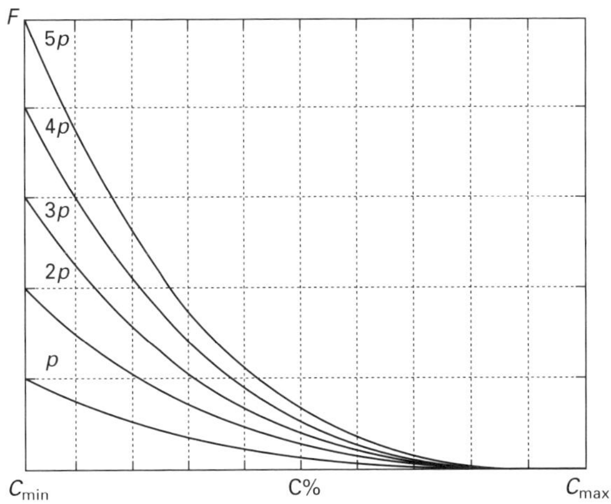

12.2 Change in force for contractions at constant pressure.

undergone by the gas. It also follows that slow (isothermal) transformations will entail smaller increases in pressure, and thus lower stiffness, than fast (adiabatic) transformations.

Pneumatic muscles can only generate pulling forces. To obtain a bidirectional 'double-acting' motion, an antagonistic set-up as shown in Fig. 12.3(a), i.e., a biologically inspired layout, can be used. Another configuration which permits rotation using a linear actuator is shown in Fig. 12.3(b); in this case, having only one muscle, the motion is unidirectional. Some of the types of pneumatic muscle that have been investigated or patented since the 1930s will be reviewed and classified below. For certain of these types, a distinction

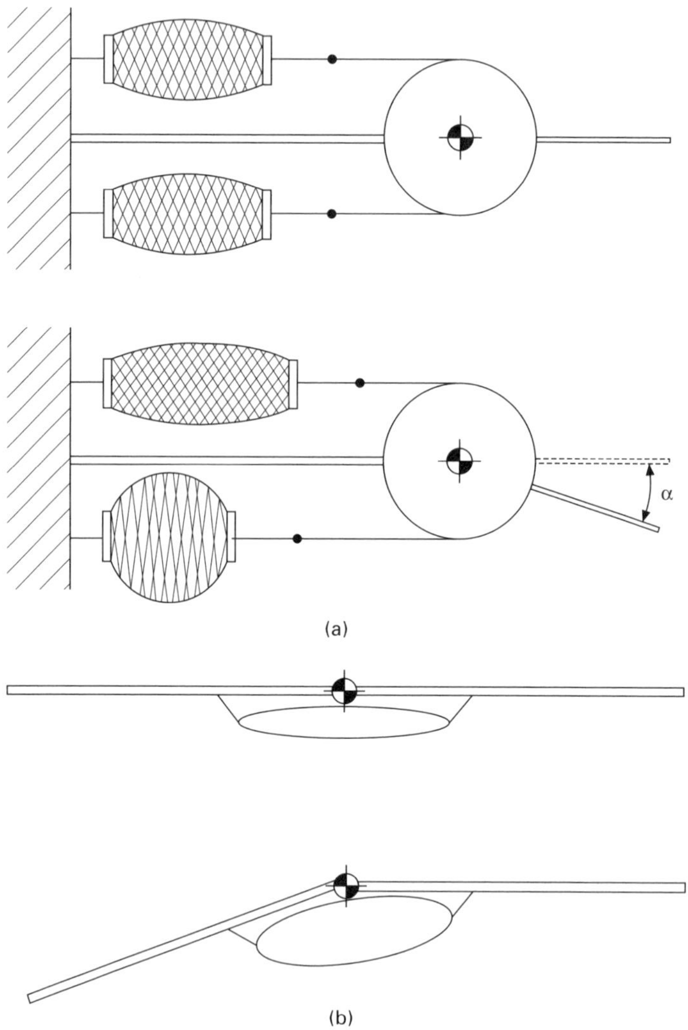

12.3 Different configurations for pneumatic muscles.

can be made between cases where the reinforcing fibers which make the membrane anisotropic are located externally to the membrane – in which case the actuator is known as a braided muscle – or are embedded in it.

McKibben muscle

These actuators are derived from a patented design by Morin [8]. According to Baldwin [9], they were introduced by J. L. McKibben as an orthotic actuator in the 1950s. They consist of a gas-tight elastic tube surrounded by a braided sleeve as shown in Fig. 12.4. The braid fibers run helically along the muscle's long axis, forming an angle called the braid angle, pitch angle or weave angle to it. When pressurized fluid is introduced in the tube, the internal pressure is balanced by braid fiber tension. In turn, the fibers are connected at the braid's end points, where the sum of all tensions on the fibers balance the external load applied to the muscle. There are two versions of this type of muscle. In the first type, generally referred to as the McKibben muscle, both the inner tube and braid are connected to fittings at both ends which seal the tube and supply gas to it. In the second type, the inner tube is in fact an unattached bladder which is not connected to the end fittings and, once inflated, serves only to put the fibers in tension.

Pleated PAM

The pleated pneumatic artificial muscle developed by Daerden [10, 11] is a membrane-rearranging actuator, meaning that the membrane's surface is rearranged rather than stretched as it is inflated, and no material strain is involved. This actuator's membrane has a number of lengthwise pleats which unfold when the muscle is inflated, allowing the membrane to expand and the actuator to contract (Fig. 12.5). This muscle is more efficient than the previous type. As a negligible fraction of the pressurized fluid's energy is needed to expand the membrane, nearly all of the energy can be used for contraction. This actuator's performance depends on the ratio of muscle length to radius.

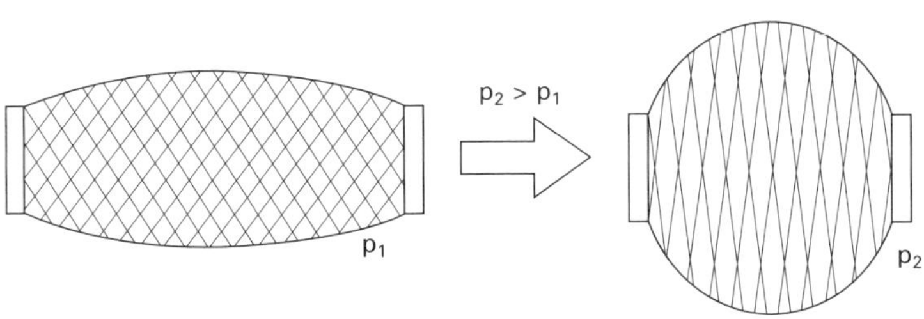

12.4 McKibben muscle.

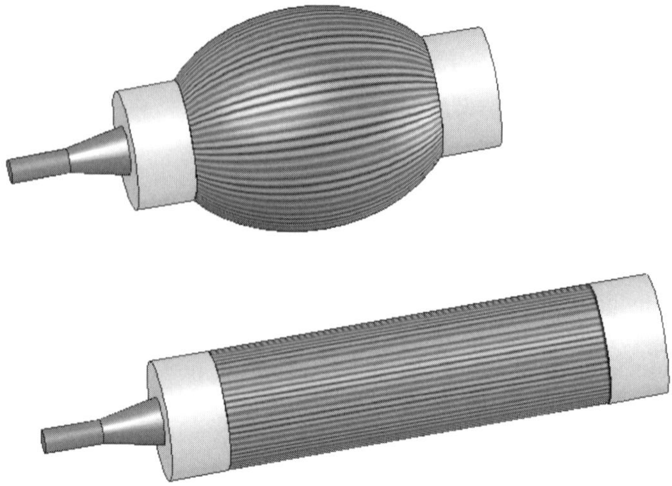

12.5 Pleated PAM.

Yarlott muscle

This actuator consists of an elastomeric bladder reinforced by a series of cords or strands running axially and connected to the end fittings. The bladder is also reinforced radially by strands to resist fluid pressure. When fully inflated, the muscle assumes a spherical shape (Fig. 12.6). A detailed description of this actuator is given in a US patent [12].

Kukolj muscle

This actuator is similar to the McKibben muscle, except that in the non-loaded condition there is a gap between the inner membrane and the outer fibers. For this actuator, the initial working condition is when load is applied and the inner membrane is fully extended. Contraction then takes place when the muscle is inflated. According to its inventor [13], the advantage of this design over the McKibben muscle is that it prevents the membrane from buckling near its ends (Fig. 12.7).

Straight fiber muscle

Many types of pneumatic muscle feature longitudinal fibers connecting the end fittings. The fittings move towards each other when a deformable inner element is inflated. Single or multi-lobed muscles can be produced by inserting circumferential stiffening rings at certain sections [14, 15]. Figure 12.8 shows a three-lobed version. Though they operate on the same principle as their single-chamber counterparts, multi-lobed actuators limit the circumferential

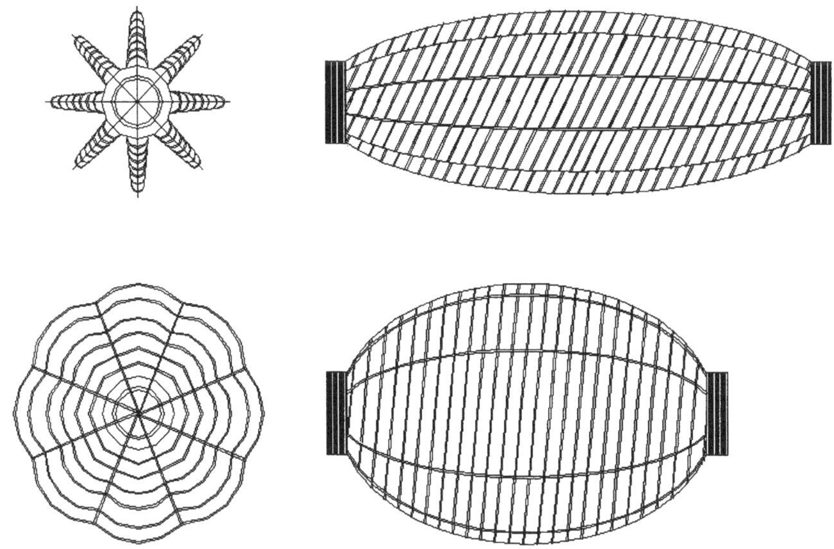

12.6 Yarlott muscle.

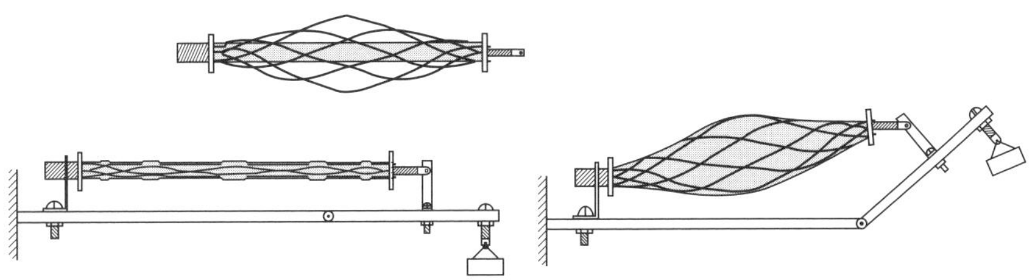

12.7 Kukolj muscle.

deformation required of the membrane for any given diameter and length. Essentially, they behave as a series of connected single-lobed actuators whose axial length, however, is a fraction of the overall length of the multi-lobed actuator.

Paynter hyperboloid muscle

A further variation in fiber arrangement is used by Paynter [16], who constructed an actuator whose membrane has the shape of a hyperboloid of revolution. The membrane is enclosed by a sleeve of inextensible, flexible threads which in the actuator's initial condition run in straight lines but form an angle to the axial direction. The result is the muscle shown in Fig. 12.9. At full contraction, the actuator expands into a nearly spherical shape.

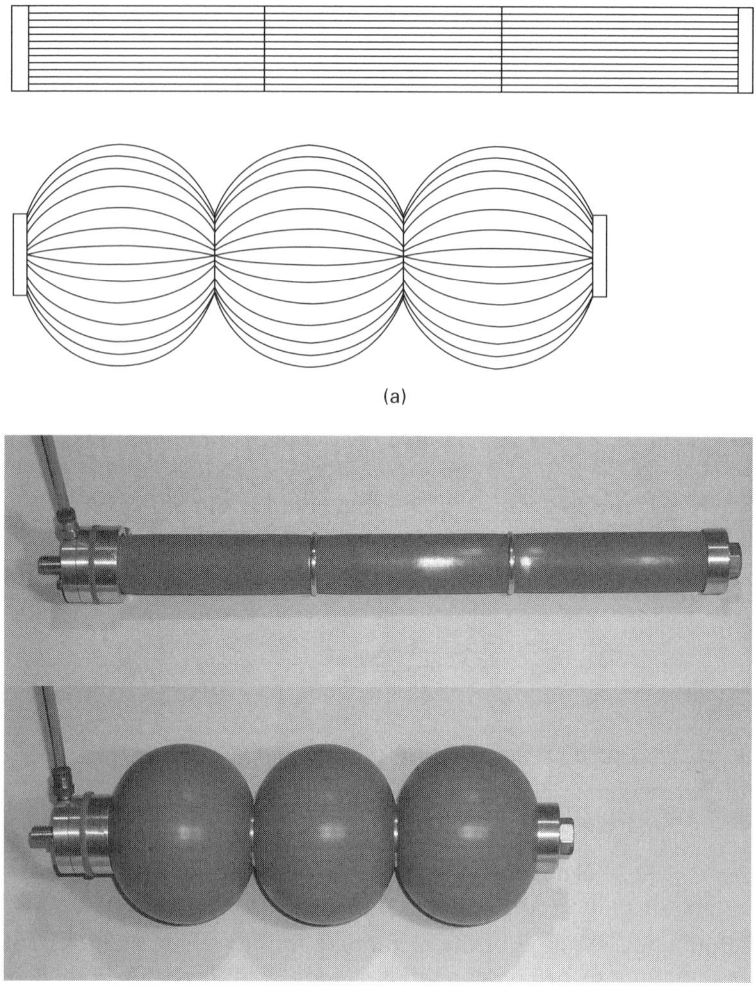

(a)

(b)

12.8 Straight fiber muscle: configuration (a) and prototype (b). Source: Raparelli T., Beomonte Zobel P., Durante F., *On the design of pneumatic muscle actuators*, 2nd Internationales Fluidtechnisches Kolloquium, 16–17 March 2000, Dresden).

Thrust actuators

Axial thrust actuators are essentially air springs. The two main types are rolling diaphragm springs and air bellows springs. In both cases, the resultant force produced by gas pressure in the spring causes an axial thrust, which is chiefly due to the spring's proportions and the shape of the membrane. Whereas for pneumatic muscles an increase in enclosed volume results in contraction, air springs will extend when their enclosed volume is increased (Fig. 12.10).

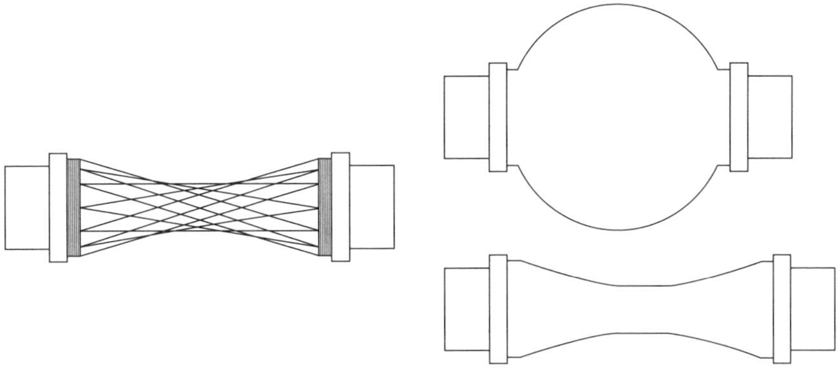

12.9 Paynter hyperboloid muscle.

Rolling diaphragm springs are suitable for relatively long axial strokes. In addition, the fact that the piston head that causes the diaphragm to roll can be shaped makes it possible to influence changes in effective area, i.e., the thrust force at constant pressure, and thus obtain (within certain limits) the spring rate curve required for the application. Bellows types, on the other hand, are subject to less membrane wear. They can develop large axial forces, especially in single-lobed versions. Using thrust actuators in appropriate configurations it is possible to create also rotational motions: an example of such a configuration is to be seen in Fig. 12.11.

Bidirectional actuators

This type of actuator [17, 18] combines the capabilities of both pneumatic muscles and air springs (Fig. 12.12). It consists of three coaxial cylindrical membranes – an outer membrane, an intermediate membrane, and a central membrane – all anchored to two end fittings at top and bottom in order to form three coaxial chambers, designated like the membranes as outer, intermediate and central. In an ideal arrangement, the three membranes have the same radius of attachment to the heads. In addition, the outer and central membranes are axially inextensible and infinitely compliant circumferentially, while the intermediate membrane is circumferentially inextensible and infinitely compliant axially.

The actuator can be used in three main supply configurations: the traction configuration, thrust configuration A, and thrust configuration B. The traction configuration is obtained by supplying both the outer and intermediate chambers, and exhausting the central chamber. The pressurized fluid thus exerts a radial force on the membranes, causing a longitudinal tensile stress to arise in each, which is then transferred to the end fittings. The axial resultant of this tensile stress thus corresponds to traction force F. Thrust

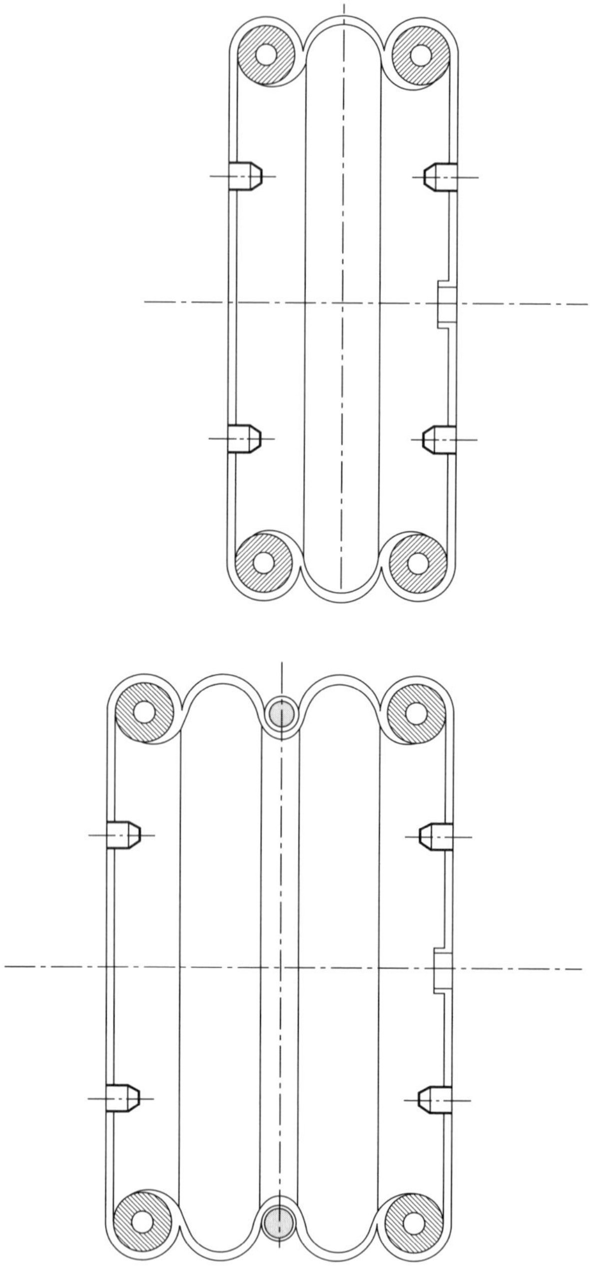

12.10 Air bellows spring.

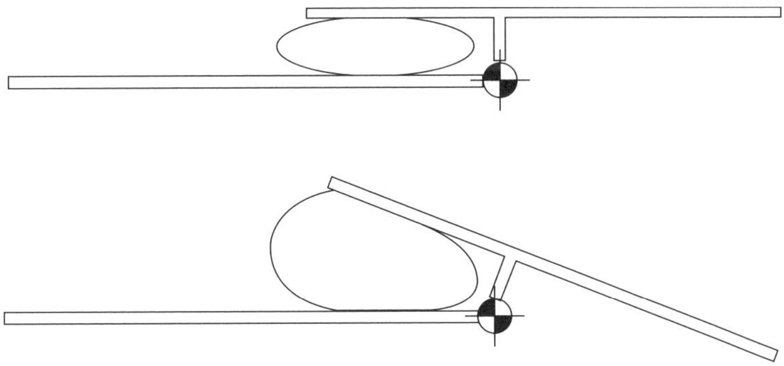

12.11 Configuration to obtain rotation with thrust actuators.

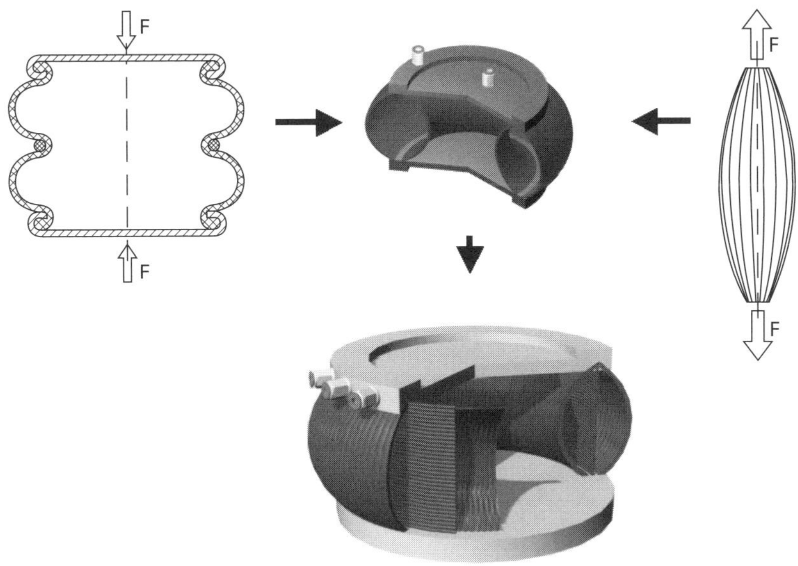

12.12 Three-membrane actuator combining the features of an air spring and a pneumatic muscle. Source: G. Quaglia, C. Ferraresi, W. Franco, *A New Fluid Power Deformable Actuator With Three Diaphragms*, 14th International Workshop on Robotics in Alpe-Adria-Danube Region, RAAD05, Bucharest, May 2005, pp. 507–512.

configuration A is obtained by supplying both the central and intermediate chambers, and exhausting the outer chamber. The intermediate membrane retains its cylindrical shape, but offers no resistance in the axial direction. Consequently, the actuator exerts a thrust force which is proportional to supply pressure and heads area. Finally, thrust configuration B is obtained by supplying all three chambers. Under these supply conditions, the thrust force, which is produced by the axial action of the pressure forces, is partially offset by the traction force exerted by the outer membrane. As a result, the overall thrust force is lower than that which can be achieved in thrust configuration A.

Flexible actuators

Flexible actuators curve when pressurized gas is introduced. As for the types discussed above, we will provide only a few examples of the many concepts that have been advanced for these actuators and the studies that have addressed them. In one design, the actuator consists of an elastomeric element divided into two sectors and provided with outer reinforcing rings in order to contain the elastomer's circumferential expansion [19]. Circumferential containment can also be achieved by means of a fabric structure wrapped around the actuator or embedded in the elastomer, and which is substantially nondeformable in the circumferential direction and highly compliant longitudinally. When a pressure differential is established between the two chambers, the actuator will bend in a plane perpendicular to the septum separating the chambers. A similar design used three sectors [20], so that the plane in which bending occurs can be selected by controlling the pressures in each chamber (Figs 12.13 and 12.14).

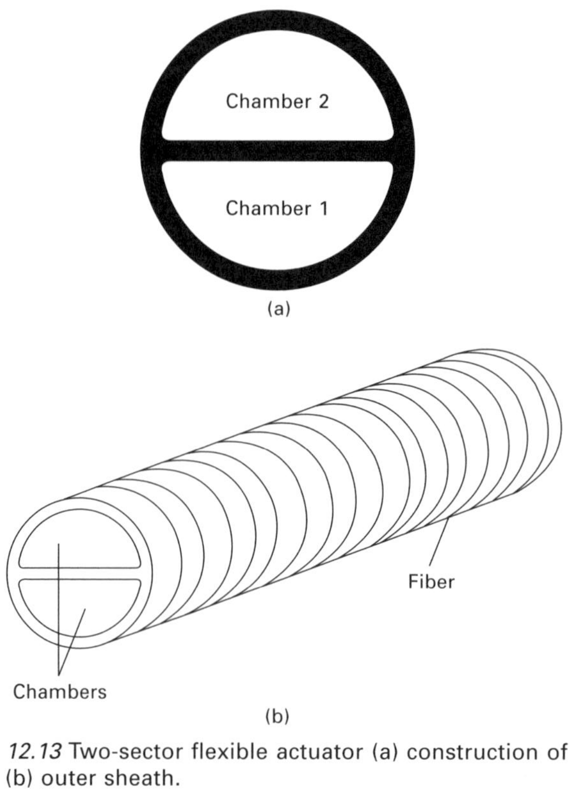

12.13 Two-sector flexible actuator (a) construction of chambers and (b) outer sheath.

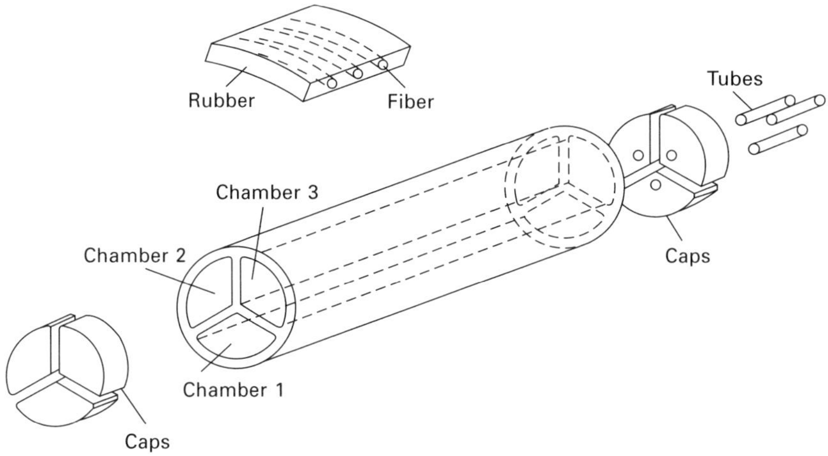

12.14 Three-sector flexible actuator schematics.

Another alternative for producing bending in a predetermined plane is the extended curved type muscle (Fig. 12.15). An actuator of this type can consist of an inner rubber tube and an outer polyester bellows [21]. To prevent axial stretching on one side, a fiber tape is applied which keeps the bellows from extending. Introducing pressurized gas causes the actuator to bend.

12.2.2 Basis of pneumatic control

Pneumatic muscles are actuated by supplying them with compressed air to produce a pressure differential. The simplest control method is to use an ON-OFF command based on two different pressure levels. Normally, the muscle operates between a zero pressure level (atmospheric pressure) at which the muscle is deactivated, and a higher pressure level, which is the operating pressure with the muscle activated.

This type of control can be achieved with a single pneumatic valve called a three-port valve which establishes connection between an outlet port connected to the muscle and either a supply port or an exhaust port. Control schematics for a muscle are shown in Fig. 12.16, where a spool valve *V* controls muscle *M*. In Fig. 12.16(a), spool S connects output 2 to a source of compressed air (muscle activated). In Fig. 12.16(b), output 2 is connected to the atmosphere (muscle deactivated).

Transitions between one operating position and the other are achieved by moving the inner spool. This movement is usually obtained by means of a manual actuation device, a pneumatic command from another valve, or an electrical signal supplied by an electronic controller. The valve shown in the figure is activated by pressing a pushbutton *B* (Fig. 12.16(a)), which overcomes

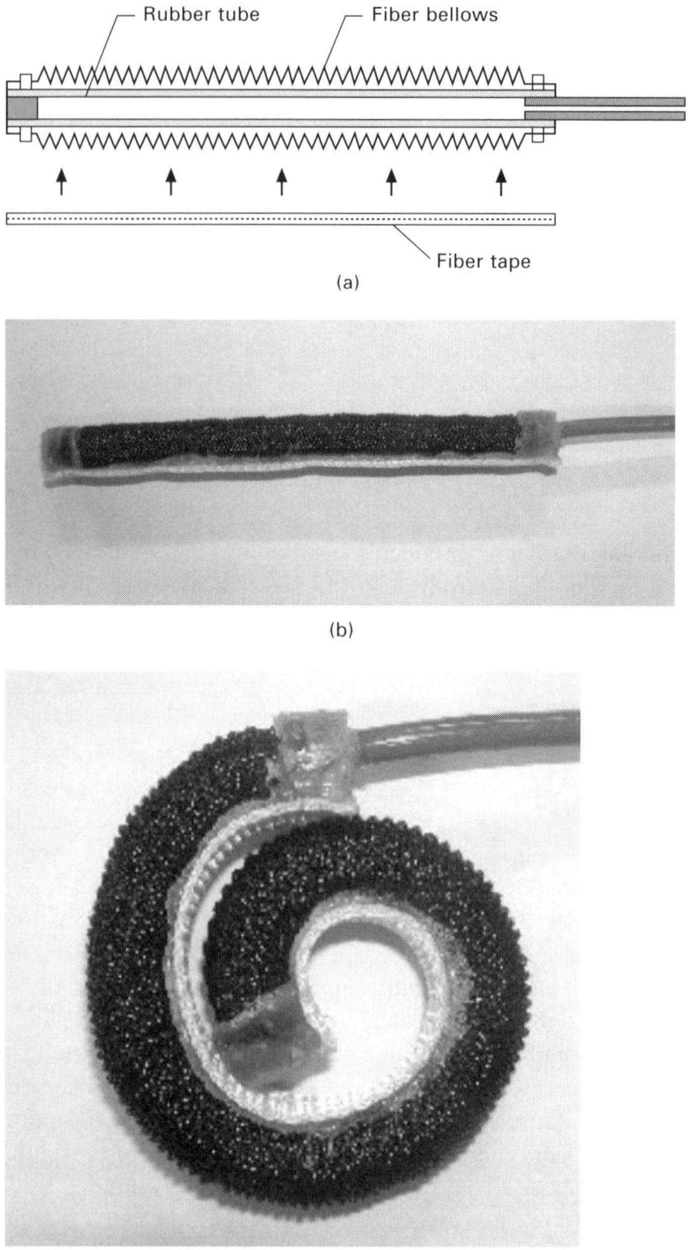

12.15 Extended curved type muscle: structure (a), extended configuration (b) and contracted configuration (c). Source: Noritsugu T., Masahiro T., Sasaki D., *Development of a pneumatic rubber artificial muscle for human support applications*, 9th Scandinavian Int. conference on Fluid Power, SICFP'05, June 1–3, 2005, Linkoeping, Sweden.

the force produced by reset spring *R*. The latter releases pressure from the muscle when it is not activated (Fig. 12.16(b)).

Naturally, varying the pressure in a pneumatic muscle will cause its extension and the force it generates to vary. To achieve efficient actuation, it is thus necessary to introduce proportional control using a circuit capable of varying the pressure delivered to the muscle. Techniques based on two different principles can be used for this purpose. The first approach employs proportional pressure regulators that can supply a variable pressure, while the second uses digital ON-OFF valves, at least one of which can connect the muscle to supply and at least another which can connect the muscle to exhaust. These valves are actuated alternately to fill the muscle in a controlled fashion, thus reaching a given internal pressure.

With the first technique, proportional solenoid valves can be used which supply an output pressure – connected directly to the muscle – that can be regulated as a function of an electrical control signal (either a voltage or a current). This approach is effective, but requires one proportional solenoid valve for each muscle. It is thus relatively costly, calls for fairly sizeable components, and requires extensive filtration for supply air. This can penalize the technique's application to muscles, which must be integrated in wearable structures and active clothing, and can be applied in varying types of situation and environments that are not strictly controlled.

A solution which is more economical and more robust than proportional solenoid valves but equally efficient is that based on digital solenoid valves. With this approach, multiple solenoid valves are connected in various ways to achieve proportional control. One way of implementing this approach is shown in Fig. 12.17. Muscle M is connected to two solenoid valves V_1 and

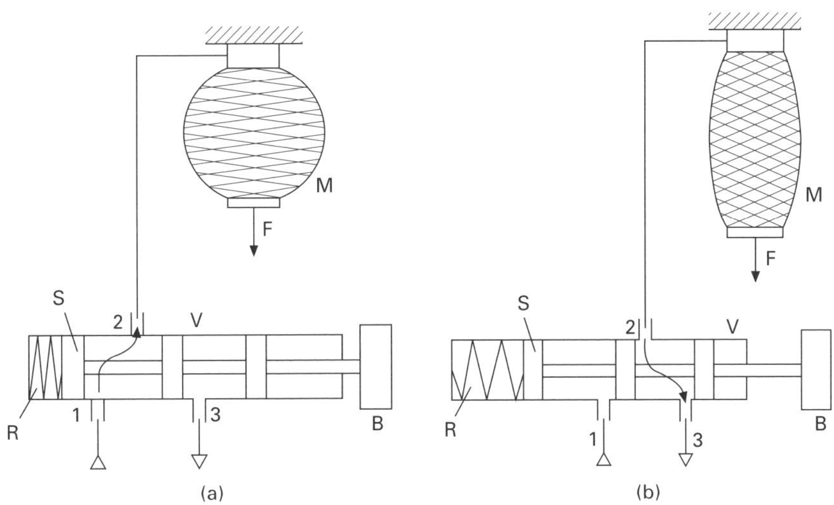

12.16 Pneumatic muscle control using a three-port valve.

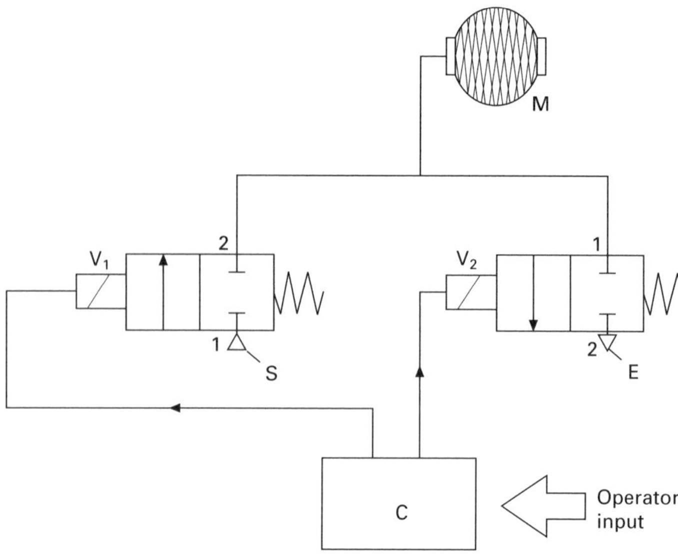

12.17 Pneumatic muscle control using modulating valves.

V_2. The latter are actuated by an electrical signal, which causes an inner spool to move and establish connection between the two inlet and outlet ports of each valve. The ports are then held closed by a spring so that there is no flow path, and no air passes.

In the figure, the valves are represented using ISO symbols, with two squares showing the two operating situations, viz., the flow path condition with electrical signal in the left square, and the condition in which the valve is closed by the spring in the square on the right of the symbol. Port 1 of valve V_1 is connected to supply *S*, and port 2 of valve V_2 is connected to exhaust *E*. Port 2 of valve V_1 and port 1 of valve V_2 are thus connected to the muscle. An electronic controller C sends intermittent command signals to the two solenoid valves. Every time valve V_1 is activated, the muscle fills, while every time valve V_2 is activated, the muscle is emptied.

This approach uses the PWM pulse width modulation control technique: signals are switched digitally on the basis of absence (signal 0) or presence (signal 1) at a fixed frequency, and the duty cycle, i.e., the ratio of total actuating signal on-time to the total period of the cycle, is varied. The duty cycle is expressed as a percentage, and can be varied from 0% (valve inactive) to 100% (valve active continuously). In commercial solenoid valves, regulation is performed at an operating frequency ranging from a few dozen to several hundred Hertz.

A second way of controlling a fabric-based artificial muscle proportionally using digital valves is the PCM, or pulse code modulation, technique illustrated in Fig. 12.18. Here, muscle *M* is connected to two sets of solenoid valves:

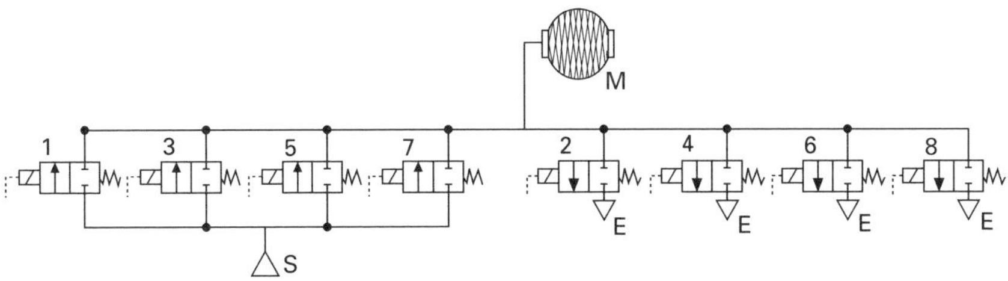

12.18 Pneumatic muscle control using the PCM technique.

two-port valves 1, 3, 5, 7 and two-port valves 2, 4, 6, 8. The first set connects the muscle to supply *S*, and the second to exhaust *E*. The valves in each set have different passage sections. In the first set, the passage section of each valve starting from the first valve 1 is twice that of the valve before it, so that its flow rate will be approximately double at any given upstream and downstream pressures. In this way, activating the valves alternately with different combinations of signals will produce different flow rates. The number of possible combinations is 2^n, where n is the number of valves. In the case in question, there are thus 16 possible regulation conditions, including the condition in which all valves are fully closed.

With this technique, the muscle's input and output flow rates can be varied separately and independently. Consequently, the muscle can be filled or emptied at varying speeds, or can be maintained with a constant mass of gas by closing all of the supply and exhaust valves. The PWM and PCM techniques control input and output flow rate; achieving pressure control requires feedback from a transducer, and a control element which receives the feedback and modulates a command signal.

An important problem is that of generating and conditioning compressed air. Wearable applications must operate with independent air generation systems, as they cannot rely on the ordinary compressed air distribution lines provided in industrial settings. Such applications, in fact, must be suitable for people using them independently in their own homes or in a workplace which may not have special equipment. Even the operating pressures used for muscles differ from those employed in industry: maximum pressures are in the neighborhood of 0.2–0.3 MPa, as opposed to the 0.6–0.8 MPa typical of industry.

Wearable applications also have completely different requirements as regards cleanliness; lubricating oils from compressors cannot be tolerated. This makes it necessary to use special compressors differing from those commonly used in industrial facilities; oil-less, silent, vibration-free. Diaphragm type compressors are particularly useful for this purpose, as they are both oil-less and operate with compression ratios, i.e., the ratio of discharge pressure p_2 and atmospheric intake pressure p_1, which are not overly high (normally $p_2/p_1 = 2–4$).

After it is produced, the compressed air must be appropriately conditioned before it is delivered to the pneumatic circuit which controls the muscles. Conditioning serves a twofold purpose: on the one hand, it is needed in order to ensure that the air is filtered and does not contain solid particles or other contaminants that could damage the valves, while on the other hand it provides the constant pressure level required to guarantee that the muscles perform under reproducible conditions. All this is achieved by means of filter-reducer units, consisting of filters to ensure that the compressed air is clean, and pressure reducers to stabilize the pressure of the air introduced to the pneumatic circuits which control the muscles. In the filter, contaminants are removed in two different ways: centrifugal action, which spins out any particles entrained in the air, and filtration through an extremely fine porous cartridge. Centrifugal action is achieved by using appropriate fins to convey the air at the filter inlet and impart a spiraling motion so that solid particles are forced against the walls of the filter bowl and then deposited on the bottom. Filtration is accomplished mechanically, as the air passes through a porous septum whose porosity is normally in the order of 10–40 μm.

The general layout of the supply and control system for a pneumatic muscle is shown in Fig. 12.19. Muscle *M* is used to power an elbow joint. The solenoid valves *V* which control the muscle, using one of the methods described above, for example, are located adjacent to the muscle. Muscle and valves must be integrated with an orthopedic brace or orthosis and inserted in appropriate clothing. The power supply unit is located in a remote position and connected to the actuation device by an 'umbilical cord'. Appropriate sensors and an electronic controller, normally a PLC, complete the system. The power unit consists of an electric motor 1 which drives a

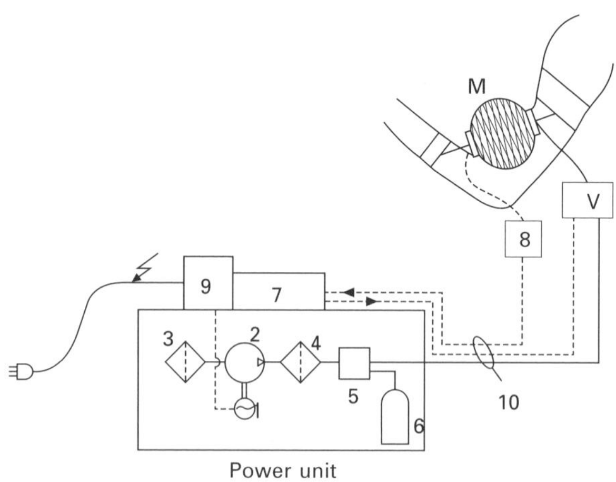

12.19 General layout of the supply and control system for a pneumatic muscle.

compressor 2. The compressed air line is provided with an intake filter 3, a delivery filter 4, a pressure reducer 5, and a compensator reservoir 6 containing sufficient compressed air to fill the muscle in the event of sudden power demands.

On the regulation and control side, the system is provided with a PLC 7, which sends electrical command signals to the solenoid valves and receives signals from sensors 8. Block 9, in addition with the cable connected to the power outlet, represents the electrical power supply of the system. The "umbilical cord" 10 may consist of a single cable containing the compressed air hose for connection between the compressor unit and the solenoid valves, one or more electrical cables for the command signals, and one or more electrical cables for the sensor signals. The sensors' structure and capabilities will depend on the functions they are required to perform. If their purpose is to monitor muscle operation, position or force sensors can be used. If their purpose is to initiate the cycle on patient command, sensors for myoelectric signals or sensors which detect the user's own muscle contractions can be used. As an alternative to an adaptive command provided by the person wearing the active clothing, it is also possible to use external means of control such as pushbuttons or joysticks which can be actuated by the wearer.

12.2.3 Energy problems

The energy consumption of a pneumatic muscle is connected to the work to be performed, which in turn depends on the forces generated and the strokes developed. In particular, the amount of work will be quite high for muscles designed to lift weights (e.g., to raise an arm, a leg or an external load), and low for muscles used in gripping operations. In the latter case, it is necessary only to open and close the fingers of an active glove or artificial hand, and guarantee a clamping force. Once the object has been grasped, the pneumatic system is capable of continuing to exert the force without expending additional energy, which is not the case for many electrically powered systems.

In a system using artificial muscles, however, it must be borne in mind that all of the compressed air contained in the muscle is discharged to the atmosphere at the end of the cycle. Consequently, the energy expended will depend on the work performed in order to compress the mass of air that filled the muscle and the portion of the pneumatic circuit which is exhausted. In the next cycle, in fact, it will be necessary to compress and use new air. All of this leads to a number of muscle design constraints and objectives. For any given cycle, the designer must keep a close eye on air consumption and operating pressure to ensure that as little energy as possible is used for compression. Naturally, the efficiency of the compressor and circuit components must also be taken into account. From the standpoint of system organization, it must be remembered that both compressed air and electrical energy are required. This means that a dual energy source must be provided.

If we take a look at the potential applications of pneumatic artificial muscles, we will note that they can be of two kinds: applications on active clothing, which is worn continuously by the user, and applications on rehabilitation equipment at specialized centers. In both cases, it is difficult to see how the system's structure can guarantee an independent energy source: the amounts of energy required and the power levels involved call for connection to a pneumatic and/or electrical supply network. One possible solution, whose structure is suitable for rehabilitation centers but also lends itself to use with active clothing in a confined area such as a home or workplace is shown schematically in Fig. 12.19. Self-contained solutions in which the power source is also installed and integrated on the active garment would not appear to be highly feasible, and would be possible only in applications involving occasional muscle use and low energy. In the latter case, rechargeable batteries could be used to supply minicompressors and small compensator reservoirs, or small high-pressure air tanks.

12.3 State of the art: applications and research

The use of pneumatic muscles in devices designed to assist people is fairly widespread, thanks to the properties that make these actuators similar to human muscles. McKibben-type muscles are chiefly used, and in most cases are retained to the limbs by means of a rigid structure such as an exoskeleton, or by appropriately positioned straps. In all cases, the aim is to produce lightweight, easily used and low-cost devices which make it possible to accomplish all natural movements; consequently, the pneumatic muscles are positioned and attached in such a way as to reproduce the forces generated by real muscles as faithfully as possible. The type of pneumatic muscle used must be suitable for the application, and will thus vary according to the movement to be produced. Several designs will be presented below which can be used for rehabilitation as well as for assistance in daily life, as they are capable of producing one or more movements any desired number of times.

12.3.1 Hand actuation

Figure 12.20 shows a schematic view (Fig. 12.20(a)) and a photograph (Fig. 12.20(b)) of the Power Assist Glove [22] developed at Okayama University. Finger bending is accomplished by curved type pneumatic rubber muscles [21] attached at the rear of the fingers, while opposable thumb movement is achieved by means of two linear type pneumatic muscles positioned at the base of the thumb, one on the back of the hand and one on the palm. The pneumatic muscles are secured to an ordinary glove, which acts as an interface

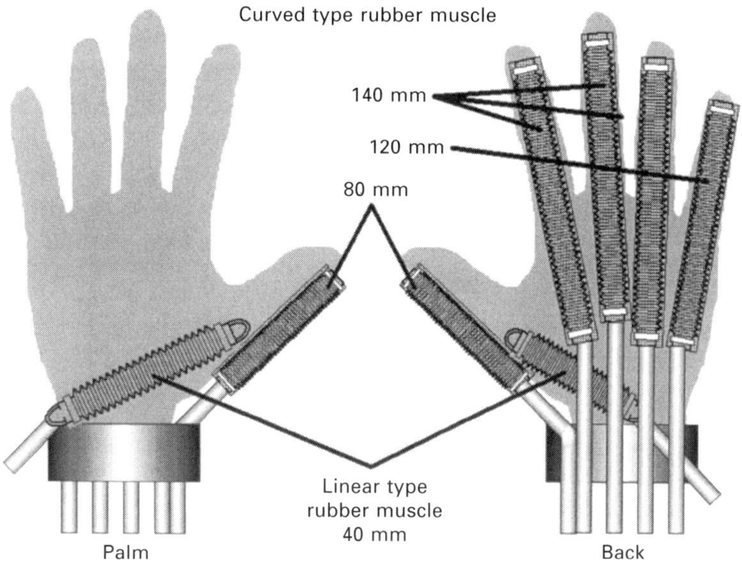

(a)

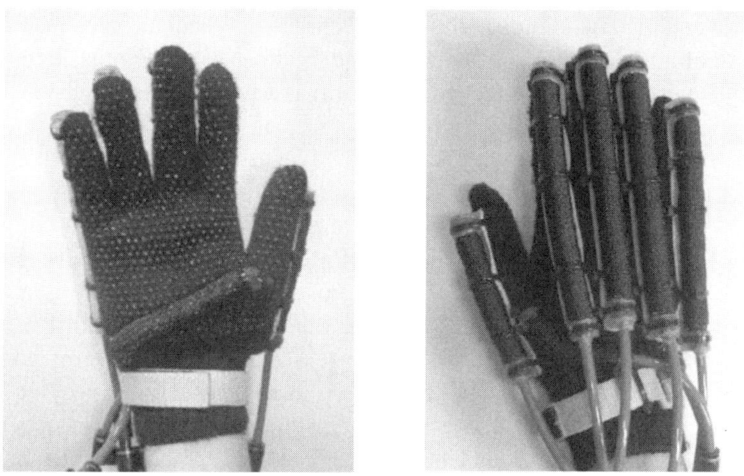

(b)

12.20 Power Assist Glove, Okayama University. Source: Sasaki D., Noritsugu T., Takaiwa M. and Yamamoto H., Wearable Power Assist Device for Hand Grasping Using Pneumatic Artificial Rubber Muscle, *Proc. of the 2004 IEEE Int. Workshop on Robot and Human Interactive Communication*, 2004.

between the patient and the device and transmits force to the fingers and thumb. The muscles are supplied at 500 kPa to achieve the approximately 20 N force required to produce movement and interact with objects. The movements that can be produced with the Power Assist Glove are sufficient for the needs of everyday life.

12.3.2 Elbow actuation

A device to assist elbow movement or aid in recovering joint function was developed at the Technical University 'Politecnico di Torino' [23] using a straight fiber pneumatic muscle as an actuator. The kinematics of this active orthosis are not strictly defined; the pneumatic muscle is constrained via formed polyethylene sleeves to the shoulder and forearm, as close as possible to the points of insertion of the biceps, thus enabling the joint to establish movement kinematics.

12.3.3 Upper limb actuation

The upper limb motion assist device [24] consists of a shoulder, an arm and a forearm, connected by two motor-driven joints (a ball joint for the shoulder and a cylindrical joint for the elbow). The kinematic architecture is such that the centers of the device's joints coincide with the centers of the natural articulations. McKibben muscles are used as actuators, and motion is transmitted by cord and pulley systems. Two pneumatic muscles installed in an agonist-antagonist set-up on the forearm are used to power elbow joint movement. The shoulder has three degrees of freedom, each powered by a pair of muscles. Flexion, adduction and rotation are accomplished respectively by a pair of muscles attached to the arm and two pairs attached at the rear of the orthosis, i.e., on the frame running along the user's trunk.

The research group at Okayama University has also developed a device for assisting upper limb motion [25], the power assist splint for upper arm shown in Fig. 12.21, which powers the wrist and elbow joints. In this case, a soft material like a glove is not sufficient as an interface with the patient. Given that the forces that the actuators transmit to the limbs are higher, greater stiffness is required. A specially designed plastic orthosis is thus used which features a hinge for the elbow joint. Elbow movement is powered by two curved type pneumatic muscles covered by a bellows provided with an axial reinforcement on one side to ensure that deformation occurs in the correct direction. The muscles are attached to the orthosis, which in addition to guiding movement, ensures that its amplitude does not exceed the limits of the natural elbow joint. The same type of actuator powers wrist joint motion. In this case, the interface consists of a fabric band that secures the device to the hand and forearm slightly below the joint.

The Science University of Tokyo is also developing a wearable device to assist upper limb motion [26, 27]. The idea here is to create a 'muscle suit' which uses the human skeleton as a support structure (an endoskeleton) and which supplies force to the limbs by means of pneumatic muscles secured to the garment. A prototype of the muscle suit is shown in Figs 12.22 and 12.23. The greatest asset of a muscle suit is 'wearing'. Wearable systems and robots normally consist of pole-like metal frames and joints, and they are

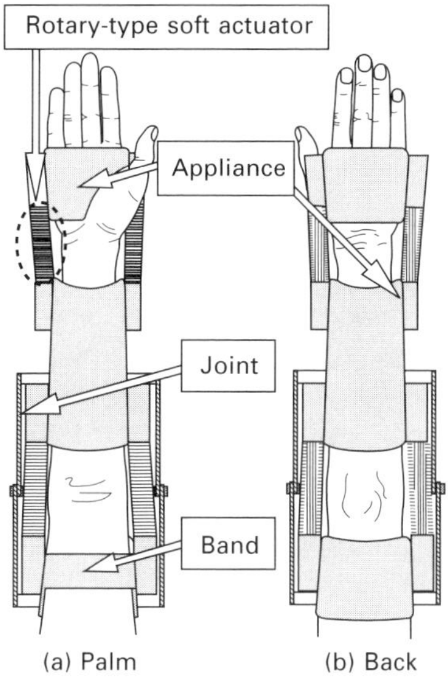

12.21 Power assist splint for upper arm, Okayama University. Source: Sasaki D., Noritsugu T., Takaiwa M. and Kataoka Y., Development of Pneumatic Wearable Power Assist Device for Human Arm 'ASSIST', *Proc. of the 6th JFPS Int. Symp. On Fluid Power*, 2005.

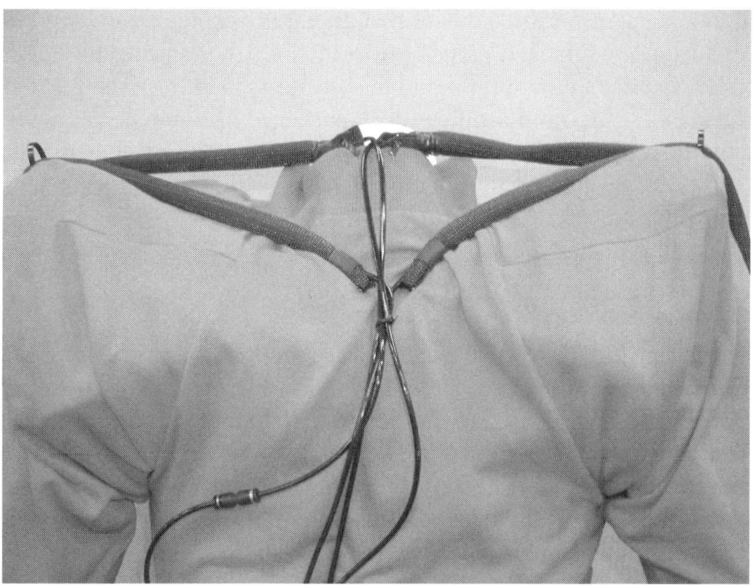

12.22 Muscle suit, Tokyo University of science. Source: www.kobalab.com.

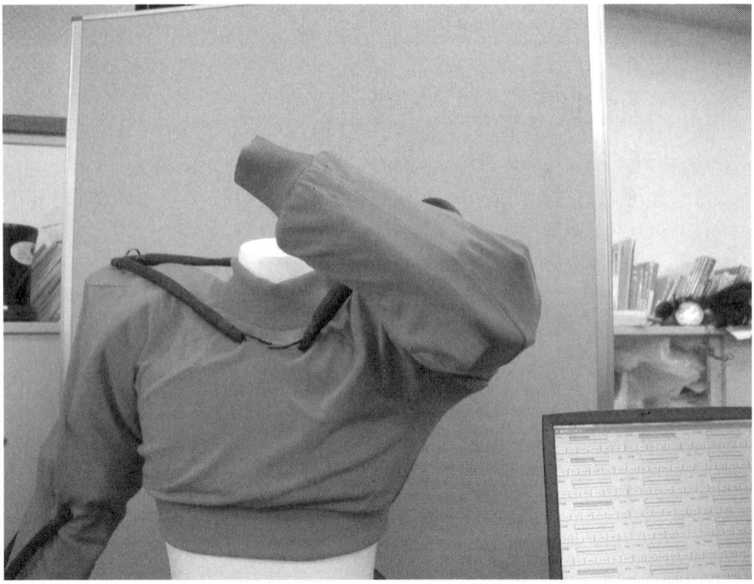

12.23 Muscle suit, Tokyo University of science. Source: www.kobalab.com.

attached to human body by band and/or hook-and-loop fasteners. A wearer suffers discomfort if the position of a joint is not precise and notices a heavy load from the attached parts. However, since the muscle suit does not have to be attached to the wearer and the wearer loaded from the inner surface of the muscle suit, no discomfort is experienced. Moreover the muscle suit is manufactured a little larger than the human limb diameter so that the wearer can move inside the muscle suit. These features make it unnecessary to adjust the muscle suit precisely to the wearer.

12.3.4 Trunk and waist actuation

The device [28] developed to assist waist motion consists of two rigid sections connected by a hinge and attached to curved type pneumatic muscles. The lower section is secured to the user's thigh and acts as a support. The upper section is secured to the waist, and is acted on by the force generated by the muscle. The device takes advantage of the lever arm given by the distance between the hinge and the end of the actuator to generate a moment that acts on the lumbar area as shown by the diagram in Fig. 12.24.

12.3.5 Lower limb actuation

Applications have also been developed for the lower limb which use pneumatic muscles as actuators powering active orthoses. An example is the lower limb

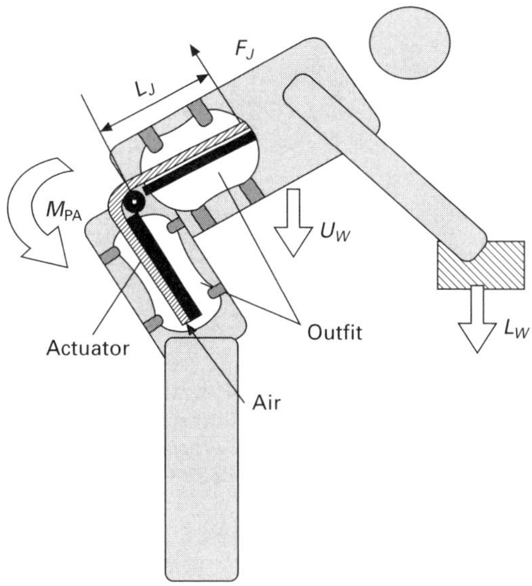

12.24 Power assist for waist, Okayama University. Source: Gao L., Noritsugu T., Takaiwa M. and Sasaki D., Development of Wearable Power Assist Device Using Curved Pneumatic Artificial Rubber Muscle, *Proc. of the 6th Int. Conf. On Fluid Power Transmission and Control*, 2005.

motion assist device [29] developed at the Università de L'Aquila. Figure 12.25 shows a prototype of this active lower limb orthosis, where the knee joint is powered by McKibben pneumatic muscles operating in parallel. The device's goal is to provide greater independence for its user; an elderly or disabled person who can walk but has difficulty sitting and rising from a seated position. Thus, the active orthosis provides assistance in rising and sitting motions. One end of the pneumatic muscle is secured to the bottom of the orthosis, while the other is connected to a cord which runs in a pulley positively connected to the top of the orthosis and transmitting motion to it. The radius of the pulley determines the relation between muscle shortening and the angular excursion between the tibia and femur. The actuation command is generated by an electropneumatic sensor that detects femoral muscle contraction, which is interpreted as indicating that the user intends to rise or sit. Both an on/off and a proportional control logic were tested; the latter provided smoother, quieter action, as the proportional valve operates continuously.

Pneumatic muscles have also been used to power the lower limb in the Hart Walker [30] developed at the Tokyo University of Science (Fig. 12.26). The device uses a conventional pneumatic cylinder to assist the user in rising from a seated position, while McKibben muscles are employed to reproduce normal gait. The ankle joint has also been studied in order to develop a

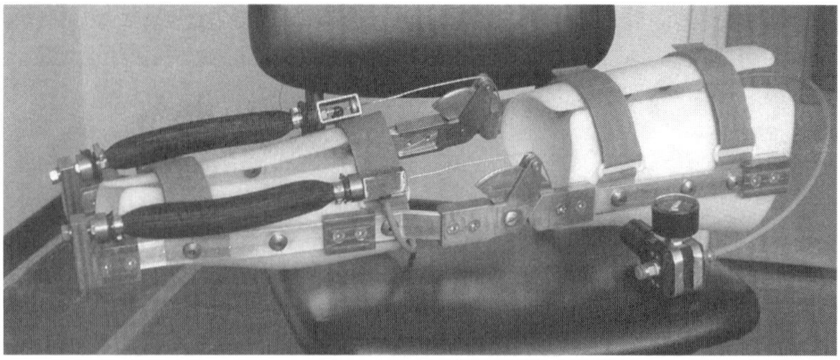

12.25 Active lower limb orthosis, Università de L'Aquila. Source: T. Raparelli, P. Beomonte Zobel, F. Durante; Powered Lower Limb Orthosis for Assisting Standing Up and Sitting Down Movements. Chapter 21 in *Designing a more inclusive world*, Eds Keates *et al.* Springer-Verlag UK, March 2004, ISBN 1-85233-819-9.

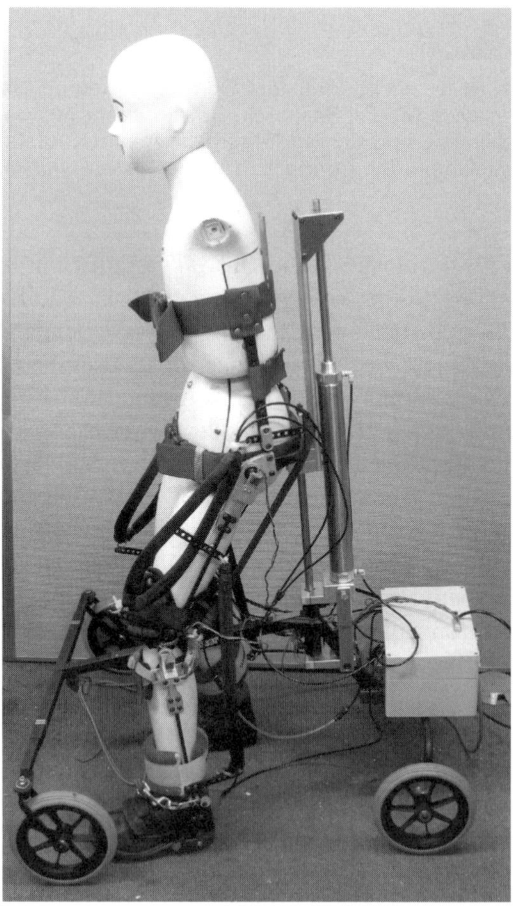

12.26 Hart Walker, Tokyo University of science. Source: www.kobalab.com.

device which can be used in rehabilitation or as a walking aid [31, 32]. McKibben type pneumatic muscles have been installed on orthoses designed to activate plantar flexion alone (one such device is shown in Fig. 12.27) or both plantar flexion and ankle joint dorsiflexion.

12.4 Future trends

The development of pneumatic muscles has stemmed from studies of a particular type of actuator whose performance capabilities differ significantly from those of the more common pneumatic cylinders. This fact has had two

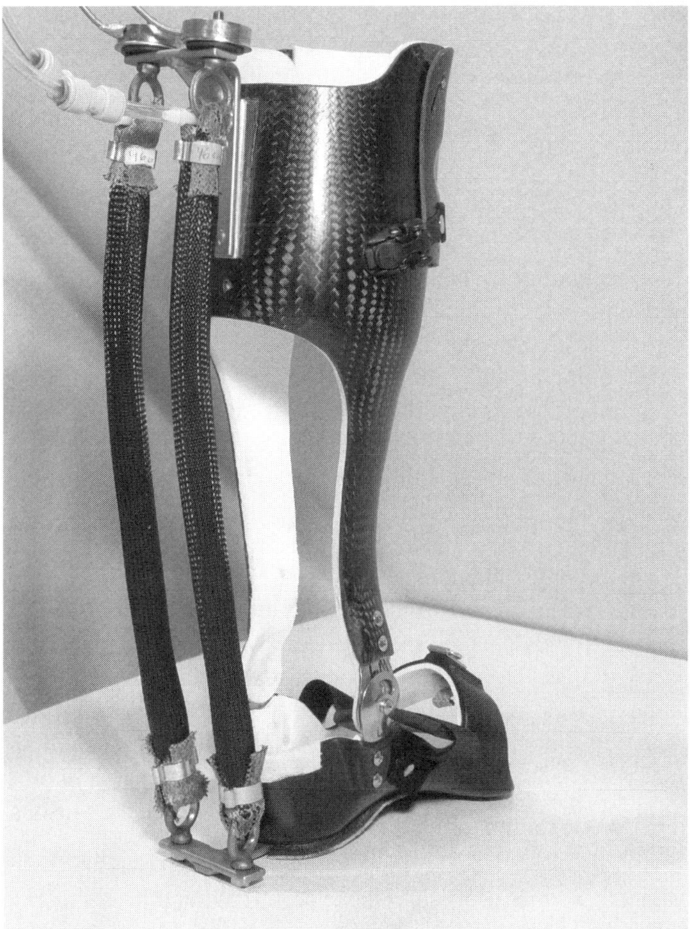

12.27 Powered ankle-foot orthosis, University of Michigan. Source: Ferris D. P., Czerniecki J. M., Hannaford B., An Ankle-Foot Orthosis Powered by Artificial Pneumatic Muscles, *J. of Applied Biomechanics*, 2005, 21, 189–197.

major consequences: first, such muscles have been presented as components to be used in automated systems on a par with many other types of drive; second, they are chiefly used in biomedicine for application on rehabilitation equipment or active orthoses. As we have seen above, pneumatic muscles can actuate a variety of mechanisms, levers and devices located off the patient, much as is done with other types of actuator. If, however, we look at the function performed by pneumatic muscles, their fabric characteristics and their behavior, we see a number of marked differences with respect to other actuators. The fact that they do not have a specific, well-defined shape of their own, the lack of rigid connection constraints, and their high adaptability to external constraints and boundary conditions all make these elements particularly suitable for installation in structures that consist of bodies that are not entirely rigid and are connected by complex constraints, as are living structures. As a result, significant advantages can accrue from installing deformable pneumatic actuators in clothing, thus converting a passive element into something active and transformable. Here, adaptability and integration are key factors.

Solving the problems involved in applications of this kind calls for addressing a variety of issues, ranging from muscle design to fabric selection and integration technologies. In addition, rotation, force and torque sensors must be provided in order to implement the sophisticated control systems needed to manage the desired laws of motion. Fabric-based wearable devices employing pneumatic muscles can adapt readily to different anthropomorphic measurements. Together with their light weight, this promotes better psychological acceptance by the wearer and makes them particularly attractive for use in rehabilitation. This, in fact, is a field where every patient must be treated individually and followed by a physiotherapist. Using active structures and clothing makes it possible to apply movements and/or forces in sequences selected by the physiotherapist, and to acquire the associated signals. As a result, exercises can be performed without direct assistance, while analyzing the recorded signals enables the physician to follow the patient's progress and order any necessary corrections in his or her activity.

This makes it possible to plan extremely flexible rehabilitation therapies which can be adapted as needed without the regular presence of specialized personnel. As a result, active clothing of this kind has excellent prospects for application. This is especially true in rehabilitation for the reasons outlined above, viz.:

- Extended exercise programs can be performed without direct intervention on the part of the physiotherapist, as appropriate software can be used to tailor exercise sequences to the individual patient.
- Cycle data can be acquired, monitoring interaction with the muscular system and permitting continual analysis and corrective action.

- Thanks to the sensors and control unit, the system can be managed in two ways. Active clothing can generate movement (with the patient passive), or can oppose movement (patient active) to exercise muscles.

Further work will be required in order to develop efficient active clothing for daily use. Much of this work must concentrate on a host of issues associated with textiles: the type of elastic-anisotropic fabric enclosing the pneumatic muscle, materials, techniques for sealing and retaining air, compatibility with the skin, wearability and appearance factors. Though there is still a long way to go, and the road ahead is challenging, the first concrete steps have been taken towards providing clothing with capabilities that will prove invaluable for therapeutic massage techniques, rehabilitation, assistance and in replacing motor and relational functions.

12.5 References

1. http://www.aging.cnr.it/atlante.htm
2. http://www.census.gov/ipc/prod/wp02/wp-02004.pdf
3. http://www.agingstats.gov
4. http://www.umbriariabilitazione.it/universita/lezioni/DiapositivedellelezioniIII.html
5. http://www.biausa.org
6. Belforte G., Gastaldi L., Sorli M., *Active Systems for Walking*, 3rd Health and Textile International Meeting, Biella, March 2003, pp. 166–169 (in Italian).
7. Belforte G., Sorli M., Testore F., Gastaldi L., *Textile drivers for rehabilitation*, World Textile Conference 4th AUTEX Conference, Roubaix, France, 22–24 June 2004.
8. Morin, A. H., *Elastic diaphragm*, US Patent No. 2 642 091, 1953.
9. Th. A. McMahon, *Muscles, reflexes, and locomotion*, Princeton University Press, 1984.
10. Daerden, F., *Conception and realization of Pleated Pneumatic Artificial Muscles and their use as compliant actuation elements*, PhD Thesis, Vrije Universiteit Brussels, 1999.
11. Daerden, F., Lefeber, D., The concept and design of pleated pneumatic artificial muscles, *International Journal of Fluid Power*, vol. 2, no. 3, pp. 41–50, 2001.
12. Yarlott, J. M., *Fluid Actuator*, US Patent No. 3 645 173, 1972.
13. Kukolj, M., *Axially contractible actuator*, US Patent No. 4 733 603, 1988.
14. Raparelli, T., Beomonte Zobel, P., Durante, F., *On the design of pneumatic muscle actuators*, 2nd Internationales Fluidtechnisches Kolloquium, 16–17 March 2000, Dresden.
15. Morecki, A., Nazarczuk, K., Some problems of bioelectric control of natural and artificial limbs, *The Active Mechanical Engineering Quarterly*, Warsaw, 1969.
16. Paynter, H. M., *Hyperboloid of revolution fluid-driven tension actuators and methods of making*, US Patent No. 4 721 030, 1988.
17. Quaglia, G., Ferraresi, C., Franco, W., *A New Fluid Power Deformable Actuator With Three Diaphragms*, 14th International Workshop on Robotics in Alpe-Adria-Danube Region, RAAD05, Bucharest, May 2005, pp. 507–512.

18. Quaglia, G., Ferraresi, C., Franco, W., *Attuatore Deformabile a Fluido a Doppio Effetto a Tre Camere*, domanda di brevetto n° TO2004A000150, Torino, 10/03/2004.
19. Cataudella, C., Ferraresi, C., Manuello Bertetto, A., Flexible actuator for oscillating tail marine robot, *Int. Journal of Mechanics and Control*, Torino, Vol. 02, n. 02, 2001, pp. 13–21, ISSN 1590–8844.
20. Suzumori, K., Likura, S., Tanaka, H., *Flexible microactuator for miniature robots*, Proc. IEEE Workshop Micro Electro Mechanical Systems, 1991, pp. 204–209.
21. Noritsugu, T., Masahiro, T., Sasaki, D., *Development of a pneumatic rubber artificial muscle for human support applications*, 9th Scandinavian Int. conference on Fluid Power, SICFP'05, June 1–3, 2005, Linkoeping, Sweden.
22. Sasaki, D., Noritsugu, T., Takaiwa, M., Yamamoto, H., *Wearable Power Assist Device for Hand Grasping Using Pneumatic Artificial Rubber Muscle*, Proc. of the 2004 IEEE Int. Workshop on Robot and Human Interactive Communication, 2004.
23. Ferraresi, C., Franco, W., Manuello Bertetto, A., *Modelisation and Characterisation of a Pneumatic Muscle Actuator for Non Conventional Robotics*, 7th International Workshop on Robotics in Alpe-Danube Region RAAD, 1998, pp. 279–284.
24. Durante, F., Raparelli, T., Beomonte Zobel, P., *A 4 d.o.f. Upper-limb Orthosis driven by Pneumatic Muscles*. 3rd FPNI PhD International Symposium on Fluid Power, June 30 July 2, Terrassa, Spain, 2004.
25. Sasaki, D., Noritsugu, T., Takaiwa, M. and Kataoka, Y., *Development of Pneumatic Wearable Power Assist Device for Human Arm 'ASSIST'*, Proc. of the 6th JFPS Int. Symp. On Fluid Power, 2005.
26. www.kobalab.com
27. www.kobalab.com
28. Gao, L., Noritsugu, T., Takaiwa, M. and Sasaki, D., *Development of Wearable Power Assist Device Using Curved Pneumatic Artificial Rubber Muscle*, Proc. of the 6th Int. Conf. On Fluid Power Transmission and Control, 2005.
29. Raparelli, T., Beomonte, Zobel, P., Durante F., Powered Lower Limb Orthosis for Assisting Standing Up and Sitting Down Movements. Chapter 21 in: *Designing a more inclusive world*. Eds Keates *et al.* Springer-Verlag UK, March 2004, ISBN 1-85233-819-9.
30. www.kobalab.com
31. Gordon, K. E., Sawicki, G. S., Ferris, D. P., Mechanical performance of artificial pneumatic muscles to power an ankle-foot orthosis, *J. of Biomechanics*, 2005.
32. Ferris, D. P., Czerniecki, J. M., Hannaford, B., An Ankle-Foot Orthosis Powered by Artificial Pneumatic Muscles, *J. of Applied Biomechanics*, 2005, 21, 189–197.

13
Wearable assistants for mobile health monitoring

T KIRSTEIN, G TRÖSTER, I LOCHER and C KÜNG, ETH Zürich, Switzerland

13.1 Introduction

The integration of electronic functionality into clothing offers new possibilities for medical monitoring. Our approach is to develop context aware textiles. Context aware means that textiles sense the state of the user and the environment and recognize situations and events. We combine electronic textile technologies with context recognition and wearable computing technologies in order to achieve an intelligent and at the same time wearable system. In the first part of this chapter we explain the vision of a wearable health assistant and our system concept. Then we describe the recent developments and achievements in the area of electronic textiles, context recognition and wearable technologies. We show how these three research fields can be combined. In the last part we present concrete applications of our wearable health assistants.

13.2 Vision of wearable health assistant

An increasingly important issue for many of today's devices and services is mobility. In particular there is a growing interest in mobile healthcare services such as portable health monitoring systems. The vision sketches personalized health services for everyone in a trusted and natural way, anywhere and at any time. Healthcare is not restricted to clinics or a stationary environment (like at home) but extended to our whole life. With this approach the current issues can be addressed:

- For many patients it is difficult to manage health problems in daily life. Generally there is a lack of motivation and advice for a continuously healthy lifestyle. Widespread problems that could be avoided are, for example, back pain, obesity and stress-related diseases.
- Physicians have only limited tools to assess patients' health status during their daily activities. Diagnosis is restricted to brief contacts with the patients.

- The costs of healthcare are increasing. The focus is on extensive professional treatment instead of illness prevention.

The wearable health assistant could help people to fight diseases by a preventive lifestyle and early diagnosis. Users could take control of their own health status and adapt a permanent healthier lifestyle. This self-management of health makes people more independent, improves their quality of life and at the same time, reduces healthcare costs.

Three main features characterize our vision of the wearable health assistant: monitoring of the physiological parameters, detection of the user's context and giving feedback to the user. Concentrating on non-invasive measuring methods, physiological parameters comprise heart rate and ECG, respiration, EMG, blood pressure, blood oximetry, skin conductance and temperature. But the meaningful assessment of these vital parameters requires the consideration of the current context of the user. For example, rapidly increasing heart rate could naturally be provoked by jumping up a staircase, but if the user has not been moving, it could indicate a dangerous health status. Context awareness includes the user's motion, activity, gestures and also the affective and emotional state like stress and depression. The user's location, both indoor and outdoor, time, weather, the illumination and noise define the environmental context. Apart from the user's activity and environment it is also important to determine the user's social context; that means his contact and communication with other people.

The combination of the vital parameters with the wearer's context, the activity and the sleep patterns together with social interactions paint a picture of the user's health status. To facilitate the feedback and interface between the individual user and the wearable health assistant we propose a 'life balance factor' (LBF) as a plain health measure and generally understandable indicator, especially for medical laypersons. The LBF summarizes the current health status; it indicates changes and calls on a consultation if health parameters are moving to a critical range.

Weiser's visionary view (Weiser, 1991) of an invisible and pervasive computing world is now coming to fruition, where tiny autonomous systems, consisting of sensors, signal processing and transmitting units, possibly as small as a grain of rice, are scattered in the environment. Radio Frequency Identification (RFID) tags are the forerunner of this vision; attached to a variety of daily artefacts, these electronic markers enable the detection of their location and also provide information about the objects to which they are attached. The impact of a computerized environment on personal healthcare varies from monitoring of people with cardiac risks (Gouaux *et al.*, 2002) to home care for elderly living alone (Korhonen *et al.*, 2003).

13.3 Approach

For the realization of continuous health monitoring we need on-body electronics (Kirstein, 2004; Lukowicz *et al.*, 2004). Figure 13.1 shows different approaches to on-body electronics, handheld electronics, electronics in accessories, electronics in clothing and finally electronic textiles. In recent years advances in miniaturization, wireless technology and worldwide networking have enabled the development of many portable (hand-held) devices such as cell phones, organizers and laptops. But until now electronic devices on the market are still bulky and inconvenient to use and especially in the medical field rather home-based than truly mobile. The first step to wearability has been made by embedding electronics into accessories like watches and belts. The HealthWear armband by BodyMedia (www.bodymedia.com) monitors, for example, the calorie balance of the user. The next step is to use clothing as a platform for electronics. This idea offers many advantages especially in the medical field because of the direct contact and continuous interaction between the garment and the user. Another important aspect is the comfort of wearing, as humans prefer to wear textiles rather than heavy and hard boxes. Clothing allows integrating the system unobtrusively and conveniently into the daily life of the user. Simply hiding electronic components in pockets or seams is a possible solution. The Lifeshirt by Vivometrics (www.vivometrics.com) is an example of medical clothing where the fabric acts as a carrier of conventional cables and electronic devices. Using the textiles themselves as electronic components goes one step further and is a new approach to the next generation of on-body electronics.

We believe that a wearable assistant as described in our vision can be achieved only by context sensitivity as described above and by a modular system concept. The modular system concept means that we use different integration methods to embed the system into the user's outfit depending on the functionality and the cost of the components. People wear many different clothes and select their outfit according to their activities. Only cheap

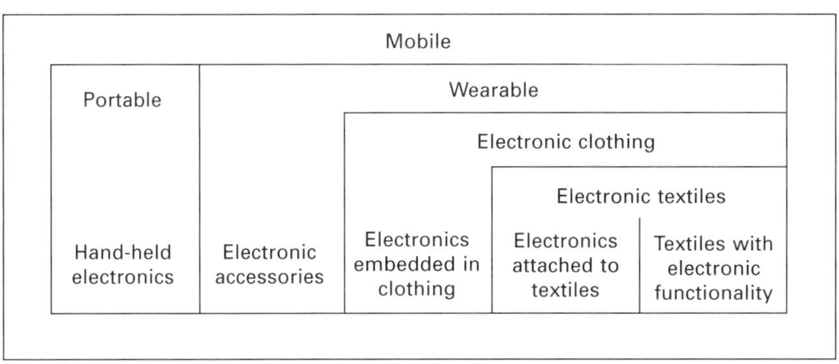

13.1 Approaches to on-body electronics.

components with task-specific functionality (e.g. sensors) should be permanently mounted into the garment whereas more expensive general-purpose devices such as processors should be detachable and usable with different outfits. For distributing sensor functionality all over the body and for having direct contact with the skin, electronic textiles offer the best solution. Therefore we embed textile sensors as well as pre-processing circuits and communication facilities into the clothing. Processing devices and components for external communication can be centralized and embedded into accessories (such as belts and watches) or hand-held devices (such as mobile phones). This combination of smart textiles with miniaturized electronics is depicted in Fig. 13.2.

13.4 Electronic textile technology

Textile technological developments have created a whole range of so-called 'smart fabrics' for many applications. The concept of smart materials describes the ability of materials to sense and react to external stimuli. However, most of the advanced textile materials like breathable, fire-resistant or substance-releasing textiles cannot be considered as smart because they do not adapt

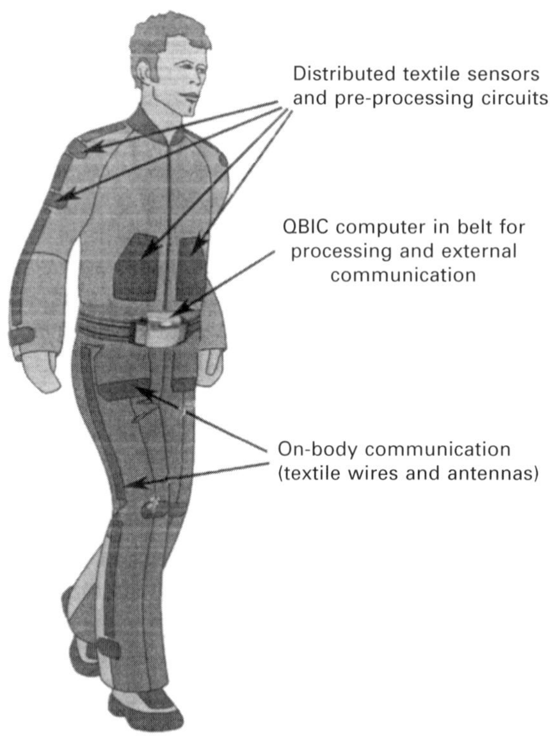

13.2 System concept of the wearable health assistant.

their functionality to the environment. Hence they are not context-aware as required for the wearable health assistant. Textile materials that can store heat when it is warm and release the heat again when it gets cold (phase change materials) react to a change in environment and therefore possess a low level of context sensitivity, but they have no active control. It is, for example, not possible to regulate the temperature of the clothing according to the user needs. Such an active control is necessary for healthcare applications but it requires an electronic system that processes the sensor data and 'decides' about the reaction. This need for electronics in textiles induced a new research field 'e-textiles'. Considering the opposed properties of electronics and textiles a merging of both seems to be impossible. Nevertheless, the first results show the potential of this idea (Kirstein *et al.*, 2005).

There are two possible ways to create textiles with electronic functionality. Miniaturized electronic components can be attached to fabrics if their size does not reduce comfort. Using electrically conductive fibres and fabrics is the second approach. In this case the textiles do not just act as a substrate but as electronic components themselves. In the following, we describe the latest developments in e-textile research.

13.4.1 Textiles for communication

Some early approaches to using textiles for communication are described in Marculescu *et al.* (2003). One of the biggest problems was that the fabrics lost much of their typical textile properties due to the embedded thick wires. Our aim was to achieve high-performance signal lines made from conductive textiles that have the same look and feel as conventional fabrics. Several types of conductive fabrics already exist and are applied mainly for shielding and antistatic applications. By developing measurement and simulation methods those textiles can now be optimized for data transmission.

The first systematic studies of the electrical properties of textile transmission lines were carried out by Cottet *et al.* (2003). The proposed textiles are fabrics with copper fibres in one or two directions and with different polyester yarn fineness. The variety of fabrics opens a wide range of possible transmission line topologies and allows finding a configuration that fits potential target applications. Using wire pair configuration the achievable characteristic impedances lie between 120 Ω and 320 Ω. To study the influence of fabrication tolerances, the textiles were modelled with an EM-field simulation tool. The simulation results showed that with the given geometry variations an accuracy of ± 5% to ± 10% for the characteristic impedances is achievable. High-frequency network analyser measurements were performed up to 6 GHz. The extracted frequency characteristics revealed that the dielectric and ohmic losses do not determine the line insertion loss. The loss is mainly influenced by a non-uniform impedance profile along the lines up to the half-wavelength and by coupling to parasitic modes above this frequency point. This results in cut-off frequencies of 1 GHz for 10 cm long lines. Good signal transmission for a 100 MHz clock signal was proved through 20 cm textile lines. Experiments showed also that a grounded copper fibre between two neighbouring lines reduced crosstalk from 7.2% to 2.8%. To conclude, conductive textiles provide potentials in signal transmission in addition to EMI shielding and power supply. Textile transmission lines can be used to create a network infrastructure in clothing and to connect different distributed components of a wearable assistant.

Another important ingredient of a wearable assistant is the connection to a wireless network. For this purpose, textile antennas were developed that guarantee flexible and comfortable embedding into clothing. Wearable antennas presented by Salonen *et al.* (2000) and by Massey (2001) are partially based on textiles possessing an inverted-F shape that results in a stiff structure. Other textile antennas described by Tanaka *et al.* (2003) and by Salonen *et al.* (2003) are designed as rectangular patches with a protruding probe feed and only linear polarization. Antennas such as presented in Salonen *et al.* (2004) utilize fabrics only as substrates whereas the patches and ground planes are copper foils.

We developed antennas that are purely textile and flat (Klemm *et al.*, 2004). Those textile patch antennas are designed for Bluetooth in the frequency range from 2400 MHz to 2483.5 MHz. The design of this antenna is inspired by the build-up of printed microstrip antennas and consists of a three-layer structure; electrically conductive fabrics act as ground plane and antenna patch and are separated with a fabric substrate. The conductive fabric should have a homogeneous resistance below 1 Ω^2. Therefore we used a metallized fabric that was plated before weaving or knitting. Using a knitted fabric leads to a highly bendable and deformable structure. From a manufacturing point of view, the knitted structure is a drawback because precise shaping as well as assembly of the antenna without warpage are difficult. The manufactured antenna shapes finally achieved a geometrical accuracy of about ±0.5 mm. Another undesired effect of the knitted fabric is a change of the sheet resistance when the structure is stretched. Conductive fabrics that are woven possess better electrical performance, but bending of such an antenna is limited. The textile substrate provides the dielectric between the antenna patch and the ground plane and needs to have a constant thickness and stable permittivity. We chose a spacer fabric with a thickness of 6 mm and performed humidity measurements covering a range from 20% to 80% relative humidity within a temperature range of 25 °C to 80 °C. The measurements showed that permittivity variations are negligible compared to measurement uncertainty. Alternative substrate materials are felts and foams.

During the design process of the antenna it was important to achieve a flat and wearable structure; that also means a planar antenna feed. We designed a microstrip feedline and applied insets in order to adjust the antenna's input impedance and to avoid losses due to mismatch between feedline and antenna. Additionally, a microstrip feedline does not increase the height of the patch antenna and maintains wearing comfort when integrated into clothing. We designed linearly and circularly polarized textile antennas and proved a good directivity that minimizes unnecessary radiation exposure to the human body and radiation losses. The textile antennas feature a 10 dB bandwidth of 200 MHz on average. Even when bent around a radius of 37.5 mm resembling a mounting on a human upper arm, Bluetooth specifications can be assured. One of the textile patch antennas is shown in Fig. 13.3.

13.4.2 Textiles for signal pre-processing (System-on-Textile)

We believe that conductive textiles offer an even greater potential than just being used as cables or antennas. Such fabrics manufactured with high precision allow complex wiring structures. Along with the proper assembly technology for electronic components and sensors, entire electrical circuits can be embedded into the fabric. We call this technology 'System-on-Textile' (SoT). Using fabrics as substrates for electronic circuits instead of rigid circuit boards enables the placement of small circuits for signal pre-processing close to the sensors. In this way we can distribute sensing functionality all over the body without affecting wearing comfort.

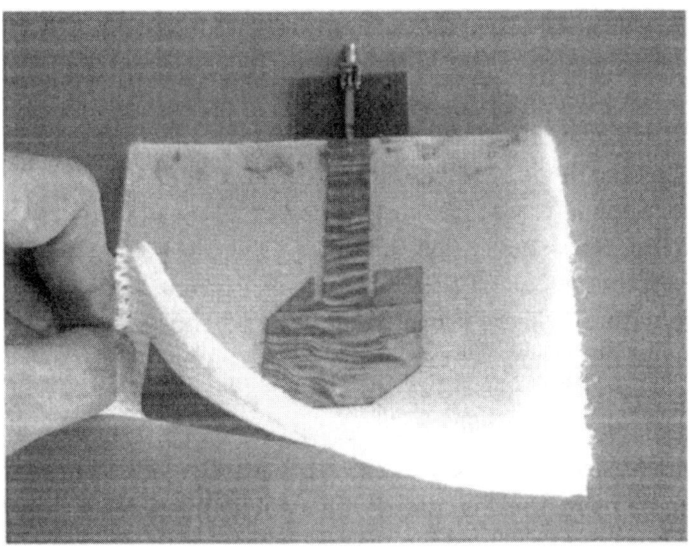

13.3 Textile Bluetooth antenna.

Suitable textile substrates must support electrical routeing structures. The newly developed woven fabric with thin insulated copper fibres provides our platform for electrical circuits. This fabric is manufactured by Sefar Inc., a producer of precision filters. From an electrical point of view, precise yarn distances within the fabric are required in order to achieve satisfactory electrical performance. Secondly, yarn distances need to be small to meet the pitches of the electrical components. On the other hand, the fabric should be fine, light and maintain typical textile properties. Nevertheless, manufacturability of the fabric with the desired materials has to be considered.

After several iterations, we achieved a hybrid fabric consisting of woven polyester yarn (PET) with an exact diameter of 42 microns and copper alloy wires with a diameter of 50 microns. The hybrid fabric with a mesh opening of 95 microns (+/– 10 microns) and an opening area of 44% is shown in Fig. 13.4. Each copper wire itself is coated with a polyurethane varnish as electrical insulation. The copper wire grid in the fabric features a spacing of 0.57 mm (mesh count in warp and in weft is 17.5 cm^{-1}). The combination of PET yarn and copper wires requires a special weaving technology, which includes two yarn systems in warp and weft direction (3 PET wires and 1 copper wire) with separate tensioning systems. We positioned our hybrid fabric with its weight of 74 g/m^2 as interlining. Its application field is therefore very versatile. The fabric represents a compromise between preserving textile properties and copper wire density, i.e., electrical connectivity. To our knowledge, such a precise hybrid fabric consisting of PET yarn and copper wire is unique.

In order to build circuits on the fabric, we need the technology to mount electrical components and interconnect them through the fabric utilizing embedded copper wires. The desired wiring structure can be established by connecting crossing copper wires at their intersections and by cutting the wires at certain locations. Since the wires are insulated against each other, the insulation needs to be removed at these intersections to enable electrical connection. Altogether, three manufacturing steps, as shown in Fig. 13.5, are required to create such an electrical connection.

1. coating removal and cutting of the copper wire using laser light at defined locations
2. assembly of the electrical components and interconnecting of the skinned wire sections with conductive adhesive
3. adding epoxy resin to the electrical components and intersections as mechanical protection.

These three steps form the building block for defined wiring structures in fabrics. They can be manufactured in automated processes using equipment for printed circuit board (PCB) fabrication. This assembly technology is described in more detail in Locher *et al.*, (2004, 2005).

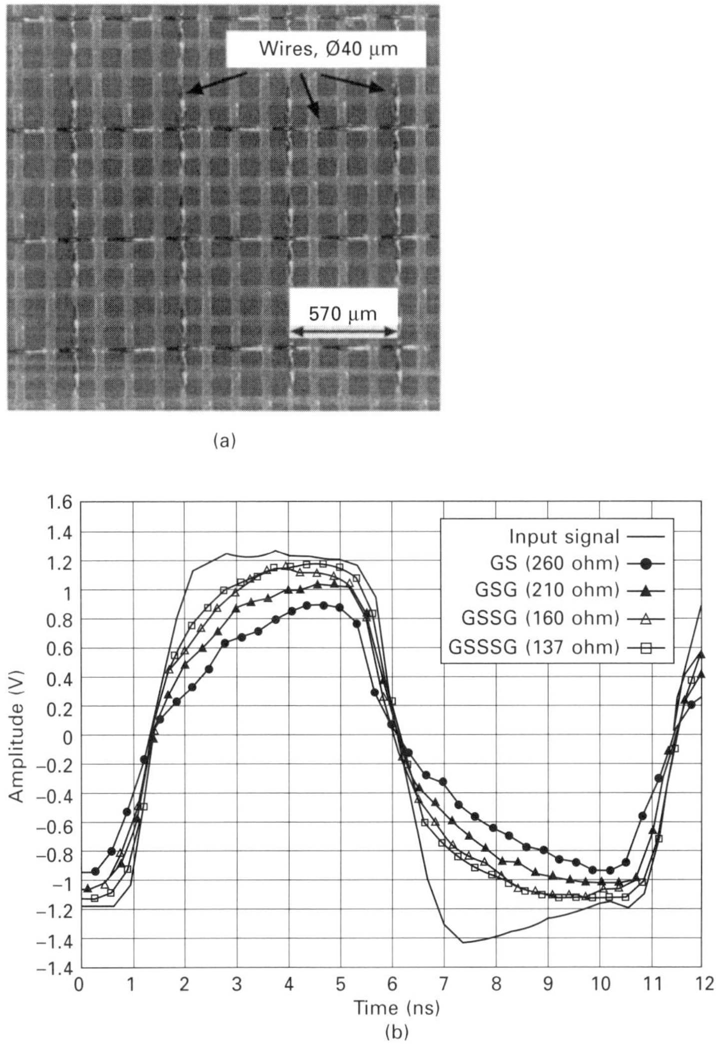

13.4 Conductive textile (by Sefar Inc.).

Electrical components usually feature a solid and rigid body whereas fabrics are soft and drapable. Thus, the placement of components onto the fabric requires special attention resulting in an additional trade-off between textile and electrical properties. From a textile point of view, the placement should be done such that drapability and softness are preserved. In other words, the components must not be placed too close together. On the other hand, the electrical wiring should be short in order to avoid electrical losses and noisy signals. In contrast to earlier developments by Virginia Tech and Infineon (Marculescu *et al.*, 2003), we were able to mount electrical components

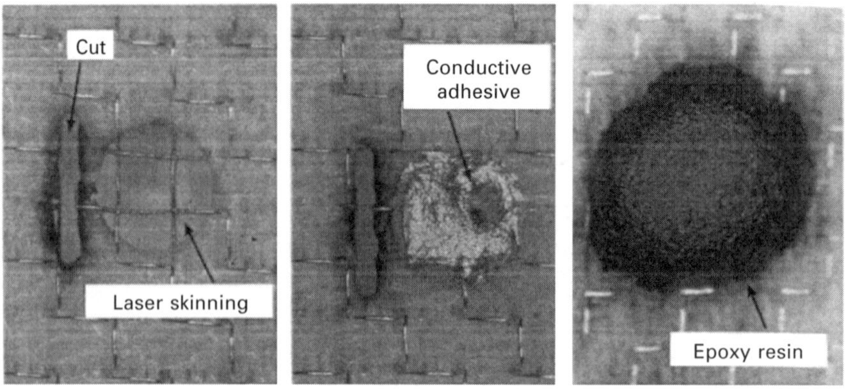

13.5 Manufacturing of wiring structures in fabrics.

directly onto the fabric and interconnect them through the fabric over an arbitrary wiring structure. Utilization of this technique is enabled only by the high precision of our hybrid fabric.

The Sefar Petex hybrid fabric combined with our assembly technology opens a promising new perspective for flexible electrical circuits in the field of e-textiles. The technology enables textiles to be used for processing and sensing tasks and for displays such as those needed in applications for medical monitoring, smart interior fabrics and drapable advertising media. Additionally, the textile properties can be adapted to the application requirements by deploying of different finishes.

13.4.3 Textiles for sensing

The next step in e-textile research is to use fibres and fabrics not just to transmit but also to transform signals. Conductive textiles that change their electrical properties due to environmental impact can be used as sensors. Typical examples are textiles that react to deformation like pressure sensors and stretch sensors and measure body movements, posture or breathing. Further parameters that can be measured with textiles are, e.g., humidity and temperature. Textile electrodes can replace conventional electrodes for heart monitoring or electrical stimulation (Kirstein *et al.*, 2003). Apart from measuring biometric or environmental data, textile sensors can also act as an input interface as, for example, textile touchpads.

Textile pressure sensor

Pressure sensors that are made from textiles have many attractive features for wearable applications. They can cover a large three-dimensionally shaped surface area and detect pressure without reducing wearing comfort. Apart from acting as input interfaces they can measure pressure distribution during sitting or lying and even detect body movements due to pressure changes in the garment.

ElekTex (www.eleksen.com) is a laminate of three textile layers. Conductive fibres in the central layer are locally compressed allowing conductive contact between the top and bottom layer. Softswitch (www.softswitch.co.uk) is made of conductive textiles with a thin layer of elastoresistive composite material (Quantum Tunnelling Composite QTC) that reduces resistance when compressed. The Sensory Fabric (patent US2003119391) contains conductive and insulating yarns in a woven structure that can create electrical contact at yarn crossing points when compressed. All these structures act as switches and do not deliver pressure values. We developed a pressure sensor mat consisting of a spacer fabric with embroidered electrically conductive patch arrays on both sides. Sitting posture and risk of bedsores (decubitus) can be detected using such a mat on seats and beds. The textile pressure sensor is shown in Fig. 13.6.

Each opposing patch pair in the arrays forms a plate capacitor whose capacity changes with compression force on the spacer fabric. Although the capacity is reciprocal proportional to the distance between the patches, the capacity versus pressure is highly nonlinear. Firstly, the compression force nonlinearly depends on the compression distance. Secondly, the permittivity of the spacer fabric (dielectric) increases when compressed since air becomes displaced. Additionally, relaxation of the spacer fabric shows a hysteresis effect as depicted in Fig. 13.7. Using the Preisach model this behaviour can

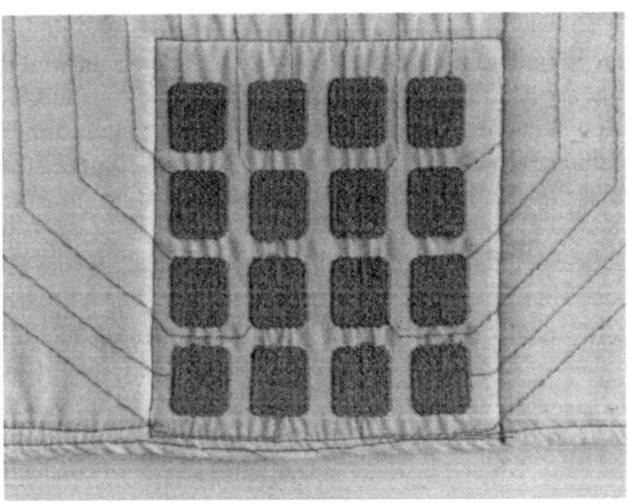

13.6 Textile pressure sensor.

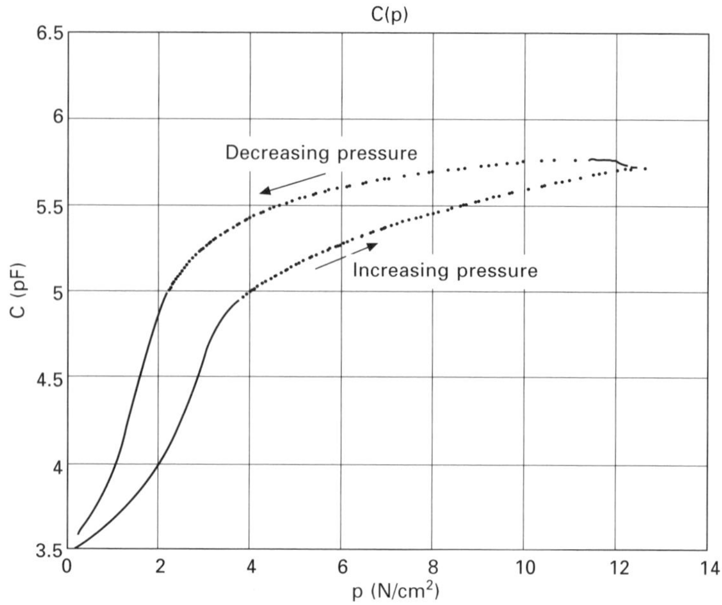

13.7 Capacity measurement hysteresis of textile pressure sensor.

be described, so that the measurement of pressure distribution over a fabric area becomes feasible.

Textile elongation sensor

Possible applications of wearable elongation sensors are, among others:

- posture and motion analysis in sports, medicine, rehabilitation or daily life
- artificial sensor skins for humanoid or animal-like mobile robots
- replacement of acceleration sensors used for context or gesture recognition.

The high range (including pre-stretch) of up to 30% strain which is needed for wearable applications as, for example, body posture monitoring, sets wearable elongation sensors clearly apart from other industrial elongation sensors. Additional requirements are comfort of wearing, the need for overstress tolerance and the fact that high elongations have to be measured without stiffening the textile too much.

The most wearable option of making elongation sensors is to use a knitted electroconductive fabric which is stretchable (Fig. 13.8). When such a fabric is stretched, the interconnect topology in the garment changes, and hence resistance changes. Some work on such fabrics can be found in the literature (Pacelli *et al.*, 2001; Scilingo *et al.*, 2003; Oh *et al.*, 2003; Wijesiriwardana

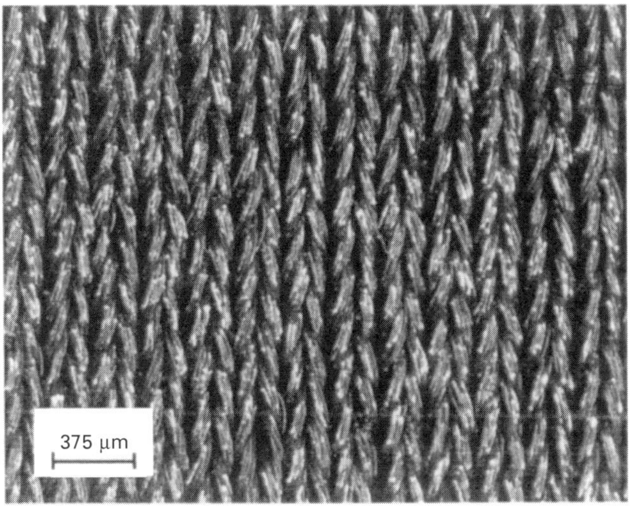

13.8 Conductive knitted fabric.

et al., 2003; Farringdon *et al.*, 1999; Bickerton, 2003). Mainly fabrics polymerized with conductive polymers, or fabrics made of conductive threads are mentioned. From what is currently published, the following is apparent: these sensors do not perform well because either the response is rather weak (polypyrrole coated threads/fabrics) or the range is too low (carbon filled rubber coated threads/fabrics). High temperature dependence and dependence of resistance on elongation rate are further problems mentioned for almost all published conductive fabrics.

We evaluated three highly stretchable electroconductive fabrics; two metallized knitted fabrics and a knitted fabric with activated carbon fibres. The general observations are the following: the fabrics show high transient times, peaks when movements start and high hysteresis. Electroconductive fabrics used as elongation sensors are wearable, but the transducer qualities are poor (see Fig. 13.9).

Another kind of wearable elongation sensors can be made by utilizing the piezoresistive effect of electroconductive elastomers. The following options were evaluated: carbon filled silicone rubber coated onto a fabric (Fig. 13.10) and carbon filled thermoplastic elastomer fibers. Carbon filled silicone rubber coated onto stretchable fabrics are extensively used at the University of Pisa (Tognetti *et al.*, 2005). Thereby, a commercial electroconductive silicone rubber product is used. This commercial product was extensively evaluated. It was found that the resistance of this material behaves in a very complex manner when the material is strained. The problems are that there is insufficient repeatability (Fig. 13.11) because the resistance depends on the strain history of the material, there is high electrical hysteresis, the resistance depends on the speed of deformation, the transient time is very high (due to the resistance

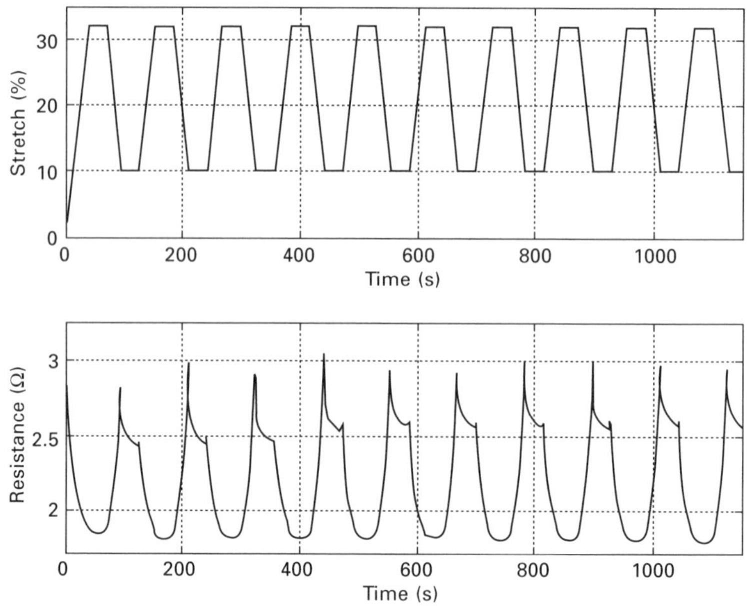

13.9 Periodic elongation and resistance change of conductive knitted fabric.

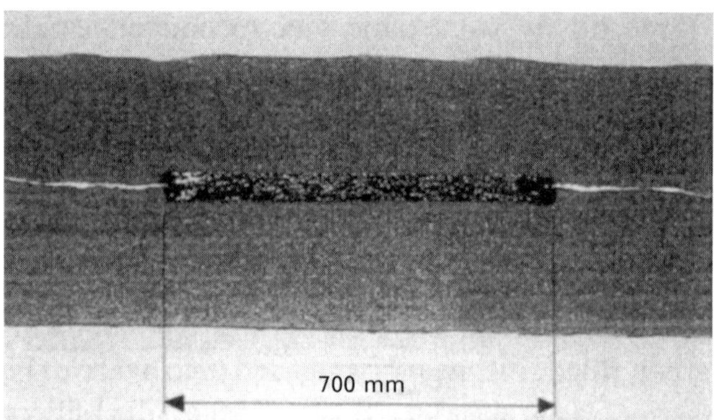

13.10 Carbon filled silicon rubber sensor.

recovery behaviour), and the general resistance level of the material depends on the applied strain. Resistance recovery is an effect observed in all particle filled elastomeric materials. After a movement, resistance is not constant, but decreases very slowly.

As an alternative to the commercial conductive rubber described above, six different compounds of carbon filled thermoplastic elastomer fibres were tested. Most of the problems mentioned above can also be found in these materials. However, for some of the compounds, the problems are much less pronounced. The hysteresis problem seems to have been removed completely,

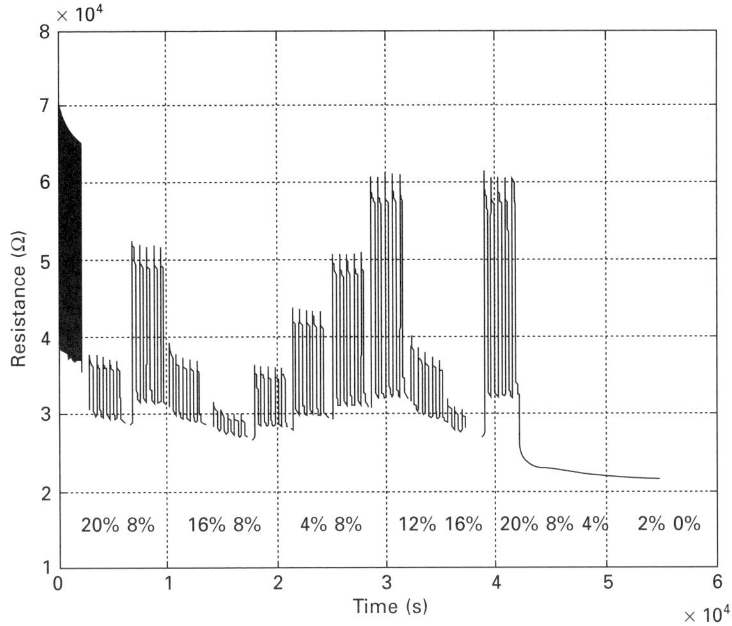

13.11 Repeated cycling of carbon filled silicon rubber sensor (with different strain levels, always starting from the pre-stretched zero position).

but resistance recovery is present as well. It is very important to understand that these kinds of materials are sensitive to all kinds of deformations. Resistance changes not only in response to elongation, but also in response to pressure, shear and bending. Therefore, it is unlikely that these materials can be used as pure elongation sensors. If these materials are integrated into a garment, they will most likely act as general deformation sensors. This is in fact how such materials are used in (Tognetti *et al.*, 2005). In these papers, some work on modelling of these materials and on how signal processing techniques can be applied to compensate the excessive transient times is presented. Summarizing, electroconductive elastomers show complex behaviour and can therefore not be applied as elongation sensors without advanced signal processing. Furthermore, it is questionable if all the unfavourable effects can be compensated through modelling and signal processing techniques.

An alternative approach to using purely textile sensors is to mount non-textile structures onto a fabric. A sensor was produced which utilizes an electroconductive fluid as the transducer medium (Küng, 2005). The fluid is filled into a rubber tube which is glued onto the textile. For the experiments an electrolyte was used. The problem with this fluid is that it diffuses from the tube very quickly. Another type of sensor makes use of the changing light transmission through a fabric when it is stretched (Schultze, 2003). A prototype was built and characterized (Küng, 2005). The results of the evaluations done with the prototype are quite promising. There are no transient times, no hysteresis, and also no dependence on elongation rate. The drawbacks of this sensor are the relatively high obtrusiveness compared to the other sensors and the possibly high power consumption due to the requirement of a light source.

Summarizing, the sensors that are made by attaching a structure to the fabric are not as unobtrusive as the sensors that are made of pure textile material. Yet, their transducer performances are better compared to the other sensors.

13.5 Context recognition technology

The recognition of context, that is, the activity of the user and the status of his environment, relies on continuously measured sensor data. In Lukowicz *et al.* (2002) recommendations are made about which sensor or which combinations of sensors are appropriate to detect specific context components. The signals of the sensor data have to be pre-conditioned, e.g., converted, amplified and filtered, before the characteristic features like signal energy or moments are extracted. Several methods and tools have been proved for the fusion of the features. The Bayesian decision theory, for example, offers a fundamental approach for fusion and assignment of predefined classes like motion, sleep, etc. Frequently used methods are the kNN-approach, Kalman and particle filter as well as the Hidden Markov Models and Neural Networks. Combining basic context classes affords the classification also of more complex user contexts like stress and depression. As described in Piccard *et al.* (2001), four wearable sensors (muscle activity EMG, blood oxygen SpO_2, skin conductance and respiration) have been applied to detect and to classify eight different motions like anger, grief, joy or hate.

13.6 Wearable components

13.6.1 Embedded microsystems

Recent developments in microtechnology have paved the way to embedding microsystems, either directly in fabrics, or in clothing components like buttons. As a design example Bharatula *et al.* (2004) (Fig. 13.12) shows an autonomous sensor, consisting of a light sensor, a microphone, an accelerometer, a microprocessor and a RF transceiver. A solar cell powers the system even for continuous indoor operation. The two holes allow this system to be sewn in clothes like a normal button.

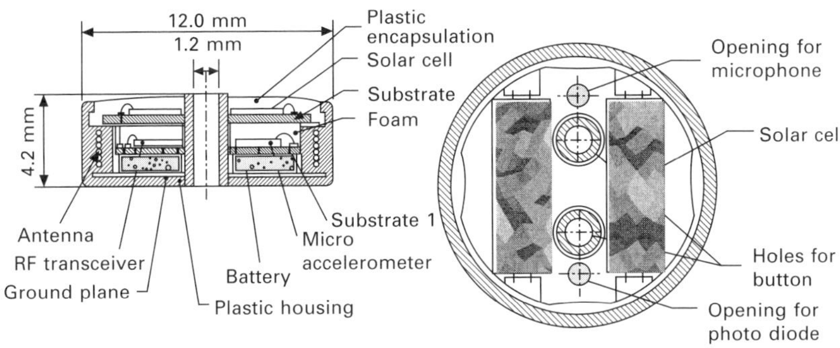

13.12 Design of an autonomous 'sensor button': cross-section and top view.

13.6.2 Accessories

The fusion of the mobile phone, personal digital assistant (PDA) and even the MP3 player into 'smart phones' offers an interface between the personal communication environment and public services. But today's 'smart phones' require manual handling and focusing on the interface. Stripped of bulky IO interfaces and large batteries, mobile computing and communication modules are small enough to be easily carried in a purse or be part of carry-on accessories such as a key chain or a belt buckle as depicted in Fig. 13.13 (Amft *et al.*, 2004).

13.7 Applications

13.7.1 Wearable back manager

Back pain is often caused by unhealthy behaviour. Personal circumstances and activities can increase the risk of musculoskeletal disorders and accidents. Many occupations are characterized by monotonic body postures, lack of body movements or high stress. European studies reveal that every third employee suffers from back pain and every second complains about exhausting and painful body postures during work. Consequences are often chronic pain, inability to work and long and expensive medical treatment. Prevention of back pain would be much more effective than therapy, but for most people it is difficult to change their behaviour. A personal wearable back manager could help an individual to adopt a healthier life-style in daily life. Using our approach of context-aware textiles the garment could monitor body posture, movements and activities, stress levels and other physiological data.

Figure 13.14 shows the concept of a wearable back manager with distributed sensors that are connected over a textile network. Combining different types of sensors enables detection of situations that are critical for the back. One example of a critical situation is lifting a heavy weight incorrectly. Bending

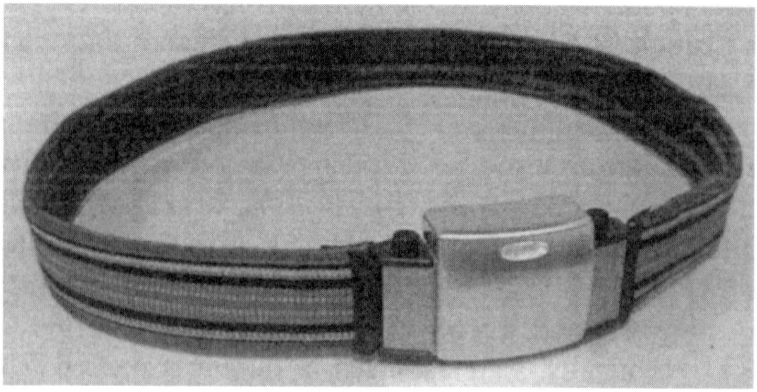

13.13 ETH-QBIC – a mobile computer (Xscale CPU, 256 MB SRAM, USB, RS-232, VGA, Bluetooth) integrated in a belt buckle; the belt houses the flexible batteries and interface connectors.

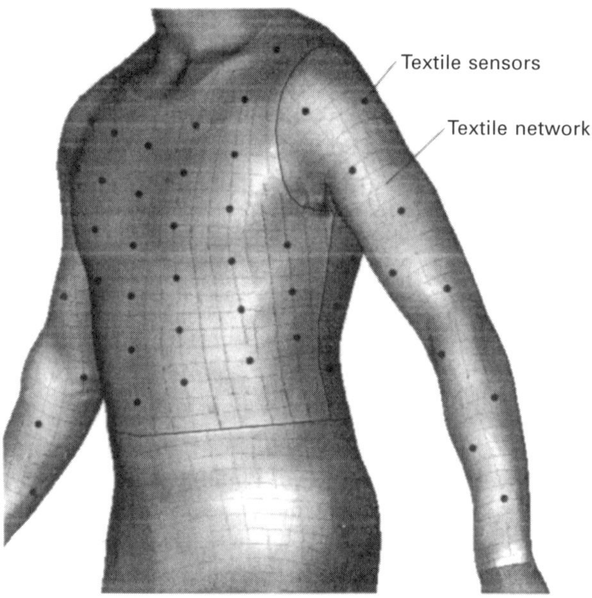

13.14 Concept of back manager.

the back instead of the knees can damage the spinal column. In order to know if the situation is critical it is necessary to detect not only the posture of the back but also the lifting movements of the arms, the weight of the object and the bending of the knee joint. Context recognition algorithms as described in Section 13.5 can be used to extract relevant information from the sensor data.

We evaluated the feasibility of measuring back postures with elongation sensors integrated into tight-fitting clothing. We identified regions of high elongations that are characteristic for specific postures (Fig. 13.15). However, existing textile elongation sensors are not suitable for this application as the back manager is intended to be used also in situations with low activity as, for example, sitting in front of a computer. During such activities the elongation does not vary dynamically, so a static sensor output is needed. The textile elongation sensors have to be optimized to fulfil this requirement. Further sensors like pressure sensors, accelerometers, gyroscopes and magnetic field sensors can provide information about the movements of the extremities and pressure changes (e.g. in the shoes). Additional data can come from the objects, for example, by labelling heavy weights with RFID-tags.

13.7.2 Wearable heart manager

The EU-funded project MyHeart (MyHeart, 2004) aims at the reduction of cardio-vascular diseases using wearable health assistants. Cardio-vascular diseases cause roughly 45% of all deaths in Europe; 4 million deaths in Europe, 1.5 million of them in the EU every year. More than 20% of all European citizens suffer from chronic cardio-vascular diseases. Assuming that (only) 5% of the EU population, namely, 19 million persons, will use the MyHeart wearable health assistant, about 60,000 deaths per year caused by

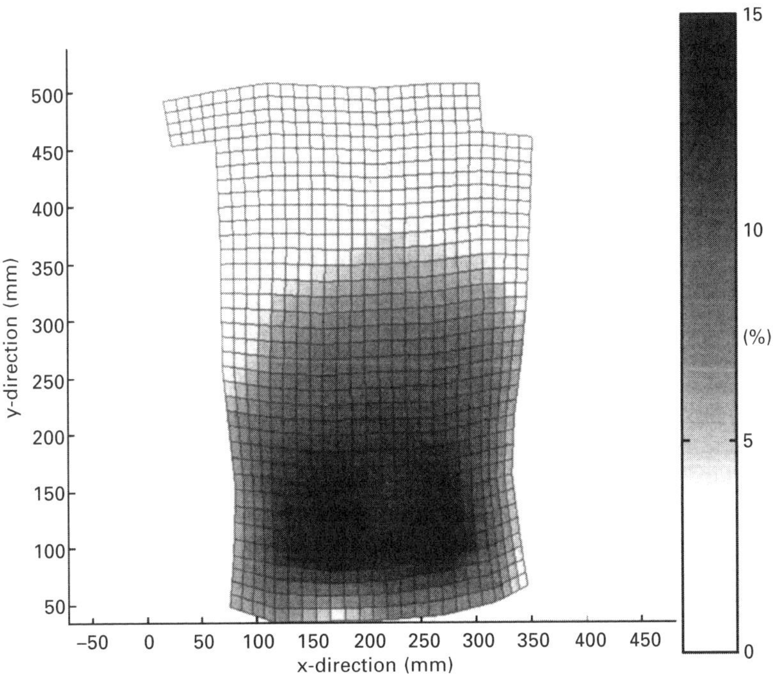

13.15 Example of a measured elongation distribution of the garment on the back.

myocardial infarctions and strokes could be avoided, saving costs in the range of 12 billion Euros per year.

The project MyHeart focuses on five application fields: improving physical activities, nutrition and dieting, sleep and relaxation phases, stress prevention and early diagnosis and prediction of acute events. The My Heart wearable health assistant comprises several 'intelligent' clothes with embedded sensors. The data communication with the family doctor, hospital or medical care centre enables an individually matched acknowledgement and health control.

13.8 Outlook

In this chapter we described how the combination of electronic textiles with context recognition technology and miniaturized wearable computers enables a wearable health assistant. Our approach is practicable in terms of modularity and also costs and will allow electronic clothing to become a mass product, one day being affordable for everyone. This trend will have a strong impact on the fashion business. It is not just a chance to strengthen the textile industry by innovation and new market potentials, it also requires a convergence between textile and the electronics industry. That means textile companies have to learn the rules for producing and marketing high-tech products, whereas the electronics companies have to understand the importance of fashion trends.

First implementations of our concept of context-aware textiles in the area of posture training and heart monitoring have been described. Further applications are foreseeable such as prevention of obesity or stress-related illnesses, assisted living for elderly or disabled people, as well as work assistance (e.g. for high-risk environments or remote working). Going one step further from wearable health assistants to even more general-purpose personal assistants will be the next challenge. Such a personal assistant not only monitors the health but also recognizes the needs of the user and provides automatic and active support like a personal servant or friend.

13.9 Acknowledgement

The authors would like to thank Jan Meyer and Corinne Mattmann for contributing their research results.

13.10 References

Amft O, Lauffer M, Ossevoort S, Macaluso F, Lukowicz P, Tröster G (2004), Design of the QBIC wearable computing platform. *Proc. 15th IEEE Application-specific systems, architectures and processors ASAP* 2004.

Bharatula N B, Ossevoort S, Stäger M, Tröster G (2004), Towards wearable autonomous microsystems. *Pervasive 2004*, Springer; 2004: 225–237.

Bickerton M (2003), Effects of fiber interaction on conductivity, within a knitted fabric stretch sensor. In *Proceedings of the IEE Eurowearable 2003*, pages 67–72, Birmingham, UK, September 4–5 2003.

Cottet D, Grzyb J, Kirstein T, Tröster G (2003), Electrical Characterization of Textile Transmission Lines, *IEEE Transactions on Advanced Packaging*, Vol. 26, No. 2, May 2003, pages 182–190.

Farringdon J, Moore A J, Tilbury N, Church J, Biemond P D (1999), Wearable sensor badge & sensor jacket for context awareness. In *The Third International Symposium on Wearable Computers*, Digest of Papers, pages 107–113, San Francisco, California, October 18–19 1999.

Gouaux F, Simon-Chautemps, Fayn J, Arzi M, Assanelli D *et al.* (2002), Ambient Intelligence and Pervasive Computing for the Monitoring of Citizens at Cardiac Risk: New Solutions form the EPI-MEDICS Project. *Computers in Cardiology*; 29; 2002: 289–292.

Kirstein T, Lawrence M, Tröster G (2003), Functional Electrical Stimulation (FES) with Smart Textile Electrodes, *Proc. Wearable Systems for e-Health Workshop*, Pisa Italy, 11–14 December 2003.

Kirstein T (2004), Medical Applications of Electronic Clothing, *Medical Device Technology*, Vol. 15, 06/2004.

Kirstein T, Cottet D, Grzyb J, Tröster G (2005), *Wearable Computing Systems – Electronic Textiles, Wearable Electronics and Photonics*, edited by X. Tao, Woodhead Publishing Ltd., 2005.

Klemm M, Locher I, Tröster G (2004), A novel circularly polarized textile antenna for wearable applications, in *Proc. 34th European Microwave Week*, pp. 137–140, October 2004.

Korhonen I, Pärkkä J, van Gils M. (2003), Health Monitoring in the Home of the Future. *IEEE Eng. Medicine and Biology Mag*. May/June 2003: 66–73.

Küng C (2005), Wearable elongation sensors for human posture analysis, diploma thesis, ETH Zürich, 2005.

Locher I, Kirstein T, Tröster G (2004), Routing methods adapted to e-textiles, in *Proc. 37th International Symposium on Microelectronics* (IMAPS 2004), November 2004.

Locher I, Kirstein T, Tröster G (2005), From Smart Textiles to Wearable Systems, *mst news*, No. 2/05, April 2005, pages 12–13.

Lukowicz P, Junker H, Stäger M, von Büren T, Tröster G (2002) WearNET: A Distributed Multi-Sensor System for Context Aware Wearables, in *Proc. of the UbiComp2002*, Springer, 2002: pages 361–370.

Lukowicz P, Kirstein T, Tröster G (2004), Wearable Systems for Healthcare Applications, *Methods of Information in Medicine*, Vol. 43, 03/2004.

Marculescu D, *et al.* (2003), Electronic Textiles: A Platform for Pervasive Computing, in *Proceedings of the IEEE*, Vol. 91, No. 12, Dec. 2003.

Massey P (2001), Mobile phone fabric antennas integrated within clothing, in *Proceedings of the 11th IEE Conference on Antennas and Propagation* (IEE Conf. Publ. No. 480), vol. 1, pp. 344–347, April 2001.

MyHeart (2004) Fighting cardio-vascular diseases by preventive lifestyle & early diagnosis. www.extra.research.philips.com/euprojects/myheart.

Oh K W, Park H J, Kim S H (2003), Stretchable conductive fabric for electrotherapy, *Journal of Applied Polymer Science*, 88: 1225–1229, 2003.

Pacelli M, *et al.* (2001), Sensing threads and fabrics for monitoring body kinematic and vital signs, in *Proceedings of Fibers and textiles for the future*, Tampere, Finland, 2001.

Piccard R, Vyzas E, Healey J (2001), Toward machine emotional intelligence: analysis of affective physiological state. *IEEE Trans. Pattern Anal. Mach. Intelligence*, vol 32, Oct 2001: 829–837.

Salonen P, Hurme H (2003), A novel fabric WLAN antenna for wearable applications, in *Proceedings of the IEEE Antennas and Propagation Society International Symposium*, vol. 2, pp. 700–703, June 2003.

Salonen P, Keskilammi M, Kivikoski M (2000), Single-feed dual-band planar inverted-f antenna with u-shaped slot, *IEEE Transaction on Antennas and Propagation*, vol. 48, pp. 1262–1264, August 2000.

Salonen P, Rahmat-Samii Y, Hurme H, Kivikoski M (2004), Dual-band wearable textile antenna, in *Proceedings of the IEEE Antennas and Propagation Society International Symposium*, vol. 1, pp. 463–466, June 2004.

Schultze C (2003), New technology for textile based monitoring of periodic physiological activity, in *Proc. Wearable Systems for eHealth*, Lucca, Italy, Dec. 11–14, 2003.

Scilingo E P, Lorussi F, Mazzoldi A, De Rossi D (2003), Strain-sensing fabrics for wearable kinaesthetic-like systems. *IEEE Sensors Journal*, 3(4), August 2003.

Tanaka M, Jae-Hyeuk J (2003), Wearable microstrip antenna, in *Proceedings of the IEEE Antennas and Propagation Society International Symposium*, vol. 2, pp. 704–707, June 2003.

Tognetti A, Lorussi F, Bartalesi R, Quaglini S, Tesconi M, Zupone G, De Rossi D (2005), Wearable kinesthetic system for capturing and classifying upper limb gesture in post-stroke rehabilitation. *Journal of NeuroEngineering and Rehabilitation*, 2(8), 2005.

Weiser M (1991), The computer for the 21st century. *Scientific American* 265, No. 3, September 1991: 94–104. Available from: URL: http://www.ubiq.com/hypertext/weiser/SciAmDraft3.html

Wijesiriwardana R, Dias T, Mukhopadhyay S (2003), Resistive Fibre-meshed transducers, in *Proceedings of the Seventh IEEE International Symposium on Wearable Computers* (ISWC'03), pages 200–209, October 21–23 2003.

14

Smart medical textiles for monitoring patients with heart conditions

O AMFT, ETH Zürich, Switzerland and
J HABETHA, Philips Research Labs, Germany

14.1 Introduction

Cardio-vascular diseases (CVDs) are a prevalent type of chronic disease with epidemic mortality rates. CVDs are a main cause of early death in developed countries. The CVD group includes high blood pressure, coronary heart disease, heart failure and stroke. The most prominent risk factors include diet, physical activity, hypertension and blood cholesterol, overweight and obesity, diabetes and stress. Each individual risk factor increases the probability for a CVD when left untreated for several years in a critical state. However, persons with a high score in the risks already suffer from a decreased quality of life, for example, obese persons have severe limitations in their ability to follow an active lifestyle. Moreover, after a cardio-vascular event patients suffer from strong reduction in quality of life. A majority of patients are afraid to take an active role in their life and potentially develop depression.

In Europe ~49% of all deaths are attributed to CVDs and more than 23% of all European citizens suffer from a chronic CVD (Petersen *et al.*, 2005). Recent numbers for the US are similar:[1] Thom *et al.* (2006) reports a mortality rate of 58% for CVD as an underlying or contributing cause and a disease prevalence of 34%. One growing cause of CVD prevalence is increasing life expectancy (ESC, 2004). With it the disease management cost rises. Currently CVDs are estimated to cost the EU economy 169 billion Euros per year, including 105 billion direct health care costs (professionals, hospital and nursing home services). However these numbers underestimate indirect costs (lost productivity, informal care) (Petersen *et al.*, 2005). The economic cost associated with CVDs in the US is estimated to be 403 billion US$,[2] including direct costs and indirect cost (Thom *et al.*, 2006). These figures indicate that it will become increasingly challenging for communities to provide its citizens with the best health care service at affordable costs.

1. Statistics based on preliminary data for the years 2002–3.
2. Cost statistics for 2006.

14.1.1 Preventive lifestyle and early diagnosis

The major CVD risk factors presented above indicate that individual lifestyle is an important disease indication. The cardiology community[3] has developed lifestyle and diet recommendations to effectively prevent CVD, identify risks and optimise post-event treatment outcomes, e.g., Lichtenstein *et al.* (2006); Kelly and Stanner (2003); Wood and EUROASPIRE I and II Group (2001); Bauman (2004).

A healthy and preventive lifestyle (primary prevention) and early diagnosis as well as optimised post-event support (secondary prevention) could save millions of life years and improve quality of life for patients. Primary and secondary prevention reduce individual risk factor scores and effectively prevent recurring of cardio-vascular events. In this way prevention can fight the origin of CVD systematically and is believed to be the solution for improving the quality of care in the future.

Prevention aiming at a healthy lifestyle is a continuous lifelong challenge for individuals. It cannot be thoroughly provided by the current medical service centres, e.g., hospitals and office-based physicians. This classic institutional point of care approach offers intermittent treatment only, focused on brief and expensive supervised episodes. However, prevention requires a continuous health care delivery emphasising a long-term change of habits. Due to the inherent cost structure, institutional care cannot achieve a cost-effective level for continuous treatment and prevention. Novel methods are needed to provide continuous and ubiquitous access to medical excellence in a cost-effective way.

The challenge of prevention stems furthermore from the difficulty of individuals to adapt to it. Knowing risks and preventive measures does not automatically lead to a successful adoption by individuals however. Wood and EUROASPIRE I and II Group (2001) indicated that even in a high-risk group the adoption of secondary prevention is rather limited. Success achieved in clinical settings could not be continued after patient discharge. Thus appropriate motivation concepts are needed to bridge the prevention gap.

In order to empower individuals to adopt prevention as a lifestyle the following challenges were identified (Schmidt and Lauter, 2005): (i) the scientific challenge to find solutions for prevention and early diagnosis, (ii) the technical challenge to develop solutions that allow ubiquitous access to medical expertise for empowering the individual to adopt a healthy life style and early diagnosing of acute events, and (iii) the psychological challenge to create pleasant and easy to use solutions that motivate people to adapt their lifestyle and improve their quality of life. The MyHeart project was initiated by Philips as an integrated project, including research and development of solutions, with the objective to address all three challenges.

---

3. European Hearts Network: http://www.ehnheart.org, British Heart Foundation: http://www.bhf.org.uk, American Heart Association: http://www.americanheart.org.

14.1.2 Solutions for prevention and early diagnosis

To accommodate the needs of individuals a segmentation of application areas and user groups was developed. The segmentation contains five application clusters and four customer groups and was chosen to simplify the design of solutions tailored to specific user groups and motivational needs. The customer groups cover (i) individuals who want to stay healthy, (ii) individuals with recognised risks for developing CVDs, (iii) individuals after a cardiac event and (iv) chronically ill patients (Lauter, 2004). The application clusters reflect main risk groups for developing CVD and address the user's need for early diagnosing to limit severity of an acute event. The following segmentation has been presented before by Schmidt and Lauter (2005) and is summarised in updated form here.

CardioActive: application cluster for improved physical activity

Sedentary lifestyle is a major risk factor for developing CVD and physical activity is widely known to decrease various CVD risks, e.g., Bauman (2004); Petersen *et al.*, (2005); Cress *et al.*, (2006). People must be made aware of this, and stimulated to be more active. For this group solutions are developed to determine the activity levels and include assessment of fitness condition of the user. The solutions include the sensing of basic vital signs like heart rate, breathing rate and activity classification as well as the determination of speed, distance and height levels. The system automatically determines the specific activity and gives feedback on the present status as well as on the achieved improvement of physical status. Specific training plans and recommendations for training will be personalised on the individual condition and the ambition level of the user. Specific attention is paid to the motivation for staying active by feedback on status, community building and virtual competition.

CardioBalance: application cluster for improved nutrition and dieting

Diet is an important health aspect and obesity the most prominent form of malnutrition. For these individuals solutions are developed to actively manage their dieting and nutrition by personalised dieting plans, continuous feedback and guided physical training plans. Special attention is paid to the motivation of the customer via community building and new methods of electronic peer pressure.

CardioSleep: application cluster for improved sleep and relaxation phases

Sleep quality and disorders such as sleep apnoea and insomnia are relevant risk areas for CVD, e.g., Coccagna *et al.*, (2006). Patients are at elevated risk to develop a CVD. Solutions are developed to assess the individual's sleep quality and diagnose sleep disorders at home. Novel methods for improving sleep quality and the therapy of sleep disorders based on biofeedback and personalised relaxation exercises are explored. Special attention is paid to diagnosing sleep quality related diseases like depression, which is a frequent complication of post-myocardial infarction patients.

CardioRelax: application cluster for improved solutions to deal with stress

Stress is a major behavioural risk factor for CVD. Solutions are developed not only for diagnosing acute stress situations and a stress meter but also for specific relaxation methods to deal with stress. Biofeedback tools are used, tailored to individual needs and enabled by Web and mobile services. The solution will limit the stress-related risk of CVD and will improve personal performance in the working environment.

CardioSafe: application cluster for early diagnosis and prediction of acute events

For early diagnosis solutions are developed to continuously analyse the vital signs of the individual in order to determine and predict acute events. A diagnosis system for the following areas has been developed: (i) myocardial infarction, (ii) stroke prevention, (iii) pump failure prevention, (iv) sudden cardiac arrest prevention and (v) hypo-hyperglycemic shock.

14.1.3 MyHeart applications

In order to tailor solutions within the application-customer segmentation scheme the notation of concepts was defined. A concept is an application solution that addresses a specific application cluster and customer group. In the first project phase individual concepts were developed and evaluated according to different criteria, including (i) application value proposition, (ii) technical feasibility and (iii) stakeholder opinion and acceptance, e.g., potential users and service providers.

At the end of the first project phase a selection and combination of individual concepts was performed and new product concepts (PCs) were established. The PCs represent combinations of concepts for specific customer groups addressing multiple application clusters. Figure 14.1 visualises the segmentation and concept approach.

14.1.4 MyHeart organisation

The MyHeart project is a joint effort of the European Commission and 33 partners from industry and academics. A partitioning in work packages and

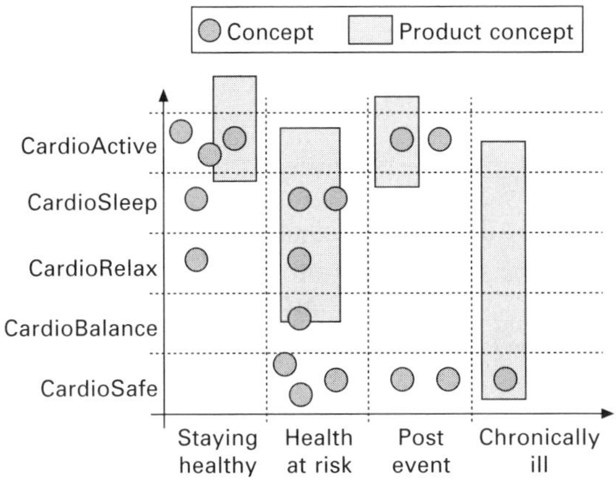

14.1 Segmentation of applications and customer groups as applied in the MyHeart concepts. The concepts (addressing individual application cluster and customer group) and product concepts (PCs) are shown. Adapted from Schmidt and Lauter (2005).

project phases is applied to structure both applications and development cycles. The project schedule is segmented into phase 1, development and evaluation of application concepts; phase 2, development of product concepts to prototypes of commercial solutions and phase 3, product concept validation. A detailed description of the project organisation is provided by Lauter (2004). The project was started in January 2004 and is scheduled to be finished by September 2007. Currently the project is in the product concept validation. However, research into novel solutions is continued and results will be integrated into the applications under evaluation when appropriate.

14.2 Personal health care: from monitoring to coaching

MyHeart aims at fighting CVD by preventive lifestyle and early diagnosis. In order to achieve this target, innovative easy-to-use solutions and tools are required. These solutions must integrate the sensing of relevant health parameters to provide the ground for a health status estimation. Based only on the estimated current status, appropriate recommendations using personal profiles can be provided therefore it is necessary to acquire sensor information and analyse health status continuously. The remainder of this section presents the technical objectives and briefly describes the MyHeart concepts (applications).

14.2.1 Technical objectives

For the continuous measurement of vital signs, electronic systems and sensors embedded into functional clothes have been developed. Sensors are partly based on textile materials. The garments are able to monitor vital signs continuously and analyse the data. Furthermore, the clothes feature a wireless transmission link to transfer the acquired and processed information to user feedback devices and, if necessary, to professional medical services. The automatic processing involves status diagnosis, trend estimation and system reactions (therapy recommendations). Additional services are available through the link to professional care suppliers. Figure 14.2 visualises the different technical objectives of MyHeart. These objectives have been presented by Schmidt and Lauter (2005) and are summarised here.

Continuous monitoring

The first basic requirement of preventive lifestyle and early diagnosis of acute events is a continuous monitoring of the cardio-vascular system. This challenge is addressed by the integration of novel sensors and monitoring systems into functional clothes. A basic set of clothes are investigated and developed that allow continuous monitoring throughout the day. Only three garments will serve the full spectrum of prevention: (i) garment for the night (nightdress, pyjamas), (ii) garment for the day (functional undergarment), and (iii) garment for sports (functional fitness dress). With this approach, a coverage of nearly 100% of a user's life is achieved.

Continuous personalised diagnosis

The intelligent biomedical clothes provide a modular basis for the pioneering of an on-body diagnosis system that allows the continuous assessment of health status and analysis in a wearable on-body system. The personal sensor signals are analysed and high-quality diagnosis of the health status is enabled. One major challenge is the development of these personalised diagnostic and

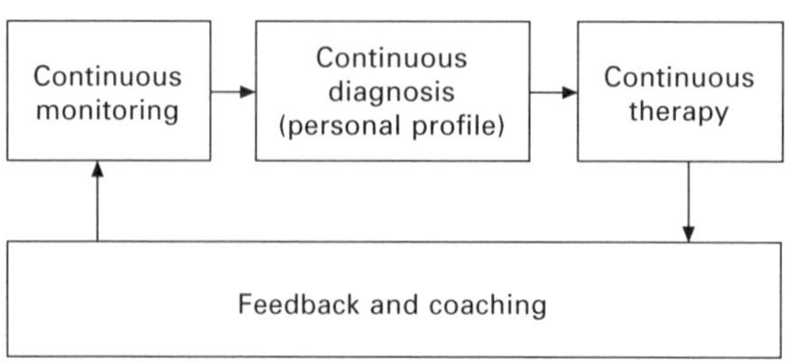

14.2 Monitoring, analysis/diagnosis, feedback cycle applied in the MyHeart project. Adapted from Lauter (2004).

trend detecting algorithms and the technology to operate the analysis algorithms in wearable electronics. By combining clinical protocols and clinical knowledge with continuous on-body diagnostic systems, access to clinical excellence is provided on a life-long timescale and in a continuous way.

Continuous therapy

Intelligent biomedical clothes provide detailed and precise information on the actual health condition. Therapy is provided in the form of specific user instructions and information. Examples are on-line recommendations during sports to adapt heart rate and breathing rate. Dynamic posture and gesture recognition allows home training and physical therapy in the home setting under the supervision of trainers. Furthermore, the recognition supports behavioural algorithms for lifestyle analysis. Biofeedback technologies are developed for stress and relaxation exercises. Personal treatment recommendations and feedback on the success of activities represent a tool to motivate the user continuing their preventive lifestyle. Opportunities for novel self-medication approaches are explored for the acute medical part, e.g., pill-in-the-pocket.

Feedback to user

User terminals are adapted that allow the visualisation of recommendations and biofeedback in the home and in the mobile setting, at any time and anywhere. Mostly existing platforms and infrastructure, e.g., GSM and UMTS networks in the mobile setting, are utilised as well as existing home infrastructure like TV, personal computers and audio-systems. Health status, instructions for adapting lifestyle and notifications of preventive actions are displayed automatically on mobile terminals and connected home devices. Concepts are developed for a health-aware home with special emphasis on ease-of-use aspects.

Remote access and professional interaction

Innovative communication systems connect the user to professional medical services and to other users in the home and mobile setting. Architectures and concepts for direct and immediate access to institutional care at any time are explored. There is a need for application-specific modules that enable professionals to interact with MyHeart applications. Moreover, tools for the management of the MyHeart system from external sites as well as interfaces of the MyHeart platform with general and third-party resources have to be developed. The systems allow the interaction with professional service providers and public emergency systems.

14.2.2 MyHeart concepts and product concepts (PC)

As presented in the introduction, MyHeart addresses various different application clusters and customer groups by implementing different concepts. In the first project phase 16 concepts were developed and evaluated where each focused on an individual application cluster and one or two user groups. Table 14.1 lists the different evaluated concepts and indicates responsible partners. These partners may be contacted for further information regarding the specific concept.

The second phase established four product concepts (PCs) to drive the development further and approach product solutions. The PCs are summarised in Table 14.2. These PCs are further developed in the current project phase. Main technical challenges originating from these applications are discussed in section 14.3.

14.3 Technical challenges for monitoring, analysis and feedback

This section provides an overview of the MyHeart application challenges from a technology viewpoint. After reviewing the overall technical approach and information flow, individual problems of sensor data acquisition in garments, on-body signal analysis and transmission as well as user feedback are discussed. Emphasis is on garment-based solutions and primarily the sensors used. References to further research work are provided where appropriate. The section is concluded by summarising the lessons learnt of wearable system design and integration.

14.3.1 Methodology

The different MyHeart applications require the integration of monitoring, analysis (mostly signal processing) and feedback facilities. A generalisation of the data flow is visualised in Fig. 14.3. While concepts share some modules not all concepts require the identical type and number of sensors, feature analysis and feedback functions.

For the monitoring task mainly wearable on-body sensors are used. This design choice is essential to achieve the project goal of continuous everyday physiological monitoring. The sensors provide the main input for the analysis step. Manual input of data is avoided as far as possible to minimise the user's burden and measurement errors. However, for some concepts an additional instrumentation of the environment is integrated to support the analysis step, e.g., for the PC activity coach information from a gym bicycle or step device is integrated to support user performance estimation. Environmental sensing support is not discussed in this work however. The analysis task refers to

Table 14.1 MyHeart concepts in the first project phase

Concept	Description and corresponding partner
Virtual trainer	Assess physical performance and assist with personalised training plans for different sports and ambition levels, ITACA, Spain.
Prevention manager	Guide and motivate runners with adaptive music to exercise at a pace that is most effective for your health, Philips Research Labs, Holland.
Outdoor rehabilitation	Solutions for different outdoor activities (e.g. biking, walking) tailored and personalised for rehabilitation needs of CVD patients, Dr. Hein GmbH, Germany.
Interactive exercises	Interactive exercises using vital signs and body motion for feedback and input, Consorzio di Bioingegneria e Infomatica Medica, Italy.
Stroke rehabilitation	Interactive stroke rehabilitation program to improve motor control physical performance, University of Pisa, Italy.
Sleep disorders	Assessment of sleep quality, early diagnosis of sleep disorders and improvement of sleep quality, Politecnico di Milano, Italy.
Depression management	Early diagnosis of recurrence of depression on the basis of sleep fragmentation, Philips Research Labs, Germany
Cardio Relax 1	Stress relaxation based on biofeedback (HRV, breathing) and audio-visual experiences, Mind Media BV, Holland.
Cardio Relax 2	Continuous stress meter and personalised mental balance indicator, Mind Media BV, Holland.
Obesity management	Concept providing obese adolescents with monitoring services and tools that help them to lose weight, reduce their cardio-vascular risk, reintegrate into a social network and rebuild confidence, Medgate AG, Switzerland.
Sleep and care	Early detection of decompensation of CHF patients by daily measurements during sleep with bed based sensors, Philips Research Labs, Germany.
MI prevention	Early detection of ischemic events based on haemodynamic indicators (myocardial infarction, MI), Philips Research Labs, Germany.
Stroke prevention	Prevention of atrial fibrillation (AF) induced strokes by early detection and treatment of AF episodes, Philips Research Labs, Germany.
My HF-web risk monitor	Detect early indicators for heart failure (HF) and if necessary direct the user to institutional points of care for further treatment, Medtronic SA, Spain.
Hypoglycemic shock prevention	The continuous measurement of ECG, breathing rate and activity will be used to develop solutions to detect and potentially also predict hypoglycemic events, University of Padova, Italy.
Post-intervention follow up	Early detection of evolving life-threatening risks associated with (i) prosthetic heart valve dysfunction and (ii) sudden cardiac death due to ventricular arrhythmia, University of Coimbra, Portugal.

Table 14.2 MyHeart concepts in the second project phase

Product concept	Description	Corresponding partner
Activity coach	Supports and motivate users in reaching and maintaining personal training goals.	University of Madrid
Take care	Screening tool for consumers which gives feedback and coaching to (self)-manage CVD risk factors and adapt a healthier lifestyle.	Philips Research Labs, Aachen
Neurological rehabilitation	Support patients and their caregivers during neurological rehabilitation exercises, of both cognitive and physical type.	Dr. Hein GmbH
Heart failure management	Early detection of decompensation of heart failure patients based on automated vital body signs trend analysis and arrhythmia detection at the patient's home.	Philips Research Labs, Aachen

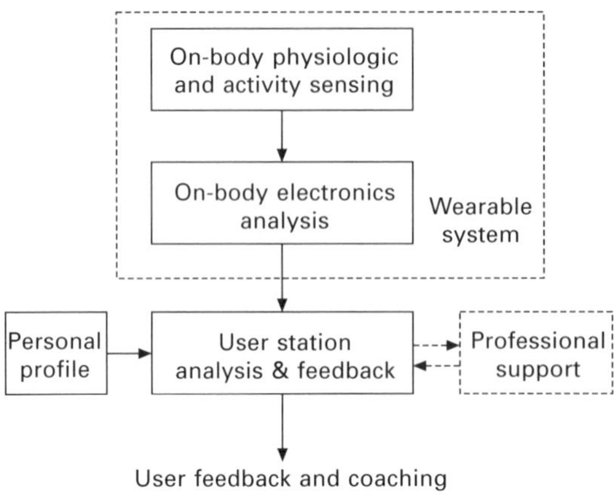

14.3 Generalised data and information flow as applied in the MyHeart concepts.

signal data acquisition, filtering and signal processing functions. The signal processing aims at deriving features as well as behavioural pattern classifications and trend estimations that can be used in feedback procedures. The wearable system is formed by the on-body monitoring and signal processing tasks.

The feedback and coaching task provides appropriate indications to the user. This is achieved by a combination of (i) presenting analysis results directly at the user station, (ii) using automated recommendation messages based on analysis results and (iii) manual or semi-automated filtering of analysis results by a professional health care centre. From the tasks described above the following basic requirements were derived: (i) the wearable solution must serve the given application robustly with high reliability in everyday situations, (ii) wearable system components worn close to the skin must be cleanable, (iii) the system must be easy to operate and control for non-trained users and finally (iv) a minimal hindrance of the normal activities of the user shall be imposed from both the wearable devices and the required system interactions.

The challenges for the on-body monitoring task can be summarised as (i) finding appropriate physiologic and activity signals and sensing locations, (ii) developing appropriate sensors and integrating the sensors into a wearable system, e.g., a T-shirt or chest band and (iii) extracting relevant features from the raw sensor data. The implementation and achieved results for the monitoring task within the MyHeart project are further detailed in section 14.3.2. Since the project focuses on wearable sensing solutions much work is targeted at preprocessing the sensor signals on the body. Hence the challenges of the analysis task can be summarised as (i) designing small and energy-efficient electronics that can process the sensor data, (ii) developing an interconnection solution between electronics and the garment sensors and (iii) adapting the signal processing algorithms to run on the constrained hardware. The implemented solutions are further discussed in section 14.3.3.

Finally, the means for feedback and the coaching concept must be developed. This includes coaching and behavioural analysis algorithms of elevated processing effort that are not provided by the on-body electronics, visualisation of analysis results and strategies to motivate the user. The feedback devices deployed for the project are discussed in section 14.3.4. The psychological theory and the applied strategies are beyond the scope of this chapter however.

14.3.2 Physiology and activity monitoring and feature extraction

The MyHeart concepts mainly require features based on the electrocardiogram (ECG), respiration and motion activity detection. Different implementation solutions and associated research issues are discussed in this section. Further monitoring approaches that are specifically tied to individual applications are summarised in the section on further research (section 14.4).

Electrocardiogram

Features continuously derived from heart activity are important information sources for all concepts, e.g., for heart failure detection, energy expenditure and stress management. The integration of different sensing approaches in textiles was tested in the first phase of the MyHeart project, including impedance cardiography, phonocardiography and ECG. The current project phase focuses on the latter and aims at improving the sensing and analysis as described below. Electric potentials of heart activity seen as an electric equivalent generator are measured by surface electrodes on the chest. These measurements provide very low voltage amplitudes (~ 1 mV for R-wave) due to the resistance of the thoracic medium and skin contact. Artefacts are introduced from other muscle activity, e.g., due to body movements. A complete cardiograph waveform provides detailed insight into the ventricle functions, e.g., the P, Q, R, S and T waves as well as the various inter-wave timings. The R-wave is usually counted over time to derive the heart rate (HR) per second. Besides the RR-timing ($HR = 1/RR$), the heart rate variability (HRV) is a relevant health status indication, e.g., for the estimation of stress level.

In continuous monitoring ECG applications alternatives to gel-based (wet) silver/silver-chloride electrodes are sought. Different dry electrode approaches have been proposed and compared (Searle and Kirkup, 2000), however the aimed-for textile integration is still an open research problem. Two main design approaches have been considered: (i) yarns made of stainless steel slivers blended with viscose textile yarn and (ii) conductive rubber thermally moulded on a textile patch. The critical issues include the quality of skin contact, selection of conductive material, yarn processing and electrode positioning. The problem of electrode positioning applies to gel electrodes as well; artefacts introduced by muscle activations during body movement or exercises must be compensated by positioning of the electrodes. With the use of textile or conductive rubber electrodes this effect is exacerbated due to potentially weaker skin contact and material conductivity. Hence these aspects require special attention in the design of textile solutions. Mühlsteff and Such (2004) reported the development of a conductive rubber electrode. For a 24-hour monitoring using a chest strap device a coverage with acceptable signal quality of ~70% was achieved (Mühlsteff *et al.*, 2004). Twelve users participated in this study.

Investigations were undertaken to compare and qualify textile electrode solutions with their gel-based counterparts. The results of these works were presented in Scilingo *et al.*, (2005); Loriga *et al.*, (2005) and Luprano *et al.*, (2006). Figure 14.4 shows the sensor layer of a prototype shirt as it is used in MyHeart with position indications for the textile electrodes. The electrodes are realised using stainless steel slivers blended in the yarn. Figure 14.5 shows different time-series plots from a simultaneous measurement using gel and textile electrodes during light physical activity. The signal waveforms correspond to the textile electrode pairs A-I, A-S, A-E and the gel electrode pairs R-L, L-F, R-F as labelled at the prototype shirt (cf. Fig. 14.4). While the gel electrodes still provide a good signal to noise ratio (SNR) in this situation, the textile electrodes knitted into the garment reflect the expected

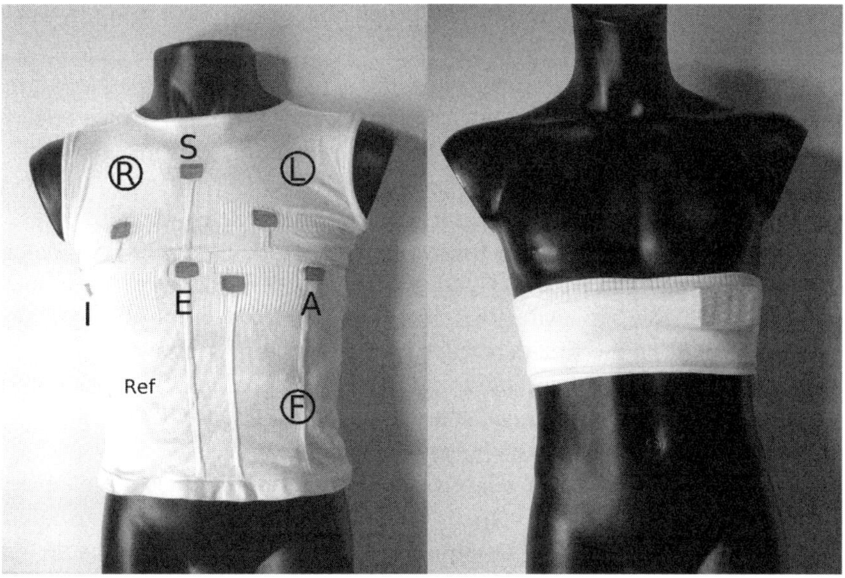

14.4 Prototypes of the MyHeart shirt and band textiles (courtesy R. Paradiso, Smartex, Italy). Textile electrode positions are indicated, see text.

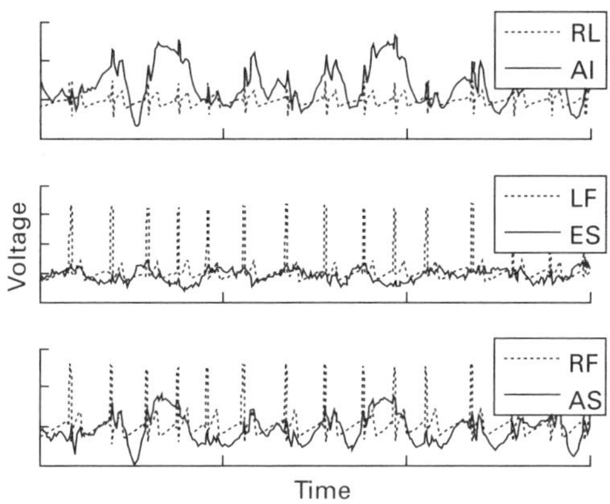

14.5 Simultaneous recording of gel and textile electrode ECG during light physical activity. Adapted with permission from Luprano *et al.* (2006).

patterns weakly. The SNR is improved by increasing electrode pressure on the skin and hence decreasing friction and movement. However, that is achieved primarily by tight fitting of the shirt and consequently decreased user comfort. One specific problem was observed with the position of electrode E at the centre of the sternum as this location has a weak skin contact depending on body shape.

Current work is aiming at improving signal processing algorithms for the feature extraction and textile sensor data quality in parallel. To ameliorate data quality different materials, embroidery and electrode locations are evaluated. Good initial results were achieved by using hydrophilic membranes (Paradiso *et al.*, 2004). The membrane is reported to decrease contact resistance and improve wearing comfort (Scilingo *et al.*, 2005).

The ECG enhancement and feature extraction is extensively researched. An overview is provided by the following works: (Xu *et al.*, (2001); Köhler *et al.*, (2002); Hamilton *et al.*, (2000). Luprano *et al.* (2006) achieved acceptable results for the R-wave extraction using textile electrodes. They used an algorithm based on the first derivative of the ECG time series supported by thresholds on the second derivative and the ECG signal itself. Additionally, the plausibility of the RR interval is tested and unlikely false beat periods are omitted. The enhancement of a complete QRS complex is achieved by replacing the original signal with an adaptive template. The template is adapted continuously from the source data. While this approach achieves a good QRS waveform it drops time variation in the complex and is not suitable for the analysis of heart pathologies.

Respiration

Respiration sensing is used in all concepts mainly to support activity and energy expenditure estimation during daytime and apnoea detection during sleeping. From the respiration signal the breath rate and variability (tidal volume) are extracted. The respiration wave is derived from the perimeter variation of the trunk due to the cyclic change of thoracic volume when breathing. Several measurement methods for the acquisition of respiration waves at the chest exist: (i) electric impedance pneumography, (ii) respiratory inductive plethysmography (RIP) and (iii) strain-sensitive chest band(s). These methods differ in the chest circumference detection principle. While the first method requires electrodes for current injection and measurement, the latter two measure the mechanical change of perimeter directly at thoracic and abdominal levels. The RIP method especially has shown good accuracy in stationary settings (Cohen *et al.*, 1997; McCool and Paek, 1993). The piezoelectric strain-gauge sensors were successfully embedded into a shirt for the IST Wealthy project[4] (Paradiso *et al.*, 2005). Since these sensors permit simple integration into a garment, respiration sensing in MyHeart follows that approach for the product concepts. However, the reliability of respiratory information derived with the strain gauge method is limited due to motion artefacts (Primiano, 1998).

4. http://www.wealthy-ist.com

Physical activity and motion

While most concepts require a categorical estimate of user motion activity, for specific applications a detailed detection of user movement is needed, e.g., the PC Neurorehabilitation to estimate the movement quality of users during training or in PC Take Care to support nutrition behaviour inference using the user's gestures. Categorical levels of motion activity are qualified as no activity to very strong activity in three to five levels or direct activities, e.g., standing/sitting, walking and lying. Here, the categorical classification is also used to determine whether the user is using/wearing the system.

Common solutions for activity level estimation integrate a two- or three-axis accelerometer (usually based on micro-electro-mechanical systems, MEMS) attached at the waist level, e.g., Bouten *et al.*, (1996); Mathie *et al.*, (2004). With the use of a shirt or chest band this position had to be shifted to an unobtrusive location on the chest. To obtain a robust system two implementations were used: (i) to sew the packaged sensor into the garment and (ii) to integrate the sensor directly into the on-body electronics. While the latter approach is technically simpler, since it avoids additional data and power transmission lines within the textiles, the first solution may provide more accurate estimation results due to improved location. In the sewn version the sensor electronics are moulded in a waterproof medical silicon material to permit normal washing of the garment. This approach is similar to the direct glob-top encapsulation of electronic packages on textiles (Peek, 2001). Package dimensions below 15 mm$\times$4 mm were achieved (Luprano *et al.*, 2006). For the automatic classification of activity levels a good fidelity is obtained. Sola *et al.* (2005) achieved an accuracy of 80% for the discrimination of no activity, walking, using stairs and running with a manually configured decision tree algorithm.

More elaborate movement detection is used in scenarios that require a detailed posture and gesture analysis of the upper body. Within MyHeart, posture detection of the upper body is used to estimate the quality of movement (Tognett *et al.*, 2005; Guilemaud *et al.*, 2004) in the PC Neurorehabilitation. Gestures are investigated to support inference of user behaviour (Amft *et al.*, 2005 a) for lifestyle coaching in the PC Take Care. Two technical solutions for motion monitoring are investigated: (i) usage of inertial sensors and (ii) utilisation of sensors based on piezoelectric materials. The first approach can be understood as a generalisation of the activity level detection, since it extends the set of sensors from one three-axis accelerometer to a combination of several acceleration, gyroscope and compass sensors. All of them are available as off-the-shelf components with a very low form factor.[5] Since piezoelectric materials respond with an electric voltage to mechanical deformation, research was done to deploy this property for the monitoring of limb movement, e.g., Edmison *et al.*, (2002).

5. Three-axis accelerometer: 7 × 7 × 2 mm (ST Microelectronics); one-axis gyroscope 7 × 7 × 3 mm (Analog Devices ADXRS); three-axis compass: 7 × 7 × 2 mm (Honeywell HMC).

Piezoelectric materials are either directly embedded into a yarn and embroidered or woven into a textile or externally attached, e.g., by coating onto a fabric. The latter method is currently being investigated in the project for upper limb postures (Lorussi *et al.*, 2005). The merit of this second approach to motion monitoring is its seamless integration into a garment while inertial sensors are robust and established devices in the sensor market are cheaply available in large quantities. Since the processing effort and energy consumption increases with the number of sensors, emphasis must be given to optimise the sensor count for continuous monitoring applications. For the discrimination of a set of dietary gestures using a hidden Markov model algorithm and inertial sensors attached to the arms, a performance of ~90% correct detections was achieved (Amft *et al.*, 2005a).

14.3.3 Signal transmission and on-body electronics

Table 14.3 summarises a typical set of sensors integrated into a MyHeart garment and their corresponding bandwidth requirements. Considering the typical set of sensors (ECG, respiration, acceleration) the sensors require a bandwidth of 5.4 kbps, amounting to ~445 MiB of data in 24 hours. An on-body processing of these signals is applied to derive relevant features before storing or transmitting the data from the body. Moreover, analog-digital conversion of the sensor signals must be done as closely as possible to the sensor to optimise signal quality, transmission lines and bandwidth usage. In the following section selected solutions for interfacing sensors in the textile and on-body processing are discussed.

Body sensor network

In order to obtain a system simple to operate and control a centralised system architecture was selected. This concept requires that all sensors communicate to a central processing master unit on the shirt. In this way individual sensors and the cleaning process are strongly simplified since individual battery, processing and transmission electronics are avoided. However, this is achieved

Table 14.3 Acquired signals and bandwidth requirements in the garment

Signal	Sampling rate	Digital resolution	Bandwidth
Electrocardiogram	250 Hz	12 bit	3 kbps (1 lead)
Respiration	50 Hz	12 bit	0.6 kbps (1 band)
Acceleration	50 Hz	12 bit	1.8 kbps (3 axis)
Total			5.4 kbps

at the expense of individual analog or digital transmission and power lines for each sensor. The main challenges for the sensor attachment are (i) selecting a flexible signal line route and (ii) interfacing the sensor with the signal line appropriately. Various approaches to establish electrical wiring structures in textiles exist. An overview is provided by Locher (2006). Textile conductivity is achieved by integrating conductive threads during the textile manufacturing process, e.g., by weaving a metal wire with the yarn, or enabled after manufacturing, e.g., by sewing or printing/plating. For the MyHeart sensor network the woven metal wire approach is most feasible. Relevant research results are available that characterise the electrical transmission properties for this approach, e.g., Locher, (2006); Cottet *et al.*, (2003); Dhawan, (2004).

Figure 14.4 introduced the sensor (skin) layer of a prototype shirt as it is used in the project. For this initial garment a solution based on the second approach was chosen to simplify reconfiguration; transmission and power lines were sewn in 'cable ducts' along textile patches. This approach, however, required including provisions for textile stretching across the body since the conductive lines cannot be elasticly elongated. Ducts and spare cable is finally covered by a top layer textile (not shown in Fig. 14.4). Wire attachments were either embroidered for the textile electrodes or included in the mould for the acceleration sensors.

On-body electronics

As shown in Fig. 14.3, the on-body processing must acquire, filter and process sensor data as well as store and forward processing results wirelessly to the user station. On-body result storage is needed for concepts that use a stationary user feedback system, e.g., placed or integrated in the user's home. In these concepts the on-body electronics must transfer the data at certain times, e.g., in the evening when the user is at home and the station is in wireless communication reach. The communication with the user station is realised by a Bluetooth connection. Critical system aspects include computational performance and power requirements as well as system size and provisions for garment cleaning. As introduced with the summary of technical challenges above, the problem of energy requirements for on-body signal processing requires a tradeoff on algorithm complexity and continuous runtime without changing/recharging batteries. Although energy requirements depend on a number of aspects, only a few main items were varied for different application-dependent implementations of the electronics, including computational performance, data storage space and number of sensor terminals. This approach allowed the establishment of common standards for wireless transmission of data to the user station, the transmission protocol, and algorithm sharing for different applications.

Three different levels of processing performance are used in the project: (i) electronics based on low-power microcontrollers, e.g., based on the TI MSP 430 family,[6] (ii) systems with medium performance, e.g., based on ARM family 7 processor[7] and (iii) systems for advanced processing and service requirements running standard operating systems. In the last category the QBIC[8] system was used (Amft *et al.*, 2004). The MSP-based systems require less energy compared to category 2 electronics, permitting highly miniaturised electronics due to smaller batteries.

Two systems from the low-power category are shown in Fig. 14.6. The system on the left was developed as a first prototype. This system is used with the band and shirt shown in Fig. 14.4. The right-hand picture shows a second-generation prototype in use with the sensor garment. These systems are capable of sampling and processing a small number of sensors and features, e.g., ECG features HR, HRV for more than 20 hours autonomously. MSP-based systems are a preferred choice for sensor nodes and have demonstrated their capabilities, e.g., even for frequency-domain feature processing of a low-bandwidth microphone (Stäger *et al.*, 2003).

The electronic system is placed into a side pocket of the garment. It must be removed before washing the textile. This approach has the advantage that the electronics do not need a waterproof seal, however, it requires a connector to the garment-based sensors that is manageable by an untrained user. The construction of textile-electronics connectors is a challenging problem since the design must be robust enough to sustain frequent connection cycles, washing and provide multiple connection lines for data and power. Some solutions for textile interfaces have been proposed by, e.g., Linz *et al.*, (2005) and Locher, (2006). Further connection approaches are currently under investigation within the project.

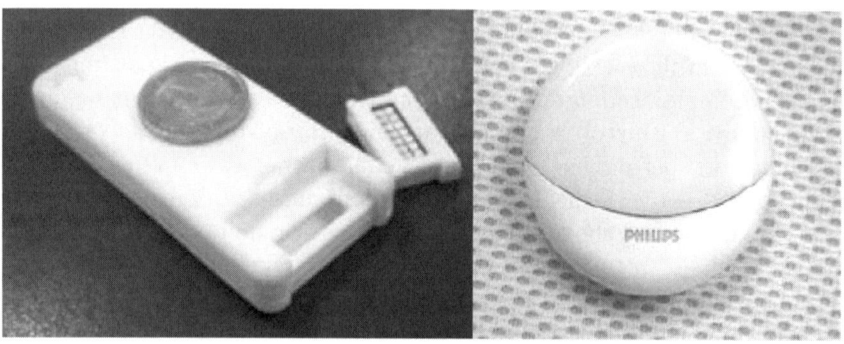

14.6 Prototypes of the MyHeart on-body electronics, left: first prototype, right: second prototype (courtesy Philips).

6. http://www.ti.com/msp430
7. http://www.arm.com/products/CPUs/families/ARM7family.html
8. Q-Belt integrated computer (QBIC), http://www.wearable.ethz.ch/qbic.html

14.3.4 User station and feedback

In the following the MyHeart feedback approach and the utilised user station solutions are briefly summarised.

Direct and indirect feedback

The user station provides direct feedback to the user, as a result of the analysis task and optionally indirect feedback which is post-processed by a professional health care service. Algorithms residing at the user station and the on-body electronics process the features for both feedback loops. While the direct feedback is intended as a regular and constant service the indirect feedback is provided on demand or as a result of detection of an abnormal trend. The direct feedback provides trend chart and statistic visualisations for different timescales as well as automatic recommendations depending on the user scenario. For example, in the PC Take Care a user may have the task assignment to review their personal activity level daily. The system provides weekly averaged trends and automatic messages, e.g., when it detects, by trend forecasting, that a defined goal cannot be reached. The indirect feedback is intended for coaching individuals or groups with special needs.

User station solutions

The choice of user station is specific for each concept, since the device must fulfil different requirements besides the visualisation of feedback information. For example, for heart failure patients a mobile phone is advisable to automatically contact medical help in case of an emergency. For the PC Take Care a stationary device in the user's home is used, which may be shared with other applications. Typical devices include personal data assistants (PDAs) or newly emerging mobile computing gadgets.

14.3.5 Summary and lessons learnt

This section provided an overview of the main technological challenges in the MyHeart project. Starting from a general monitoring, analysis and feedback methodology specific problems for garment-based health monitoring and analysis were presented and relevant sources for further information were indicated. Emphasis was given to common problems for all MyHeart concepts.

From the technical experience gained in the completed project phases several practical issues have been identified that need further evaluation. Relevant items for the garment system part include the improvement of textile electrodes and their positioning, the textile-based network and the wearing comfort of the garment. To achieve good electrode contact a tight fitting was aimed for. This raised the difficulty of donning and doffing the garment. Furthermore, the textile strain sensors for the detection of postures and gestures need further investigation to simplify the interface to a high number of signalling lines, the resistance adaptation method for the electronics and to evaluate applications with regard to the intrinsic sensor hysteresis problem, e.g., found in Amft *et al.*, (2006) for a standard type of textile strain sensor. For the inertial sensing approach, issues with the use of compass sensors (disturbances of the magnetic field orientation) have been identified in the literature (Miller *et al.*, 2004). From the experiments of the authors it was found that even a table or chair constructed from metal parts interferes with the orientation estimation. This requires careful algorithm design when using these sensors.

In the forthcoming project phase a clinical trial will be started. This unveils new challenges for the entire wearable system, e.g., the production of more than 200 wearable systems for different body sizes and both genders, medical certification of the systems and support of the subjects using the devices in the trial.

14.4 Evolution of MyHeart approach and related work

This section summarises further development within MyHeart. Moreover, a brief summary of commercial and research works related to MyHeart are presented. The section is concluded by summarising related projects supported by the European Commission.

14.4.1 Research in sensing and analysis

After introducing the technical objectives of MyHeart in section 14.2, the technical approach and associated challenges for frequently applied sensing and analysis methods was discussed in section 14.3. The following sections review further wearable and textile monitoring and analysis approaches that are currently being investigated within the project and provide references to the performed research.

Heart activity

Continuous monitoring of heart activity clearly provides the most important information for determining actual cardiac status. Current works aim at the further analysis of features related to heart activity, e.g., interrelation and prognostics in chronic heart failure patients (Maestri *et al.*, 2005) and further parameters (Folino *et al.*, 2005; Guasti *et al.*, 2005b) as well as the relation of cardiac status to lifestyle, e.g., Quaglini *et al.*, (2005). The integration of analysis algorithms into wearable systems is a technical objective of MyHeart and addressed by, e.g., Milanesi *et al.*, 2005 and Brito *et al.*, (2005).

Sleep and stress

As mentioned earlier, sleep and stress are two important aspects of quality of life and linked to CVD. MyHeart aims at providing prevention solutions that are applicable during the night too; current work studies sleep behaviour, e.g., Ferini-Strambi *et al.*, (2005) and the interrelation to wearable systems (Puzzuoli *et al.*, 2005; Mendez *et al.*, 2005). Furthermore, the relation to stress was analysed by Guasti *et al.*, (2005a).

Virtual activity trainers

Virtual sport trainers address the physical activity improvement in the CardioActive application cluster. Sala *et al.*, (2005) presented a wearable solution.

Neurological rehabilitation

The integration of activity sensing solutions into garments promises convenient textile solutions. Current work aims at optimising textile strain sensors for posture detection and compensating for sensor limitations, e.g., Giorgino *et al.*, (2006) and Lorussi *et al.*, (2005).

Nutrition behaviour

Dietary behaviour is strongly interrelated to malnutrition and CVD. Wearable solutions are sought that provide behavioural statistics and are capable of analysing the eating microstructure on the body. Sensing approaches are evaluated that provide such information, e.g., the analysis of chewing activity (Amft *et al.*, 2005b) and gestures associated with foodstuff intake (Amft *et al.*, 2005a). Furthermore, the combination of different information sources is investigated (Amft and Tröster, 2005).

Feedback and professional interaction

Besides the challenges in establishing psychological effective solutions to continously motivate the user, further solutions simplifying the interaction with professional medical services are required. Villalba *et al.*, (2006) presents an approach to establish a heart failure management system, integrating information acquisition, database management as well as processing and retrieval functions. The system provides interfaces for the patient and professionals.

14.4.2 Related works and projects

Related work

Commercial heart rate and Holter monitoring systems have been developed, e.g., by Polar[9] or Schiller[10]. Reima[11] developed belts and garments for communication and outdoor sports. Complete sensing shirts, integrating various physiological signals are developed by Vivometrics[12] and Sensatex[13]. The Vivometrics' Lifeshirt system is available for research purposes, Sensatex announced field tests of their SmartShirt for 2006. Various other smart textile systems, e.g., Smart Bra,[14] Burton Amp Jacket[15] and carry-on devices, e.g., Body Media Armband[16] have been investigated. Most of the systems and devices realised to date relied on the sensing and processing of physiological data. In many cases the monitoring systems are limited either in duration of continuous usage, number of analysed parameters, functionality or wearing comfort. Besides resolving these restrictions, MyHeart aims at providing personalised feedback, including long-term plans and recommendations. Moreover, in MyHeart the preventive effectiveness of derived information is evaluated.

Related European activities

The MyHeart project is embedded into the smart fabrics interactive textile (SFIT) cluster of research and development projects founded by the European Commission.[17] The SFIT cluster targets the realisation of the 'e-textile' paradigm by further integration of micro- and nano-technologies into textile solutions. The developed systems shall seamlessly integrate sensing, actuating, processing, communication and power sources. MyHeart was launched,

9. http://www.polar.fi
10. http://www.schiller.ch
11. http://www.reima.com
12. http://www.vivometrics.com
13. http://www.sensatex.com
14. University of Wollongong, http://www.uow.edu.au
15. http://www.apple.com; http://www.burton.com
16. http://www.bodymedia.com
17. Information about the SFIT activities was presented by A. Lymberis at the Pervasive Health Conference, 2006, Lucerne, Switzerland and was provided to the authors for further dissemination.

building partly on the results of Wealthy,[18] a project of the European Commission's fifth framework programme addressing the simultaneous recording of vital signs from textile sensors. A number of projects related to MyHeart were initiated aiming at exploring different applications and future business opportunities, e.g.:

- PROETEX: development of protection e-textiles for emergency and disaster wear[19]
- STELLA: development of stretchable electronics for large textile area applications[20]
- BIOTEX:[21] development of bio-sensing textiles to support health management using chemical sensors
- CONTEXT: contact-less sensors for continuous heart and muscle monitoring incorporated in textiles
- OFSETH:[22] integration of optical fibre based sensors into functional textile for extending the capabilities of wearable solutions in health monitoring
- MERMOTH:[23] development of a generic medical monitoring system using smart bio-sensors.

14.5 Sources of further information

Further information on MyHeart can be found on the Internet pages.[24] Information on related projects in the sixth framework programme are available from the European Commission.[25]

14.6 Acknowledgements

The authors would like to thank all MyHeart project partners for their contribution to this work. MyHeart is a European project funded by the European Commission in the sixth framework programme (IST-2002-507816). This work was supported by the Swiss State Secretariat for Education and Research (SER).

18. http://www.wealthy-ist.com
19. http://www.proetex.org
20. http://www.stella-project.eu
21. http://www.biotex-eu.com
22. http://www.ofseth.org
23. http://www.mermoth.org
24. http://www.hitech-projects.com/euprojectsw/myheart
25. http://www.cordis.europa.eu/ist/health; http://www.cordis.europa.eu/ist/mnd

14.7 References

Amft, O., Tröster, G., September 2005. Automated human dietary monitoring by fusing physiologic information. In: CIHP2005: *Symposium of the Centre for Integrative Human Physiology*.

Amft, O., Lauffer, M., Ossevoort, S., Macaluso, F., Lukowicz, P., Tröster, G., September 2004. Design of the QBIC wearable computing platform. In: ASAP2005: *Proceedings of the 15th IEEE International Conference on Application-specific Systems, Architectures and Processors*. pp. 398–410.

Amft, O., Junker, H., Tröster, G., October 2005a. Detection of eating and drinking arm gestures using inertial body-worn sensors. In: ISWC2005: *IEEE Proceedings of the Ninth International Symposium on Wearable Computers*. pp. 160–163.

Amft, O., Stäger, M., Lukowicz, P., Tröster, G., September 2005b. Analysis of chewing sounds for dietary monitoring. In: Beigl, M., Intille, S., Rekimoto, J. (eds), *UbiComp 2005: Proceedings of the 7th International Conference on Ubiquitous Computing*. Springer: *Lecture Notes in Computer Science*, pp. 56–72.

Amft, O., Junker, H., Lukowicz, P. Tröster, G., Schuster, C., April 2006. Sensing muscle activities with body-worn sensors. In: BSN 2006: *International Workshop on Wearable and Implantable Body Sensor Networks*. pp. 138–141.

Bauman, A. E., April 2004. Updating the evidence that physical activity is good for health: an epidemiological review 2000-2003. *J Sci Med Sport* 7 (1 Suppl), 6–19.

Bouten, C. V., van de Venne, W. P. V., Westerterp, K. R., Verduin, M., Janssen, J. D., August 1996. Daily physical activity assessment: comparison between movement registration and doubly labeled water. *J Appl Physiol* 81 (2), 1019–1026.

Brito, M., Henriques, J., Gil, P., Antunes, M., September 2005. A predictive adaptive approach to generic ecg data compression. In: *Proceedings of the IEEE International Workshop on Intelligent Signal Processing*. pp. 32–37.

Coccagna, G., Pollini, A., Provini, F., 2006. Cardiovascular disorders and obstructive sleep apnea syndrome. *Clin Exp Hypertens* 28 (3-4), 217–224.

Cohen, K. P., Ladd, W. M., Beams, D. M., Sheers, W. S., Radwin, R. G., Tompkins, W. J., Webster, J. G., July 1997. Comparison of impedance and inductance ventilation sensors on adults during breathing, motion, and simulated airway obstruction. *IEEE Trans Biomed Eng* 44 (7), 555–566.

Cottet, D., Grzyb, J., Kirstein, T., Troster, G., May 2003. Electrical characterization of textile transmission lines. *IEEE Transactions on Advanced Packaging* 26 (2), 182–190.

Cress, M. E., Buchner, D. M., Prohaska, T., Rimmer, J., Brown, M., Macera, C., DePietro, L., Chodzko-Zajko, W., May 2006. Best practices for physical activity programs and behavior counseling in older adult populations. *ER Age PhyAct* 3 (1), 34–42.

Dhawan, A., November 2004. Woven fabric-based electrical circuits: Part ii: Yarn and fabric structures to reduce crosstalk noise in woven fabric-based circuits. *Textile Research Journal* 74 (11), 955–960.

Edmison, J., Jones, M., Nakad, Z., Martin, T., October 2002. Using piezoelectric materials for wearable electronic textiles. In: *ISWC 2002: Proceedings of the Sixth International Symposium on Wearable Computers*. pp. 41–48.

ESC, 2004. Cardiovascular diseases in europe 2004. http://www.escardio.org/knowledge/ehs/reports/, european Society of Cardiology.

Ferini-Strambi, L., Fantini, M. L., Zucconi, M., Castronovo, V., Marelli, S., Oldani, A., Cappa, S., December 2005. Rem sleep behaviour disorder. *Neurol Sci* 26 Suppl 3, s186–s192, neurological sciences : official journal of the Italian Neurological Society and of the Italian Society of Clinical Neurophysiology.

Folino, A. F., Tokajuk, B., Porta, A., Romano, S., Cerutti, S., Volta, S. D., April 2005. Autonomic modulation and clinical outcome in patients with chronic heart failure. *Int J Cardiol* 100 (2), 247–251.

Giorgino, T., Quaglini, S., Lorussi, F., De Rossi, D., April 2006. Experiments in the detection of upper limb posture through kinestetic strain sensor. In: BSN 2006: *Proceedings of the International Workshop on Wearable and Implantable Body Sensor Networks*, pp. 9–12.

Guasti, L., Simoni, C., Mainardi, L., Crespi, C., Cimpanelli, M., Klersy, C., Gaudio, G., Grandi, A. M., Cerutti, S., Venco, A., June 2005a. Global link between heart rate and blood pressure oscillations at rest and during mental arousal in normotensive and hypertensive subjects. *Auton Neurosci* 120 (1–2), 80–87.

Guasti, L., Simoni, C., Mainardi, L. T., Cimpanelli, M., Crespi, C., Gaudio, G., Clersy, C., Grandi, A. M., Cerutti, S., Venco, A., June 2005b. Circadian blood pressure variability is associated with autonomic and baroreflex-mediated modulation of the sinoatrial node. *Acta Cardiol* 60 (3), 319–324.

Guilemaud, R., Caritu, Y., David, D., Favre-Reguillon, F., Fontaine, D., Bonnet, S., 2004. Body motion capture for activity monitoring. In: Lymberis, A., de Rossi, D. (eds), *Wearable eHealth Systems for Personalised Health Management: State of the Art and Future Challenges*. Vol. 108 of Studies in Health Technology and Informatics. IOS press, pp. 286–291.

Hamilton, P., Curley, M., Aimi, R., Sae-Hau, C., September 2000. Comparison of methods for adaptive removal of motion artifact. In: *Proceedings of the Computers in Cardiology Conference*, pp. 383–386.

Kelly, C. N. M., Stanner, S. A., August 2003. Diet and cardiovascular disease in the UK: are the messages getting across? *Proc Nutr Soc* 62 (3), 583–589.

Köhler, B.-U., Hennig, C., Orglmeister, R., 2002. The principles of software qrs detection. *IEEE Eng Med Biol Mag* 21 (1), 42–57.

Lauter, J., 2004. Myheart: fighting cardiovascular disease by preventive lifestyle and early diagnosis. In: Lymberis, A., de Rossi, D. (eds), *Wearable eHealth Systems for Personalised Health Management: State of the Art and Future Challenges*. Vol. 108 of Studies in Health Technology and Informatics. IOS press, pp. 36–42.

Lichtenstein, A. H., Appel, L. J., Brands, M., Carnethon, M., Daniels, S., Franch, H. A., Franklin, B., Kris-Etherton, P., Harris, W. S., Howard, B., Karanja, N., Lefevre, M., Rudel, L., Sacks, F., Horn, L. V., Winston, M., Wylie-Rosett, J., July 2006. *Diet and lifestyle recommendations revision 2006: a scientific statement from the American heart association nutrition committee. Circulation* 114 (1), 82-96, American Heart Association Nutrition Committee.

Linz, T., Kallmayer, C., Aschenbrenner, R., Reichl, H., October 2005. Embroidering electrical interconnects with conductive yarn for the integration of flexible electronic modules into fabric. In: ISWC2005: *Proceedings of the Ninth IEEE International Symposium on Wearable Computers*. pp. 86–89.

Locher, I., 2006. *Technologies for system-on-textile integration*. Ph.D. thesis, ETH Zürich.

Loriga, G., Taccini, N., De Rossi, D., Paradiso, R., September 2005. Textile sensing interfaces for cardiopulmonary signs monitoring. In: *EMBS 2005: 27th Annual International Conference of the Engineering in Medicine and Biology Society*. pp. 7349–7352.

Lorussi, F., Scilingo, E. P., Tesconi, M., Tognetti, A., De Rossi, D., September 2005.

Strain sensing fabric for hand posture and gesture monitoring. *IEEE Trans Inf Technol Biomed* 9 (3), 372–381.

Luprano, J., Sola, J., Dasen, S., Koller, J., Chetelat, O., April 2006. Combination of body sensor networks and on-body signal processing algorithms: the practical case of myheart project. In: BSN 2006: *Proceedings of the International Workshop on Wearable and Implantable Body Sensor Networks*. pp. 76–79.

Maestri, R., Pinna, G., Allegrini, P., Balocchi, R., Casaleggio, A., D'Addio, G., Ferrario, M., Menicucci, D., Porta, A., Sassi, R., Signorini, M., La Rovere, M., Cerutti, S., September 2005. Linear and non-linear indices of heart rate variability in chronic heart failure: mutual interrelationships and prognostic value. In: *Proceedings of the Computers in Cardiology Conference*. pp. 981–984.

Mathie, M. J., Celler, B. G., Lovell, N. H., Coster, A. C. F., September 2004. Classification of basic daily movements using a triaxial accelerometer. *Medical & biological engineering & computing* 42 (5), 679–687.

McCool, F. D., Paek, D., May 1993. Measurements of ventilation in freely ranging subjects. *Res Rep Health Eff Inst* 59, 1–17; discussion 57–69.

Mendez, M., Villantieri, O., Bianchi, A., Cerutti, S., September 2005. Sleep analysis for wearable devices applying autoregressive parametric models. In: *EMBS 2005: Proceedings of the 27th Annual International Conference of the Engineering in Medicine and Biology Society*. pp. 7353–7356.

Milanesi, M., Vanello, N., Positano, V., Santarelli, M., Paradiso, R., De Rossi, D., Landini, L., September 2005. Frequency domain approach to blind source separation in ecg monitoring by wearable system. In: *Proceedings of the Computers in Cardiology Conference*. pp. 767–770.

Miller, N., Jenkins, O., Kallmann, M., Mataric, M., November 2004. Motion capture from inertial sensing for untethered humanoid teleoperation. In: *RAS 2004: Proceedings of the 4th IEEE/RAS International Conference on Humanoid Robots*. Vol. 2. pp. 547–565.

Mühlsteff, J., Such, O., September 2004. Dry electrodes for monitoring of vital signs in functional textiles. In: *Engineering in Medicine and Biology Society. EMBC 2004. Conference Proceedings*. Vol. 3. pp. 2212–2215.

Mühlsteff, J., Such, O., Schmidt, R., Perkuhn, M., Reiter, H., Lauter, J., Thijs, J., Msch, G., M., H., September 2004. Wearable approach for continuous ECG and activity patient-monitoring. In: *EMBS 2004: Proceedings of the IEEE Conference of Engineering in Medicine and Biology*. pp. 2184–2187.

Paradiso, R., Loriga, G., Taccini, N., 2004. Wearable health care system for vital signs monitoring. In: *Medicon 2004: Proceedings of the Mediterranean Conference on Medical and Biological Engineering*.

Paradiso, R., Loriga, G., Taccini, N., September 2005. A wearable health care system based on knitted integrated sensors. *IEEE Trans Inf Technol Biomed* 9 (3), 337–344.

Peek, R., 2001. Liquid encapsulation protects electronic components. *EP&P magazine* 217, 170–180.

Petersen, S., Peto, V., Rayner, M., Leal, J., Luengo-Fernandez, R., Gray, A., February 2005. *European cardiovascular disease statistics*, 2nd edn. British Heart Foundation.

Primiano, F. P., 1998. *Medical Instrumentation: Application and Design*, 3rd edn. John Wiley and Sons, Inc., Ch. Measurements of the Respiratory System, pp. 372–439.

Puzzuoli, S., Marcheschi, P., Bianchi, A., Mendez Garcia, M., De Rossi, D., Landini, L., September 2005. Remote transmission and analysis of signals from wearable devices in sleep disorders evaluation. In: *Proceedings of the Computers in Cardiology Conference*. pp. 53–56.

Quaglini, S., Stefanelli, M., Boiocchi, L., Campari, F., Cavallini, A., Micieli, G., March 2005. Cardiovascular risk calculators: understanding differences and realising economic implications. *Int J Med Inform* 74 (2–4), 191–199.

Sala, P., Traver, M., Romagnoli, M., V.Traver, Guill, S., September 2005. Virtual trainer using smart wearable devices. In: *Conference Proceedings of Ambience05: Intelligent Ambience and Well-Being*. Tampere.

Schmidt, R., Lauter, J., 2005. Myheart: fighting cardio-vascular diseases by preventive lifestyle and early diagnosis. In: Nugent, C. D., McCullagh, P. J., McAdams, E. T., Lymberis, A. (eds), *Personalised Health Management Systems: The Integration of Innovative Sensing, Textile, Information and Communication Technologies*. Vol. 117 of Studies in Health Technology and Informatics. IOS press, pp. 51–59.

Scilingo, E. P., Gemignani, A., Paradiso, R., Taccini, N., Ghelarducci, B., Rossi, D. D., September 2005. Performance evaluation of sensing fabrics for monitoring physiological and biomechanical variables. *IEEE Trans Inf Technol Biomed* 9 (3), 345–352.

Searle, A., Kirkup, L., May 2000. A direct comparison of wet, dry and insulating bioelectric recording electrodes. *Physiol Meas* 21 (2), 271–283.

Sola, J., Chetelat, O., Celka, P., Dasen, S., November 2005. Very low complexity algorithm for ambulatory activity classification. In: *EMBEC 2005: Proceedings of the European Medical and Biological Engineering Conference*. Prague, CZ.

Stäger, M., Lukowicz, P., Perera, N., von Büren, T., Tröster, G., Starner, T., October 2003. Soundbutton: Design of a low power wearable audio classification system. In: *ISWC 2003: Proceedings of the 7th IEEE International Symposium on Wearable Computers*. pp. 12–17.

Thom, T., Haase, N., Rosamond, W., Howard, V. J., Rumsfeld, J., Manolio, T., Zheng, Z.-J., Flegal, K., O'Donnell, C., Kittner, S., Lloyd-Jones, D., Goff, Jr, D. C., Hong, Y., members of the Statistics Committee and Stroke Statistics, Subcommittee, Adams, R., Friday, G., Furie, K., Gorelick, P., Kissela, B., Marler, J., Meigs, J., Roger, V., Sidney, S., Sorlie, P., Steinberger, J., Wasserthiel-Smoller, S., Wilson, M., Wolf, P., January 2006. Heart disease and stroke statistics – 2006 update. *AHA Circ* 113 (6), e85–e151.

Tognett, A., Lorussi, F., Tesconi, M., Bartalesi, R., Zupone, G., De Rossi, D., 2005. Wearable kinesthetic systems for capturing and classifying body posture and gesture. In: *EMBS 2005: Proceedings of the IEEE Conference of Engineering in Medicine and Biology*.

Villalba, E., Arredondo, M., Hoyo-Barbolla, E., Guillen, S., April 2006. A new solution for a heart failure monitoring system based on wearable and information technologies. In: *BSN 2006: Proceedings of the International Workshop on Wearable and Implantable Body Sensor Networks*. pp. 150–153.

Wood, D., EUROASPIRE I and II Group, March 2001. Clinical reality of coronary prevention guidelines: a comparison of EUROASPIRE I and II in nine countries. EUROASPIRE I and II group. European action on secondary prevention by intervention to reduce events. *Lancet* 357 (9261), 995–1001.

Xu, X., Schuckers, S., CHIME Study Group, 2001. Automatic detection of artifacts in heart period data. *J Electrocardiol* 34 (Suppl), 205–210, collaborative Home Infant Monitoring Evaluation.

Index